AF568115

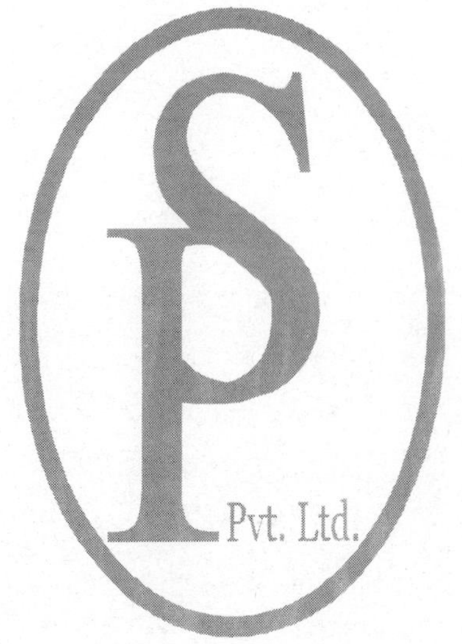
SP
Pvt. Ltd.

Biotechnology Series: **Vol. 2**

MONOCLONAL ANTIBODIES
Application in Disease and Health

G. Dhinakar Raj, J. Seshu, P.P. Bhat and P.N. Bhat

Centre for Integrated Animal Husbandry Dairy Development,
Flat No. 205, Block No. F – 64/C9,
Sector – 40, Noida – 201 301

2012

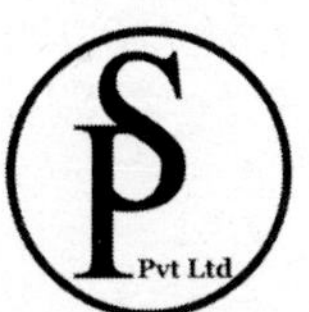

Studium Press (India) Pvt. Ltd.

Biotechnology Series: Vol. 2

MONOCLONAL ANTIBODIES
Application in Disease and Health

Series ISBN: 978-93-80012-49-0
ISBN: 978-93-80012-27-8

Published by:

Studium Press (India) Pvt. Ltd.
4735/22, 2nd Floor, Prakash Deep Building
(Near Delhi Medical Association),
Ansari Road, Darya Ganj, New Delhi-110 002
Tel.: +91-11-43240200-15 (15 lines); Fax: +91-11-43240215
E-mail: studiumpress@gmail.com

Printed at:

Salasar Imaging Systems, Lawrence Road, Delhi-35

ABOUT THE SERIES

It was realized by 1985 that the available diagnostics and vaccines used in Animal Health Protection were not giving the kind of protection, which was required for a country of the size of India. It was also realized that in addition to artificial insemination, country has to undertake research and development in embryo transfer and associated technologies in cattle for which technologies had been developed and standardized in scientifically advanced countries. And these to be researched in the buffalo, a species contributing 65% of the total milk in the country, and standardized particularly when this could be used as an adjunct to progeny testing programme in livestock species.

In order to enhance the genetic improvement in cattle and buffaloes and other species of livestock the embryo transfer and associated technologies were considered vital and critical if the gains obtained from crossbreeding of cattle were to be sustained.

Dr S. Ramachandran, the then Chairman, National Biotechnology Board (NBTB), Department of Science and Technology in Ministry of Science and Technology, was convinced that if animal biotechnology had to assist India to sort out the problems of enhancement of food, we had to put a two pronged attack to solve the problems. He used to tell that after all the Americans are not going to solve the problems of basic reproduction in buffaloes. It is our animal and we have to solve these problems. The board considered several projects on the basic and applied animal biotechnology including a mission mode project for Embryo Transfer Technology (ETT) and associated reproductive technologies.

By 1986 the Cabinet approved the creation of a new science department of biotechnology with Dr S. Ramachandran as its secretary. Dr Ramachandran established a task force on animal biotechnology in Department of Biotechnology (DBT), which was charged with responsibility of creating the structural plan for the Animal Biotechnology Sector with Prof. (Dr) P.N. Bhat, as the Chairman. One of gaps that was realized near total absence of trained manpower in the sector, except for a few laboratories, on biotechnology applications no research or development was being done in the country, hence it was necessary that apart from introducing short term training programmes, it was necessary to initiate a master's level programme in biotechnology with specific emphasis on application. One such centre was established at Indian Veterinary Research Institute (IVRI) as a part of a National Centre on Animal Biotechnology along with R & D Project on Embryo transfer technology for training the manpower. All the short-term training programmes had mandatory arrangements for producing training manuals. A similar project on producing training manuals for master's degree programmes was also initiated.

These manuals have been in use since 1987 in various areas of animal biotechnology at IVRI and other institutions around the country. In several courses, foreign faculty members were associated.

There was great interest at IVRI in this new area of biology which had tremendous application in diagnostics/vaccines/reproductive biotechnology/genetic improvement of livestock. The British Council supported two major projects under their programme (i) Recombinant DNA technology and its application for producing recombinant vaccines, and (ii) Embryo transfer technology and associated reproduction technologies. All had emphasis on human resource development and publication of workable monographs.

The present project with Studium Press (India) Pvt. Ltd. publication is the culmination of the idea of Dr S. Ramachandran in order to develop text books based on Indian experience, which has made a remarkable progress. Prof. Pran P. Bhat was the group leader of a group of young scientists, students and faculty who joined hands with support from undersigned to convert these monographs into as the texts for the students. This new scientific endeavor has had support from DBT and the publication house.

In tune with this thinking, it was decided to bring out a series of books for under graduate and post graduate scholars in Biosciences, Animal, Veterinary Sciences and Agriculture in seven (7) volumes under the Chief editorship of Professor (Dr) P.N. Bhat, Former Vice Chancellor and Director of Indian Veterinary Research Institute, Izatnagar 243122 (Uttar Pradesh) and Former Animal Husbandry Commissioner of India and Deputy Director-General (Animal Science) of Indian Council of Agricultural Research, Ministry of Agriculture, Krishi Bhawan, New Delhi. The basic idea of the series is to provide first rate text books to students and scholars in developing countries based on the experiences of India with special focus on Indo-Pak sub-continent in conformity with standards laid out by regulatory agencies in India (VCI, ICAR, UGC, AICTE, IMC, CSIR) and similar agencies in other developing countries.

The series includes books on

1. Animal Cell Culture
2. Hybridoma Technology and Antibody Engineering
3. Cell and Molecular Biology
4. Genetic Engineering
5. Microbial Fermentation
6. Feed Biotechnology
7. Embryo Biotechnology

It is hoped that in next 2–3 years these books will be available for the benefit of students, teachers and professionals in this area and fill the gap which is becoming wide.

Prof (Dr) Pushkar Nath Bhat
Chairman-World Buffalo Trust
and
Centre for Integrated Animal Husbandry & Dairy Development
and
Chief Editor

ABOUT THE AUTHORS

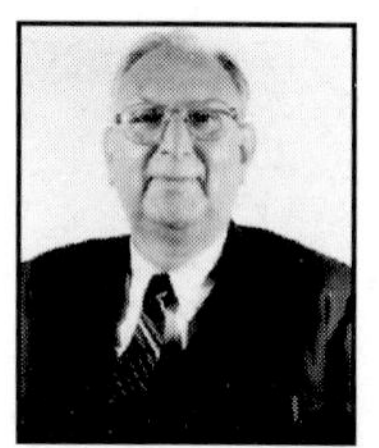

Prof (Dr) P.N. Bhat got his Ph.D in population genetics from Institute of Population Genetics Purdue University, West Laffayette, Indiana, USA in the year 1965 followed by several post doctoral assignments and visiting professorship in genetics, biotechnology, livestock production systems. He returned to India and joined Punjab Agricultural University at Hisar–Ludhiana followed by several professional assignments in India and abroad. He joined as Project co-ordinator (Animal Breeding) and subsequently as Head, Division of Animal Genetics at Indian Veterinary Research Institute in 1971. He was responsible for establishing coordinated projects on cattle, buffalo, sheep, goat, pigs and poultry during 1970–74. He was founder Director of Central Institute for Research on Goats. In 1984 he became Vice-Chancellor and Director of IVRI. He joined as Deputy Director-General (Animal Science) in May, 1992 and Animal Husbandry Commissioner in December, 1992. He is fellow of several National and International Science Academies.

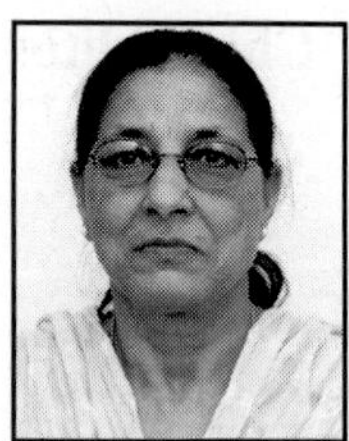

Dr P.P. Bhat got her PhD in Animal Genetics in 1971. She joined as Assistant Professor Animal Genetics at IVRI and subsequently as Scientist S3 at CIRG, Course coordinator and Principal Investigator-Animal Biotechnology, educational programme of Department of Biotechnology and established National Biotechnology Centre at IVRI, Principal Scientist (Education Division, ICAR), Principal Scientist (AG&B), Animal Science Division ICAR, Assistant Director General (AP&B) ICAR. She was recipient of PAU Fellowship Award 1966–70, Lal Bahadur Shastri Award for excellence in Science (Biotechnology) by Prime Minister 1988, Dr R. Eswaran Memorial Medal 1993, Award of gold Record of Achievement from American Biographical Institute Inc. USA 1996. Kashmir Education, Cultural and Science Society Award 2003, ICAR National Fellowship in 1995. She is Fellow of New York Academy of Science, National Academy of Agricultural Sciences. She is associated with R&D in Animal Genetics and Breeding, Animal Biotechnology (Production and Health).

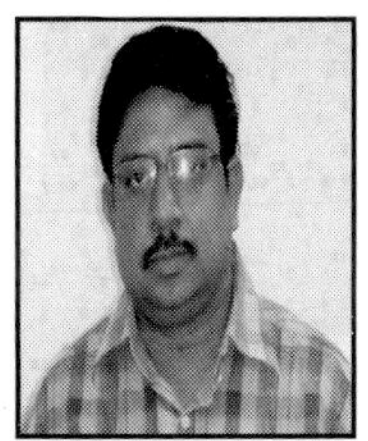

G. Dhinakar Raj did his B.V.Sc degree at Madras Veterinary College, Chennai, India in 1986 and obtained University first with four gold medals. He obtained his Master's degree in Biotechnology at the Indian Veterinary Research Institute, Izatnagar, UP (1986–1989) and Ph. D from the University of Liverpool, United Kingdom (1994–1997) under the Commonwealth Fellowship Programme. He has also undergone post doctoral training programmes at the University of Nebraska, USA (2001) and at the Institute for Animal Health, UK (2008). His field of speciallization is Animal Biotechnology with special reference to Molecular diagnostics and Immunology. He has developed diagnostic tests/kits for Egg drop syndrome (EDS), Peste des petits ruminants (PPR) and rabies. He was involved in understanding the molecular epidemiology of viruses affecting livestock and poultry circulating in India such as egg drop syndrome, PPR, infectious bronchitis and rabies viruses. He was also involved in genotyping of Chikungunya viruses involved in outbreaks in 2006–2007 in Tamil Nadu. He has applied flow cytometry in animal science research in several fields such as buffalo lymphocyte subset analysis in tuberculosis positive buffaloes, rabies antigen and antibody detection, apoptosis induction by mycotoxins and lymphocyte subset alterations after tick infestation in sheep. He has developed and validated PPR vaccine, immunology teaching and diagnostic kits, recombinant PPR virus nucleoprotein based flow through assays and biomarker for chickens. He is presently involved in elucidating the role of innate immunity in genetic resistance of Indian breeds of goats and buffaloes. He has guided 9 M.V.Sc, 4 M. Phil students and 2 Ph. D students. He has been granted one Indian Patent for the PPRV strip test. He has presently 90 international and 30 national publications in various peer-reviewed journals with high impact factors.

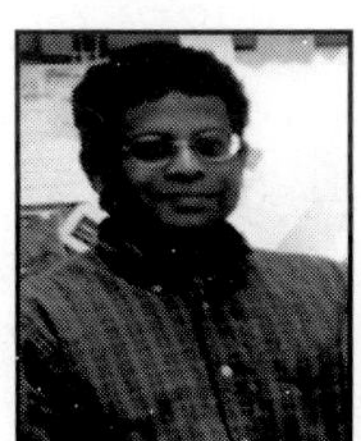

J. Seshu, Associate Professor, Bacterial Pathogenesis, Department of Biology, University of Texas at San Antonio, USA. A brief profile–JS did his B. V. Sc degree at Madras Veterinary College, Chennai, India in 1987 and obtained his Master's degree in Biotechnology at the Indian Veterinary Research Institute, Izatnagar, UP (1988–1990) and Ph.D from the Washington State University, Pullman, USA. He is presently Associate Professor, Bacterial Pathogenesis, Department of Biology, University of Texas at San Antonio, USA. His field of specialization is on the pathogenesis of two infectious diseases, Lyme disease and Q fever. He has several publications in high impact factor journals and has guided more than 10 post graduate students.

PREFACE

This book on *Hybridoma Technology and Antibody Engineering* is intended as an introductory book for those who are new to cell culture, whether undergraduates, graduates, technicians or scientists who want to move into the general area of biotechnology.

The aim of this text book is to drive home to the readers the basic concepts of all facets of monoclonal antibody technology platform and antibody engineering methods and engineered products. Our target audience is students in biotechnology, microbiology, immunology and all other facets of biological sciences. Our aim is to introduce students to these concepts with live examples and problems. The book stems from pedagogic material used for teaching Immunobiotechnology course to Master's and M. Phil degree students.

Monoclonal antibody technology is one of the epoch-making, un-patented technologies of the last century. In fact, this technology lead to production of specific reagents, that facilitated the dissection of the immune responses in terms of the cell types involved and the molecules they produce. Thirty-six years later, this technology has no parallel and refinements to this technology are still brought about through antibody engineering methods.

Interdisciplinary approaches between biological sciences and engineering are predicted as the happening of the next decade. Already we see its output in terms of phage display technology, alternate hosts for monoclonal antibody production, aptamers, engineered antibodies, transgenic animals and plants producing antibodies etc.

As researchers who have both spent much of their time at the bench, performing cell culture, and hybridoma technology and antibody engineering we recognize the need for an inexpensive, introductory text for the first timers who study biotechnology for research or as a profession. Many comprehensive works are already available in this field, but the sheer number and variety of current techniques has resulted in long and expensive texts. This book is not meant to give a comprehensive list of every available protocol, it aims to explain why and how the basic techniques are used, and their applications in modern molecular biology and biotechnology.

Molecular biology and immunology are growing rapidly with technological innovations being produced by the hour. However, understanding of basic concepts is important so that the improvements in these fields are better understood and applied. Molecular biology is more about 'visualization' while immunology is more about 'conceptualization'. You can see DNA as bands on agarose gel electrophoresis, but antibodies are visualized only indirectly. If you see a precipitin line on agar gels, we must conceptualize that the antigen and antibody has reacted and produced this line. Thus, it is all the more important that immunology concepts are made clearer. One of the important requirements for this is to forget the 'Y' shape of the antibody and conceptualize antibodies as globular proteins in a highly folded form with antigen-binding sites exposed on the outside.

The initial chapters describe the basic methodologies needed for culture of cells, including laboratory design, sterilization techniques, media preparation and guidelines for the correct use of equipment. The basics of techniques on primary as well as established cell lines are described, together with the essentials of dealing with contamination. The storing of hybridomas cells by cryopreservation completes the knowhow of basic and essential techniques. Armed with this necessary background, these techniques can be applied to the cloning of cells, the separation of lymphocytes from various sources and the use of these in cell fusion, cytotoxicity assays and the immortalization of various cells.

No effort is 'fool-proof' and there is always scope for improvement. The readers should feel free to comment on the contents, point out mistakes, if any and suggest methods for further improvement.

It is hoped that this book may act as a stimulus for further, more detailed, reading. Theoretical considerations have been included where necessary for a better understanding of the techniques described. Much of what is contained in this book is the result of accumulated knowledge and experience of countless researchers who have refined techniques to the point from where they can give reliable results even in the hands of inexperienced workers. We hope that with feedbacks from the students/scientists who use this text, the subsequent editions will be reorganized based on their experiments.

New Delhi
10th August, 2011

G. Dhinakar Raj
J. Seshu
P.P. Bhat
P.N. Bhat

CONTENTS

LIST OF FIGURES

Chapter 1 Introduction

Chapter 2 Requirements of a Hybridoma Laboratory

Chapter 3 Production of Monoclonal Antibodies

Chapter 7 Cryopreservation of Hybridomas

Chapter 8 Conjugation of Monoclonal Antibodies

Chapter 9 Application of Monoclonal Antibodies

Chapter10 Antibody Engineering

Chapter 11 Alternatives to Monoclonal Antibodies

LIST OF TABLES

CHAPTER 1

INTRODUCTION

1.1 History of Hybridoma Technique

The discovery by J.W. Littefield (1964) that when two clonal lines of mouse fibroblasts, each containing a drug-resistant marker, are grown together, hybrid cells can be detected under selective media conditions 'sowed the seed' for the future development of hybridoma technology. This was followed by another discovery by Schwaber and Cohen (1973) who reported the isolation of a hybrid clone, resulting from fusion of mouse myeloma cells secreting immunoglobulin A and human peripheral blood lymphocytes not secreting detectable immunoglobulins. The hybrid cells continue secretion of mouse immunoglobulin and initiate synthesis and secretion of human immunoglobulin. All these landmark discoveries culminated in the production of monoclonal antibodies (mAbs) by Kohler and Milstein (1975).

They described the derivation of a number of hybrid cell lines which secrete anti-sheep red blood cell antibodies. The cell lines are made by fusion of a mouse myeloma and mouse spleen cells from an immunized donor. To understand the expression and interactions of the Ig chains from the parental lines, fusion experiments with known mouse myeloma lines were carried out. They pioneered continuous culture of fused cells secreting antibodies of predefined specification using inactivated Sendai virus as the fusing agent. Later Pontecorvo (1976) showed that polyethylene glycol (PEG) could be used in place of Sendai virus in production of somatic cell hybrids.

Cesar Milstein, a biochemist at Cambridge in England was working on tumours produced by plasma cells while Georges Kohler in Basel, Switzerland was studying normal antibody-producing cells in tissue culture, which had a very limited life span. Their combination succeeded in converting the undesirable feature of continuous proliferation of tumour cells into a beneficial feature to the short-living lymphocytes. The hybrid cells created by fusion of the tumour and lymphocytes had eternal life and also the capacity to produce the very same antibody in large quantity. Kohler and Milstein called these hybrid cells hybridomas, and as all cells in a given hybridoma come from one single hybrid cell, the antibodies made are monoclonal. George Kohler and Cesar Milstein shared the Nobel Prize in Physiology or Medicine in 1984 (along with Niels Jerne for the discovery). The hybridoma technique discovered by Kohler and Milstein is considered one of the major unpatented methodological advances in medicine during this century.

1.2 Principles of Monoclonal Antibody Production of Pre Defined Specificity

The primed B-cells with a finite life span are obtained from the spleen of mice following repeated immunization of mice with the antigen of interest. They are fused using a fusing agent with the myeloma cells which has the property of infinite life span.

Following fusion of spleen lymphocytes and myeloma cells the following types of fused and unfused cells are possible.

- Unfused myelomal cells (parent cells)
- Unfused lymphocytes (parent cells)
- Myeloma × myeloma fused cells
- Lymphocyte × lymphocyte fused cells
- Myeloma × lymphocyte fused cells.

It is the last group of cells that we need and only these cells would possess the characteristics of both the parents. Unfused lymphocytes and lymphocyte × lymphocyte fused cells have a finite life span and would die after 10–14 days.

However, the myeloma parent cells and myeloma × myeloma fused cells have infinite life span and hence this property can not be used to differentiate them from our required fused cells between lymphocyte and myeloma cells. A new technique HAT (Hypoxanthine-Aminopterin-Thymidine) selection method is used to differentiate parent myeloma cells from fused lymphocyte and myeloma cells. This technique depends on synthesis of ribonucleotides and deoxy ribonucleotides.

There are two pathways available for synthesis of ribonucleotides and deoxy ribonucleotides from purines and pyrimidines, the *de novo* pathway and salvage the salvage pathway operates to save the cells from possible death. The salvage pathways require hypoxanthine and thymidine and the enzymes hypoxanthine salvage pathway can not operate in the myeloma parent cells since they are deficient in (HGPRT) and thymidine kinase (TK). The slavage pathway can not operate in the myeloma parent cells since they are deficient in HGPRT enzyme, even if hypoxanthine and thymidine are provided in the form of HAT medium. So, when the *de novo* pathway is blocked by the presence of aminopterin, the myeloma parent cells and myeloma and myeloma × myeloma fused cells die out since they can not survive using the salvage pathway.

However, the myeloma × lymphocyte fused cells can survive because these fused cells have obtained the HGPRT enzyme from the spleen lymphocyte partner and can operate the salvage pathway using this enzyme, in the presence of hypoxanthine and thymidine. This by itself is not enough. Our requirement is that these fused cells should have the capability of secreting antibodies of our desired specificity against the antigen of interest. This can be achieved only by screening the supernatant of the cells surviving in the HAT medium (myeloma × lymphocyte fused cells) as to whether they are secreting the antibodies of our interest by appropriate screening assays.

After identifying such supernatants these cells in that particular wells have to be brought down to the level of a single individual cell and then multiplied from that individual cell to produce a clone of that particular antibody secreting cell. This is achieved by a process of sub cloning by limiting dilution–making a dilution with a theoretical possibility of having a single cell per well and then expanding the same and also ensuring that the expanded cells produce antibodies of the desired specificity.

Each lymphocyte is capable of making an antibody of a single specificity. The resultant is a clone of identical cells each capable of producing antibodies of the desired specificity as screened in our assay. Such antibodies are called as monoclonal antibodies (mAbs)–antibodies of a single specificity produced by a single clone of lymphocytes.

Thus this process has resulted in the:

- Fusion of lymphocyte × myeloma cells thereby giving the lymphocyte an infinite life span
- Single clone of lymphocyte producing antibodies of the desired specificity
- Such mAbs are directed against a single epitope, belonging to a particular class and subclass and have a particular affinity.

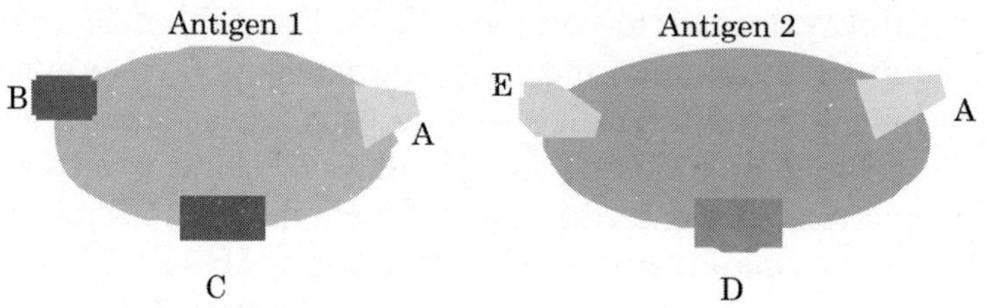

Fig. 1.1. Potential cross reaction between two dissimilar antigens

Polyclonal serum raised against antigen 1 would show partial cross reactions with antigen 2 since determinant A is shared but the other two epitopes are not shared. Monoclonal antibodies to determinant A would cross react 100% with antigen 2. However mAbs to epitopes B and C would not cross react at all with antigen 2.

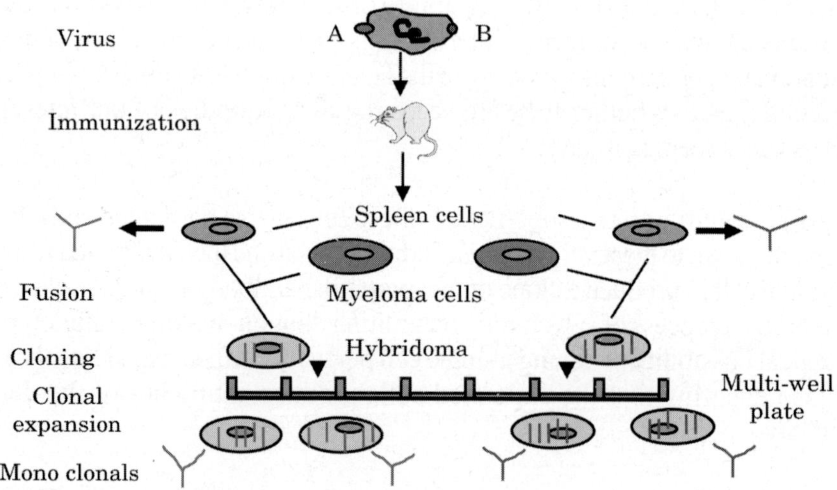

Fig. 1.2: Overview of monoclonal antibody production

Table 1.1: Comparison of Polyclonal and Monoclonal Antibodies

Characteristic	*Polyclonal serum*	*Monoclonal antibodies*
Specificity	Against many epitopes	Against single epitope
Affinity	Variable with every bleed	Can be selected during cloning
Isotype	Variable antibodies belong to different classes and subclasses	Antibody belong to a single class and subclass
Host species	Any species of animal	Predominantly in mouse systems, may be rat and humans and now with rabbits and chickens too

Table 1.1: (*Contd...*)

Table 1.1: (*Contd...*)

Characteristic	*Polyclonal serum*	*Monoclonal antibodies*
Cross reactivity	Variable with every bleed, cross reactions can be adsorbed out	Governed by nature of cross reacting epitope present in other related or unrelated antigen
Contaminating host immunoglobulins	Contaminated with all the host fluids	None in culture; 10% in ascitic
Yield	1–10 mg/ml	100 ì g/ml in culture or 20 ì g/ml in ascitic fluids
Cost	Cheaper	Capital intensive

Polyclonal serum has antibodies against all the epitopes on the antigen while mAbs has antibodies against a single selected epitope. This specificity of mAbs has both advantages and disadvantages depending on the context of application of mAbs. Cross reactions can occur with the use of polyclonal serum and 2 proteins which have similar determinants. This could be avoided by the use of mAbs that has been produced to bind to an epitope unique to the desired antigen. By using mAbs it is possible to distinguish between two closely related organisms (that may be difficult to achieve using polyclonal serum). A typical example is peste des petits ruminants (PPR) and rinderpest (RP) viruses.

They are two closely related viruses belonging to the Moribilli virus genus and family *Paramyxoviridae* that infects small and large ruminants respectively. It is difficult to distinguish these two viruses by the use of polyclonal serum since both these viruses share common epitopes and antibodies to these epitopes would be present in polyclonal serum.

These two viruses also possess some unique epitopes and mAbs produced against these epitopes can be used to differentiate these two viruses. For example the nucleoprotein (N) of these two viruses is sufficiently different to target epitopes on this protein for use in discrimination of these two viruses.

Although this exquisite specificity is advantageous it could be disadvantageous when it is not ensured that all the isolates of the virus does not possess the same epitope. For example, some portions of the nucleoprotein of PPRV is also very variable between isolates and if mAbs are directed against an epitope present in this region, although it is useful to differentiate between PPR and RP viruses, it may end up in not picking up all PPR viruses circulating in the field. In such instances a polyclonal serum could have been useful since even though one epitope would have mutated in a particular virus, there would be antibodies to other epitopes that would still aid in diagnosing the virus infection.

The choice hence depends on the final application of the mAbs. May be a poly monoclonal antibody that is a mixture of some well defined mAbs would provide a via media between a mAbs that is too specific and polyclonal serum that is too variable.

As a reagent, mAbs is only too superior to polyclonal serum since they are well defined, not variable with bleed or with individual animals and would produce always reproducible results in any laboratory using it. The isotype of mAbs can also be selected based on the final application.

For example, if the mAbs has to be used in an agglutination assay, an IgM type of mAb would be preferable since it is a better agglutinating antibody by virtue of its valency of 10 mAbs should not be thought of as a total alternative to the conventional polyclonal serum but it is for the reader and researcher to know clearly the pros and cons of each system and decide the requirement of each system. Many of the immunocapture enzyme linked immunosorbant assay (ELISA) kits for diagnosis of diseases utilize a combination of both, a polyclonal serum to capture the pathogen (broader specificity) and mAbs as a detection reagent (finer specificity) thereby taking advantage of both the systems.

1.3 Monoclonal Antibodies–An Overview

An *in vivo* response to an antigen is polyclonal–the particular antigen binds to a B-cell with membrane IgM of IgD receptor complementary to the antigen, from a whole repertoire of about 10^{13} B cell specificities pre existent in our body (clonal selection theory). Afterwards the B cell undergoes clonal expansion and differentiation in to plasma cells to secrete more antibodies of the same specificity. Since the antigen involved is multi-epitopic, the same process would be occurring for each epitope on the antigen. Next step is switching of isotype resulting in conversion of isotype of antibody to other classes and subclasses while retaining the same epitope specificity. The affinity maturation occurs by somatic hyper mutation thereby increasing affinity of the antibody.

What if one event is dissected out from this complex response. That is, one B-cell that possesses a membrane receptor complementary to one of the epitopes on the antigen is separated out and then allowed to expand *in vitro*. These cells would all be secreting antibody of the same specificity capable of binding to the same epitope. The advantage of this separation is that we will have particular pre defined antibody specificity against a single epitope. However, the B-cells are having a finite life span and thus the secreted antibody may be of limited quantity. Thus if this particular B-cell secreting antibody of a single specificity is immortalized then it would be a continuous source of antibody of a desired specificity. A series of discoveries culminated in this discovery by Kohler and Milstein in 1975 with a paper in *Nature*.

DNA, RNA and proteins are the major bio-molecules controlling majority of life processes. While DNA tells us what we can do, it is the protein molecule that actually does the functions.

1.4 On Proteins *vs* Nucleic Acids

The main functions of proteins include:

- Catalysis
- Movement
- Regulation
- Storage
- Structure
- Defense
- Transport
- Stress response

Amino acids are building blocks for proteins. A protein chain consists of amino acid monomers connected by covalent amide linkages called peptide bonds. All amino acids have a general structure with an á carbon atom at the centre, to its right is an acidic carboxyl group (COO-, when ionized) and to its left is the basic amino group (NH_3^+, when ionized). A hydrogen atom and the side chain group (R) connect to the alpha carbon atom from the two other sides (Fig. 1.3).

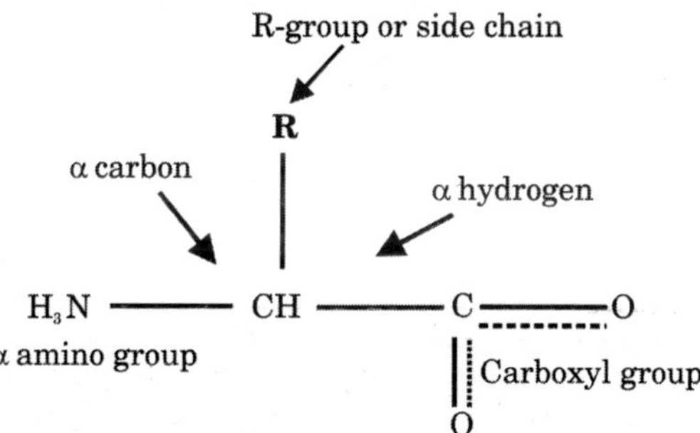

Fig. 1.3: Structure of amino acid

The amino acids have the same core structure but differ in the composition of the R side chain. Normally twenty different amino acids form proteins.

The α-C is chiral (except glycine); proteins contain only L-isoforms. Amino acids are ampholytes, pKa of α-COOH is ~2 and of α-NH_2 is ~ 9.01. At physiological pH most amino acids occur as zwitterions.

Amino acids are classified as polar or non-polar (Timberlake, 1992) and further sub classified as acidic-polar (side chain containing a carboxylic acid) and basic polar (side chain containing an amino group). The classification of amino acids is given in Table 1.2.

Table 1.2: Classification of Amino acids

Classification	*Amino acids*
Non polar	Glycine, alanine, vline, leucine, isoleucine, proline, methionine, phenyl alanine, tryptophan
Polar	Serine, threonine, asparagine, glutamine, cysteine, tyrosine
Acidic (polar)	Aspartic acid, glutamic acid
Basic (polar)	Lysine, arginine, histidine

Another method of classification based on structural lines (Devlin 1992) is given in Table 1.3.

Table 1.3: Classification of Amino acids Based on Structural Lines

Super structure	*Structure*	*Amino acids*
Monoamino, moncarboxylic		Glycine, alanine
	Unsubstituted	Valine, leucine, isoleucine
	Heterocyclic	Proline, phenylalanine
	Aromatic	Tyrosine, tryptophan
	Thioether	Methionine
	Hydroxy	Serine, threonine
	Mercapto	Cysteine
	Carboxamide	Asparagine, glutamine
Monamino, dicarboxylic		Aspartate, glutamate
Diamino, monocarboxylic		Lysine, arginine, histidine

A third classification is based on the structure of the side chain (Koolman and Rohm 1996) is given in Table 1.4.

Table 1.4: Method of Classification of Amino acids Based on Structure of side Chain

Classification	*Amino acids*
Alphatic (do not contain N, O, S in side chain)	Glycine, alanine, valine,leucine, isoleucine
Sulphur-containing	cysteine, methionine
Aromatic (benzene ring in side chain)	Phenylalanine, tyrosine, tryptophan
Neutral (hydroxyl or amide groups in side chain)	Serine, threonine, asparagine, glutamine
Acidic (carboxylate groups in side chain)	Aspartic acid, Glutamic acid
Basic	Lysine, arginine
Imino acid (special case)	Proline

The side chains of amino acids and its structure at neutral pH is given in Table 1.5.

Table 1.5: Side Chains of Amino acids

Amino acids	*Structure at neutral pH*
Non-polar (hydrophobic) R groups	
Glycine	H | H_3N^+ — CH — CO_2
Alanine	CH_3 \\ H_2N^+ — CH — CO_2

Table 1.5 (*Contd...*)

Table 1.5 (*Contd...*)

Amino acids	*Structure at neutral pH*
Valine	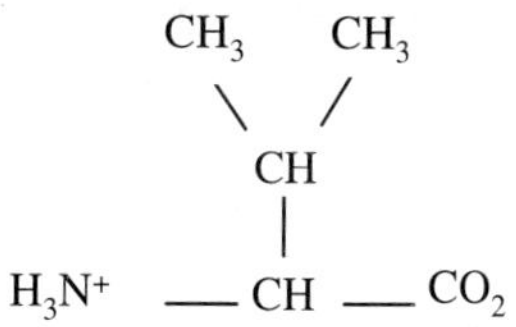 CH_3 CH_3 \ / CH | H_3N^+ — CH — CO_2
Leucine	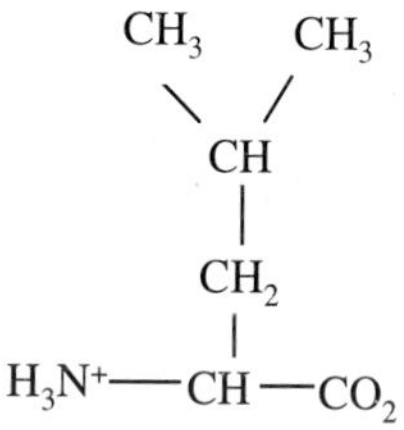 CH_3 CH_3 \ / CH | CH_2 | H_3N^+—CH—CO_2
Isoleucine	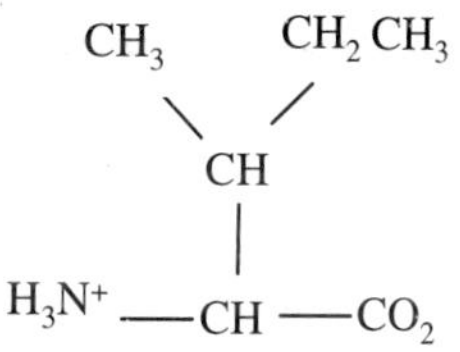 CH_3 $CH_2\,CH_3$ \ / CH | H_3N^+ —CH —CO_2
Proline	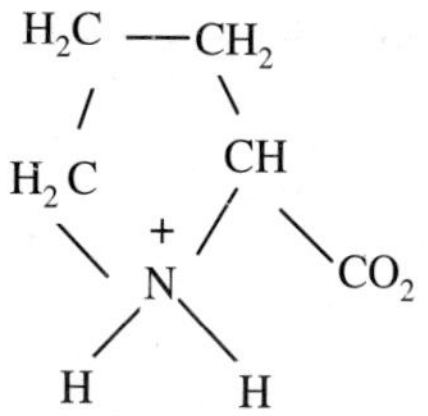 H_2C —CH_2 / \ H_2C CH \ + / \ CO_2 N / \ H H
Methioine	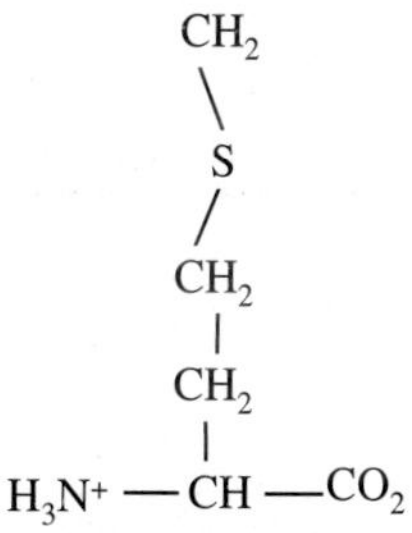 CH_2 \ S / CH_2 | CH_2 | H_3N^+ —CH —CO_2
Phenyl alanine	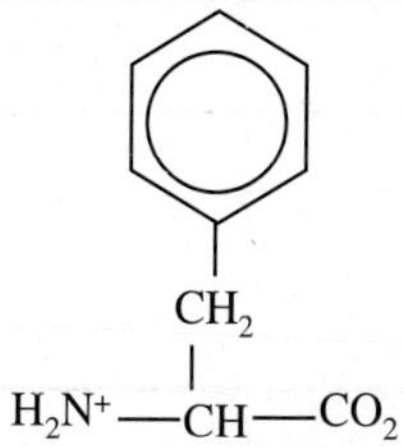 | CH_2 | H_2N^+—CH—CO_2

Table 1.5 (*Contd...*)

Table 1.5 (*Contd...*)

Amino acids	*Structure at neutral pH*
Polar (hydrophilic) R groups	
Serine	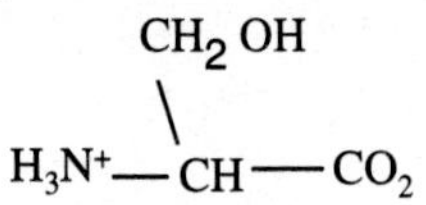 $H_3N^+—CH(CH_2OH)—CO_2$
Tryptophan	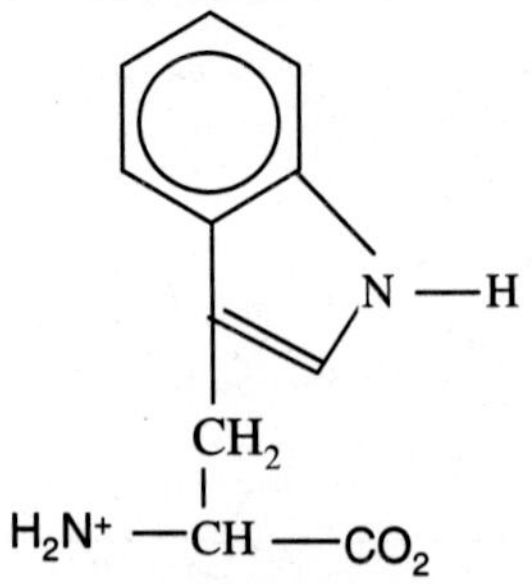 $H_2N^+—CH(CH_2\text{-indole, N—H})—CO_2$
Threnine	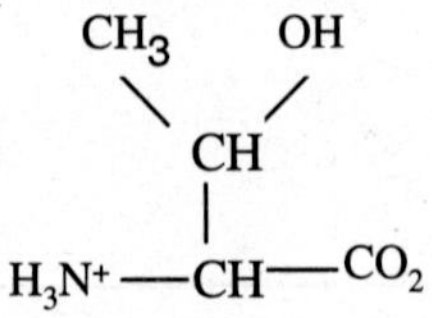 $H_3N^+—CH(CH(CH_3)(OH))—CO_2$
Tyrosine	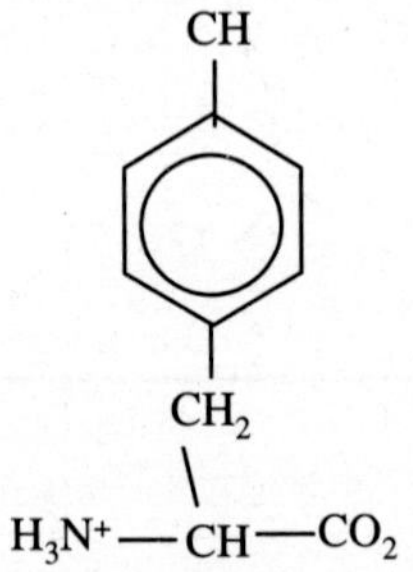 $H_3N^+—CH(CH_2\text{-C}_6\text{H}_4\text{-CH})—CO_2$
Asparagine	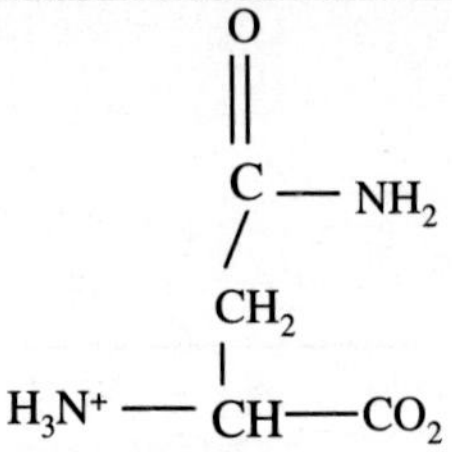 $H_3N^+—CH(CH_2—C(=O)—NH_2)—CO_2$
Cysteine	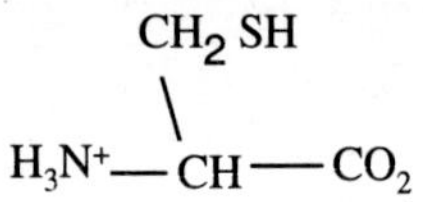 $H_3N^+—CH(CH_2SH)—CO_2$

Table 1.5 (*Contd...*)

Table 1.5 (*Contd...*)

Amino acids	*Structure at neutral pH*
Negatively charged R groups	
Aspartic acid	CO_2 / CH_2 / H_3N^+—CH—CO_2
Glutamic acid	CO_2 / CH_2 / CH_2 / H_3N^+—CH—CO_2
Positively charged R Group	
Lysine	NH_3^+ / CH_2 / CH_2 / CH_2 / CH_2 / H_3N^+—CH—CO_2
Arginine	NH_2 / C=NH_2 / NH / CH_2 / CH_2 / CH_2 / H_3N^+—CH—CO_2
Histidine	N, N, —H, H / CH_2 / H_2N^+—C —CO

A carboxylic acid condenses with an amino group with the release of water to form a peptide bond (Fig. 1.4).

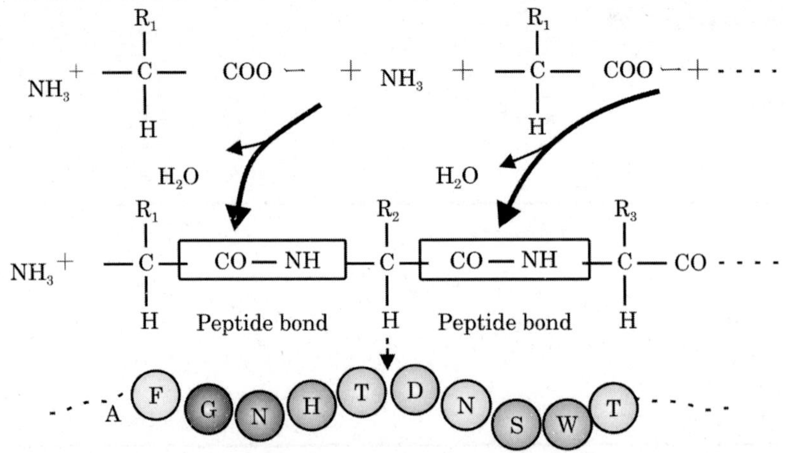

Fig. 1.4: Formation of peptide bond

DNA is composed of nucleotides made of a pentose sugar, hetero cyclic base and phosphate group. The base is attached to the sugar through the glycosidic bond. The bases are adenine, guanine, cytosine, thymine and uracil. Uracil does not occur in the DNA. The phosphate group is covalently linked to the sugar. Adjacent nucleotides are bound by the covalent phospho di ester bonds between the 3' carbon of one nucleotide and the 5' carbon of the adjacent nucleotide.

The structure of the nucleotide is given in (Fig. 1.5).

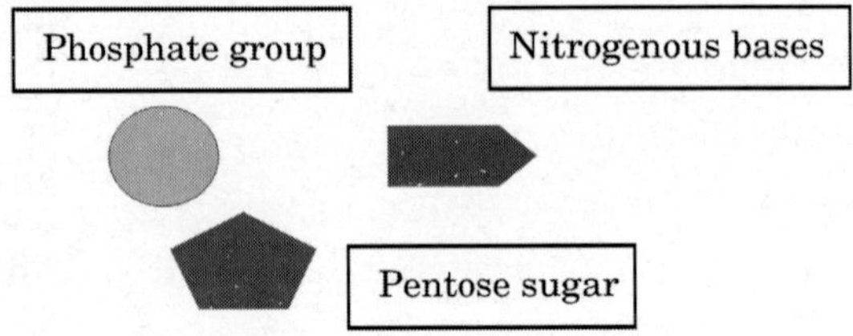

Fig. 1.5: Nucleotide structure of DNA

The structure of the sugars and bases are shown in Fig. 1.6, 1.7, 1.8 and 1.9

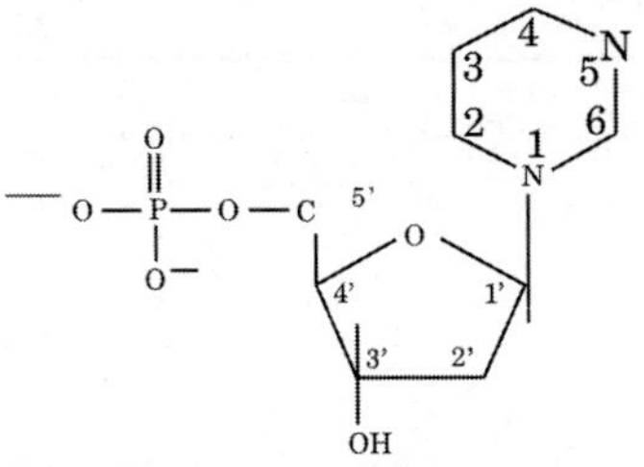

Fig. 1.6: Structure of sugars and bases

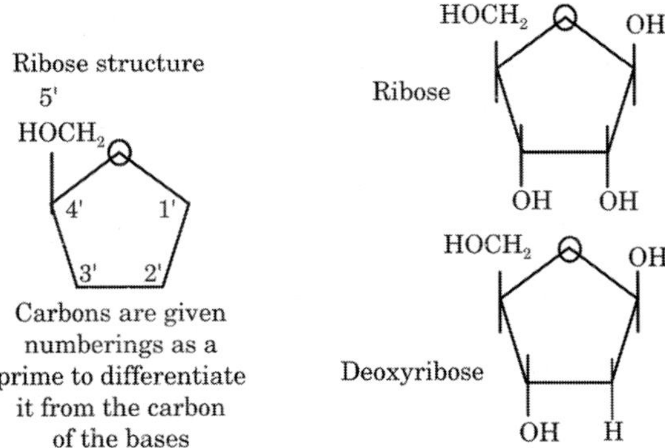

Fig. 1.7: Structure of sugars in nucleic acid

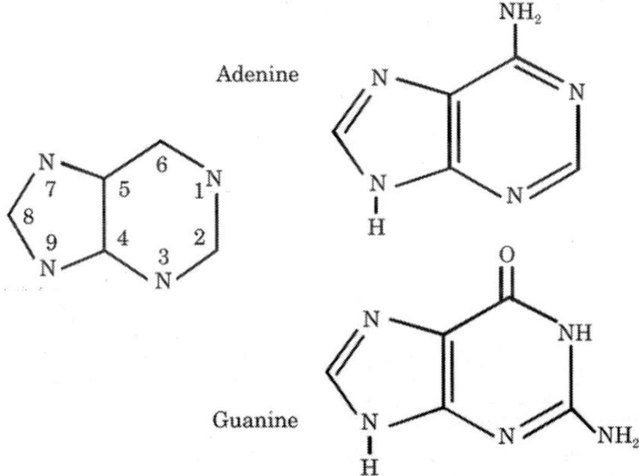

Fig. 1.8: Structure of purines

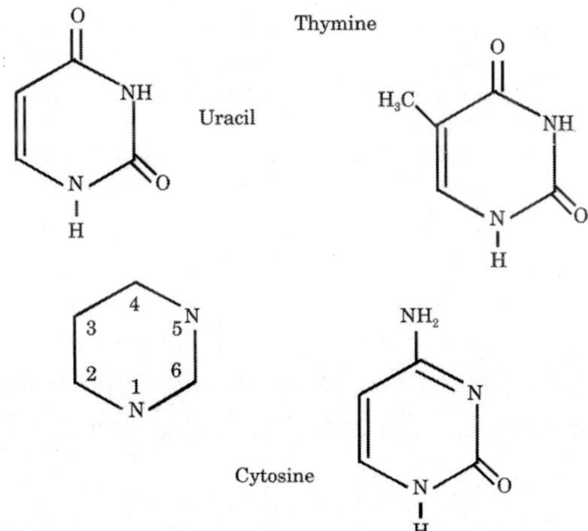

Fig. 1.9: Structure of pyrimidines

The DNA has a 5'–3' polarity with a free phosphate group at the 5' end and a free hydroxyl group at the 3' end DNA base pairing is anti-parallel. DNA has 10 base pairs per turn. Each base pair is 0.34 nm thick. 10 base pairs would be 0.34 nm × 10 = 3.4 nm length. If you are given the length of a segment of DNA you can calculate the number of base pairs. If a DNA molecule is 1 mm

$$1\mu = 1000 \text{ nm}$$

$$1000 \text{ nm}/0.34 \text{ nm/bp} = 2941 \text{ base pairs}$$

The proteins have an amino terminal with a free amino group and a carboxyl terminal with a free carboxyl group.

5' mRNA sequence 3'
AUG AAC AAU GCG CCG GAG GAA GCG GAG
Met -----Asn -----Asn -----Ala -----Pro -----Glu -----Glu -----Ala ----Glu
N-terminus Protein sequence C-terminus

The genetic code is shown in Table 1.6.

Table 1.6: Genetic code

First letter		Second letter								Third letter
		T		**C**		**A**		**G**		
T	TTT	Phe	TCT	Ser	TAT	Tyr	TGT	Cys	T	
	TTC		TCC		TAC		TGC		C	
	TTA	Leu	TCA		TAA	Stop	TGA	Stop	A	
	TTG		TCG		TAG		TGG	Trp	G	
C	CTT	Leu	CCT	Pro	CAT	His	CGT	Arg	T	
	CTC		CCC		CAC		CGC		C	
	CTA		CCA		CAA	Gln	CGA		A	
	CTG		CCG		CAG		CGG		G	
A	ATT	Lle	ACT	Thr	AAT	Asn	AGT	Ser	T	
	ATC		ACC		AAC		AGC		C	
	ATA		ACA		AAA	Lys	AGA	Arg	A	
	ATG	Met	ACG		AAG		AGG		G	
G	GTT	Val	GCT	Ala	GAT	Asp	GGT	Gly	T	
	GTC		GCC		GAC		GGC		C	
	GTA		GCA		GAA	Glu	GGA		A	
	GTG		GCG		GAG		GGG		G	

DNA also has 3 different conformations, A, B and Z DNA

B-DNA is the most stable form, predominating in biological organisms. It is right-handed, approximately 20Å diameter, double-helix, with 10 base-pairs/turn giving a pitch of 34Å.

A-DNA occurs when DNA is dehydrated. It closely approximates the conformation of RNA helices. It is right-handed, approximately 26Å diameter, double-helix, with 11 base-pairs/turn giving a pitch of 28Å.

Z-DNA occurs in short stretches of DNA acting as a regulatory switching element, but biological existence uncertain. It is left-handed, approximately 18Å diameter, double helix, with 12 base-pairs/turn giving a pitch of 45Å.

1.5 Structure of Proteins

Proteins have a primary structure consisting of the linear sequence of amino acids. The bonds that make up the primary structure are the peptide bonds between each amino acid.

The secondary structure refers to the shape the protein made by hydrogen bonds that form between the side chains of the amino acids. The three common shapes formed are α-*helix*, the β-*pleated sheet* and the *triple helix*. They represent the conformation of the peptide bonds in short sections of the peptide backbone.

The *tertiary structure* of proteins is the result of further bonding between side chains within the protein and with any water molecules that may be present around the protein. Polar amino acids move to the outside of the protein and non-polar amino acids are buried inside when placed in a polar solution. The bonds in the tertiary structure include:

Bonds formed between non-polar side chains, disulphide bonds formed between sulphur atoms in cysteine side chains, ionic bonds formed between acidic and basic side chains, and hydrogen bonds formed between carbonyl groups and hydroxyl or amino groups. The tertiary structure is the three dimensional arrangement of the main polypeptide chain and side chains.

The quaternary structure is the three dimensional arrangement of the subunit chains of the protein. The bonds formed are the same as those found in the tertiary structure of proteins.

The primary structure of insulin consists of an A chain of 21 amino acids and a B chain of 30 amino acids. The secondary structure of the A chain consists of 2 sections of alpha helix (A2 Ile A8 Thr and A13 Leu A19 Tyr) with flat ribbon structures in between them. The B chain, wraps around the A chain and consists of a larger section of alpha-helix (B9 Ser-B19 Cys). In addition, the smaller glycine residues at 20 and 23 allow it to fold into V shape. This brings the C terminal residues B24 Phe and B26 Tyr into Van der Waals contact with B15 Leu and B11 Leu of the alpha-helix. The tertiary structure of insulin is stabilized by disulphide bridges, 2 between the A and B chains (between A7 and B7, and A20 and B19), and one within the A chain (A6 and A11). Insulin can form into granules consisting of hexamers (6 insulin molecules grouped around 2 zinc ions) due to interactions between hydrophobic surfaces.

The shape of proteins which determines its function is governed by the bonds that form between the side chains of amino acids. Thus the primary purpose of the side chains in amino acids is to give proteins their shape.

1.5.1 Protein Quantification and Detection Methods

- Spectroscopic procedures for characterizing protein samples
- Amino acid analysis
- Radiolabelling of proteins
- Measurement of the total protein content by colorimetry
- Edman degradation.

1.5.1.1 *Spectrophotometric measurement of proteins*

Most proteins have an absorption maximum at 280 nm due to the phenolic group of tyrosine and indolic group of tryptophan. Measuring the concentration of the protein using this method is inaccurate unless the protein is pure and its extinction coefficient is known. Purine and pyrimidine rings that absorb at 280 nm interferes with the measurement and hence a correction factor is used.

$$\text{Protein (mg/ml)} = 1.55\,A_{280} - 0.76\,A_{260}$$

In addition, the peptide bonds have well defined absorption maxima at 191–194 nm. Measurement is made at 205 nm and this method is less dependent on amino acid composition. Correction is made for the tyrosine and tryptophan content measurement at 280 nm.

$$E_{205}^{1mg/ml} = 27.0 + 120 \times \frac{A\,280}{A\,205}$$

1.5.1.2 *Colorimetric detection of proteins*

1.5.1.2.1 *Biuret method*

The assay is based on polypeptide chelation of cupric ion (colored chelate) in strong alkali. Compounds containing two or more peptide bonds react with cupric ions (Cu^{2+}) in alkaline solution to produce a complex of reddish-purple colour.

Reagent: alkaline Copper sulphate
Sensitivity -1 mg, peptide bonds (A = 550 nm)

1.5.1.2.2 *Lowry method*

Lowry-Folin-Ciocalteau reagent consists of phosphomolybdate and phosphotungstate with oxidize metal constituents. The assay is a colorimetric assay based on cupric ions and Folin-Ciocalteau reagent for phenolic groups (A = 650 nm). The reagent reacts at susceptible amino acid residues in proteins, *e.g.*, phenolic group of Tyr; Indole of Trp; -SH of Cys. Thus, the phosphomolybdate–phosphotungstate is reduced to blue-coloured salts (molydenum blue-type salts).

Most proteins contain little Trp or Cys. Therefore, the colour here is largely due to Tyr content. Sensitivity-A few micrograms but very different with various proteins.

1.5.1.2.3 *Bis-cinchoninic acid (BCA) reagent for proteins*

The BCA assay for total protein is a spectophotometric assay based on the alkaline reduction of the cupric ion to the cuprous ion by the protein, followed by chelation and color development by the BCA reagent. (A = 562 nm). Cu^{2+} ions reduced to Cu^{1+} ions by aromatic amino acids in protein. Cu^{1+} ions + bicinchoninic acid® complex gives an intense absorption maximum at 562 nm. BCA assay has a good combination of sensitivity and simplicity.

1.5.1.2.4 *Bradford method*

This assay is based on the measurement of bound Coomassie dye (Brilliant blue G250) (A = 595 nm).

1.6 DNA and Protein Electrophoresis

The charge on the DNA is negative by virtue of its phosphate group and its charge mass ratio is always constant. Thus if we load a sample of DNA in the negative side of a gel and pass current, it would move towards the positive side because of the net negative charge and the separation is based on the size of the DNA.

In proteins, the charge is not only dependant on the side chains of the amino acids but also on the surrounding medium (pH of the solvent).

As the pH falls the amino acids become more positively charged (HOOC-R-NH_3^+) and as it increases the amino acids become more negatively charged ($^-$OOC-R-NH_2).

At the isoelectric point (pI) the positive and negative charges balance out and there is no net charge on the protein making it immobile at that pH.

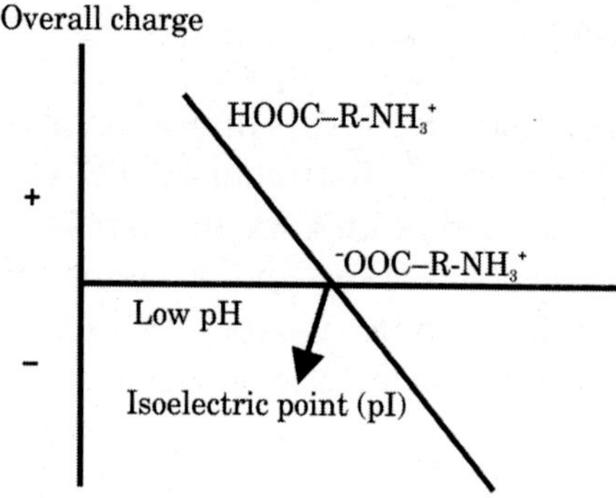

Fig. 1.10: Ionization of amino acids based on pH

The pKa of the amino acids are given in Table 1.7.

Table 1.7: Three Letter, Single Letter Code and pKa of Amino acids

Amino acid	*Single letter code*	*Molecular weight (daltons)*	*COOH*	*NH_3^+*	*R*
Ala	A	89	2.35	9.87	–
Arg	R	174	1.82	8.99	12.48
Asn	N	132	2.10	8.84	–
Asp	D	133	1.99	9.90	3.90
Cys	C	121	1.92	10.78	8.33
Glu	E	147	2.10	9.47	4.07
Gln	Q	146	2.17	9.13	–
Gly	G	75	2.35	9.78	–
His	H	155	1.80	9.33	6.04
Ile	I	131	2.32	9.76	–
Leu	L	131	2.33	9.74	–
Lys	K	146	2.16	9.18	10.79
Met	M	149	2.13	9.28	–
Phe	F	165	2.16	9.18	–
Pro	P	115	1.95	10.65	–
Ser	S	105	2.19	9.21	~13.0
Thr	T	119	2.09	9.10	~13.0
Trp	W	204	2.43	9.44	–
Tyr	Y	181	2.20	9.11	10.13
Val	V	117	2.29	9.74	–

Which direction the protein migrates under the influence of the electric current depends on the net charge on the protein, if it is negative charge it would move towards the positive charge and *vice versa*. The other influencing factor in electrophoresis is the gel matrix. The most common is agarose and polyacrylamide.

Agarose polymer consists of multiple units of agarbiose molecules linked together. This is a disaccharide of β-d-galactose and 3, 6, anhydroα, 1 galactose. Agarose exists in random coils when mixed in buffer but after boiling and cooling the chains become double helices giving the gel matrix useful for electrophoresis.

The agarose gel structure is held together by non-covalent interactions like hydrogen bonds and electrostatic interactions. Heating the solution breaks these non-covalent interactions and separates the strands. Then as the solution cools, these non-covalent interactions are re-established and the gel forms. So agarose (and agar) gels are formed by gellation and not through polymerization.

Although agarose has higher pore sizes, chemically modified agarose with smaller pore sizes are also available such as Nusieve® and Metaphor®

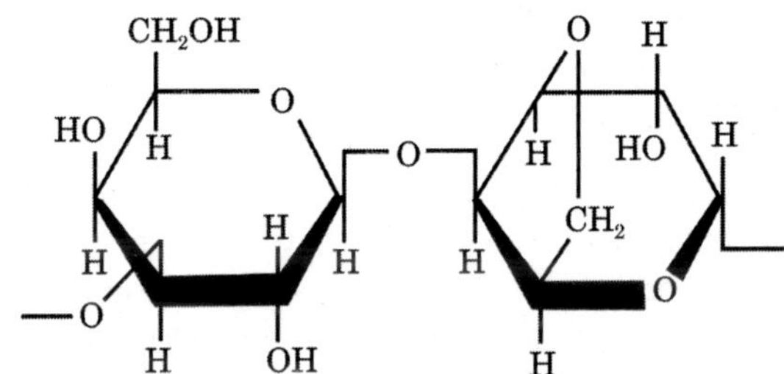

Fig. 1.11: Agarose of structure

Polyacrylamide gels are formed by copolymerization of acrylamide and bis-acrylamide (N,N'-methylene-bisacrylamide). The reaction is a vinyl addition polymerization initiated by ammonium persulphate and TEMED (tetramethy-lethylenediamine) through a free radical-generating system. TEMED accelerates the rate of formation of free radicals from persulphate which converts acrylamide monomers to free radicals which react with unactivated monomers to begin the polymerization chain reaction. The elongating polymer chains are randomly cross linked by bis, resulting in a gel with a characteristic porosity which depends on the polymerization conditions and monomer concentrations.

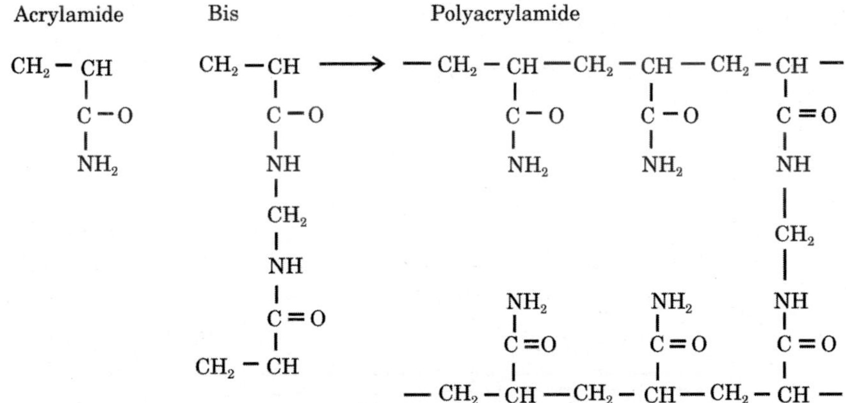

Fig. 1.12: Acrylamide bis polyacrylamide

Riboflavin (or riboflavin-5'-phosphate) may also be used as a source of free radicals, often in combination with TEMED and ammonium persulphate. In the presence of light and oxygen, riboflavin is converted to its leuco form, which is active in initiating polymerization. This is usually referred to as photochemical polymerization. It is generally considered that agarose is used for DNA and polyacrylamide for proteins. But there are exceptions, for example agar gel precipitation test or immune electrophoresis uses agarose or agar for separating proteins and polyacrylamide gels are used for sequencing or micro satellite analysis. Then what governs this choice? It is the size of the molecule.

The DNA is the larger molecule than the proteins. The average molecular weight of the amino acid is only 110 daltons while the molecular weight of a nucleotide is 660 daltons.

The average protein is 30–50 KDa while the average nucleic acid is > 2000 KDa. The agarose gels have more pore size than polyacrylamide gels. Hence it is used for separation of the large DNA or the larger protein molecules such as immune complexes. The size of pores in a 1% agarose gels is 150 nm and in 0.15% agarose gels is 500 nm.

The polyacrylamide gels have smaller pore sizes and are used for the smaller protein molecules and the smaller DNA fragments such as micro satellites or sequencing where even a single base pair difference needs to be shown up.

Electrophoresis is dependent on size, shape, charge and the porosity of the gels. Two molecules A and B are electrophoresed. A is large but highly charged; B is small and less charged. Then which of the two molecules would move faster?

In a gel with larger pores (low percentage gels) the molecule A would move faster since there is no sieving effect of the gel, so size does not matter, a larger molecule also would move fast. Hence, the charge on the molecule A would drive faster despite it being larger in size.

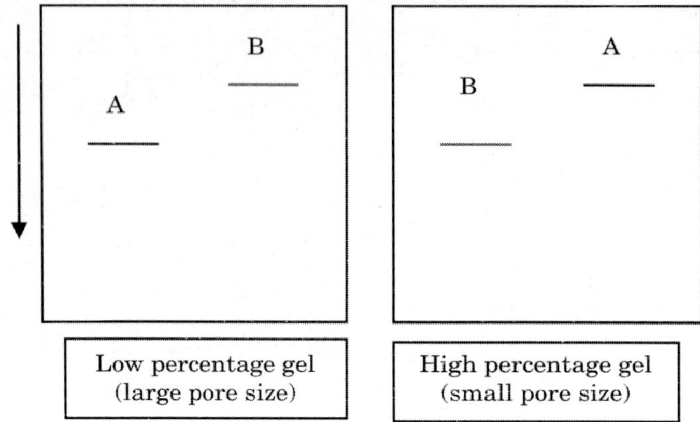

Fig. 1.13: Movement of molecules is dependent on the porosity of the gel.

In a gel with small pores (high percentage gels), the molecule B would move faster since the sieving effect of the gel would retard the larger molecule (A) despite being highly charged (Fig. 1.13).

The direction of movement of proteins depends on the net charge on the protein. Hence to achieve unidirectional movement of the proteins from negative to positive side (like DNA) the charge on the proteins should be made negative irrespective of the original intrinsic charge on the molecule.

This could be achieved by two ways. One is simply to increase the pH of the buffer in which the electrophoresis is run so that the amino acids ionize into a negative charge. This is followed in such cases as counter immuno electrophoresis (Fig. 1.14) where a high pH buffer is used (barbital buffer) and the antigen is loaded on the negative side from where it moves to the positive side. The antibody would move in the opposite direction due to electro endosmosis leading to the formation of a precipitin line due to antigen antibody interaction and immune complex formation.

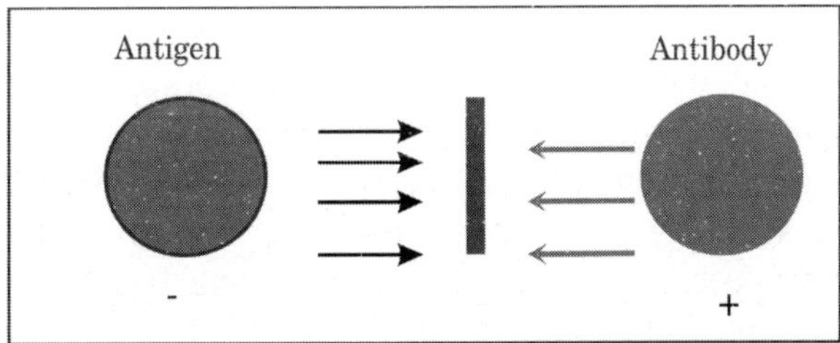

Fig. 1.14: Movement of antigen in high pH buffer (counter current electrophoresis)

The other approach is to coat the protein with an anionic detergent such as sodium dodecyl sulphate (SDS) so that the intrinsic charges on the denatured protein are covered with the 'blanket' of negative charges. Now the protein is made to behave like a DNA and it moves unidirectionally based on the porosity of the gels (Fig. 1.15).

Before coating the protein with SDS, it is denatured using heat and reducing agents such as 2-mercaptoethanol or dithiothreitol. The denatured protein molecules get a linear shape facilitating maximal and reproducible detergent binding.

The proteins are also classified as fibrous or globular. Fibrous proteins like collagen, keratin and silk fibroin exist as insoluble aggregates of many polypeptide chains. Globular proteins are spherical in shape and are soluble in the cytosol.

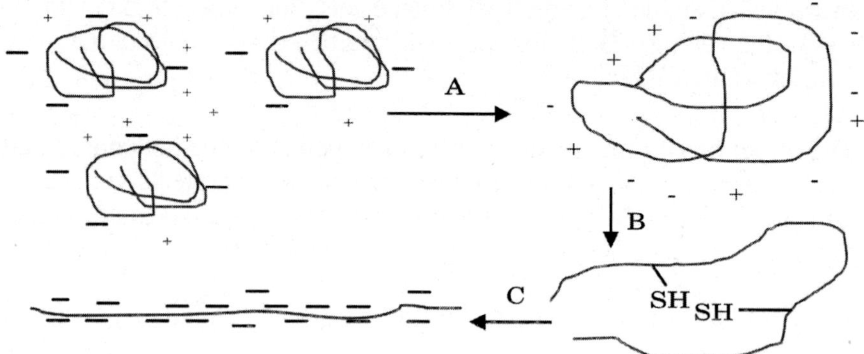

Fig. 1.15: Denaturation and coating of proteins with SDS. **A:** Dissociation of protein sub units, **B:** reduction of disulphide bonds; **C:** SDS coating

DNA functions as the hereditary molecule which stores the genetic information for making proteins. Proteins function as enzymatic, structural and other defense functions.

One of the molecules playing a role in defense is the antibodies. Antibodies are globular proteins that exist in three dimensional conformation determined by their primary amino acid sequences, the interaction between side chains of amino acids and pH of buffer in which they are present. For convenience purposes antibodies are shown as Y-shaped linear molecules. However, it is for the student to conceptualize that proteins exist in a three dimensional format and what is shown as antigen-antibody interactions is actually protein-protein interaction.

What is specificity in molecular terms is that amino acid side chains in the protein are at particular places that aid bond formation. For an empirical example, if in an antigen epitope an acidic amino acid is at position 5 and a basic amino acid is at position 9, then the combining site on the antibody molecule should have a basic amino acid at position 5 and an acidic amino acid at position 9. This would facilitate ionic bond formation between these two polypeptide chains. Then these two polypeptide chains may be considered specific.

The following types of bonds may occur between any two polypeptide chains. Covalent bonds arise when two atoms share electrons. Cysteine is the sole amino acid whose side chain can form covalent bonds, yielding disulphide bridges with other cysteine side chains:

$$-CH_2\text{-}S\text{-}S\text{-}CH_2\text{-}$$

Ionic bonds are formed as amino acids bearing opposite electrical charges are juxtaposed together. Ionic bonding in the interior is rare because most charged amino acids lie on the protein surface. They are potent electrostatic attractions that can approach the strength of covalent bonds.

Hydrogen bonds are formed due to the attraction of two negatively charged atoms for hydrogen. They are formed by the sharing of a proton between donor and acceptor groups. The strength is around 2-5 kcal/mol and the ideal distance is 2.8–3 Å.

Van der Waals forces are weak attractive force between the electron cloud of one atom and protons of another molecule.

Hydrophobic force is the attraction between non-polar groups, tends to exclude water. Hydrophobic interactions are not attractive interactions, but results from the inability of water to form hydrogen bonds with certain side chains.

1.7 Antigens and Antibodies–Structure and Functions-A Recap

Antigen is a substance that reacts with the products of specific immune response. Immunogen induces a specific immune response. Haptens are non-immunogenic but which can react with products of a specific immune response. Haptens are antigenic but not immunogenic.

- Epitope or antigenic determinant is that portion of an antigen that combines with the products of a specific immune response.
- Antibody is a glycoprotein that are produced in response to an immunogen and which reacts with an antigen.
- Antigens can be proteins, polysaccharides or lipo polysaccharides, nucleic acids and to a lesser extent lipids.
- The immunogenicity of a molecule is determined by the features of the immunogen, the host and the delivery system.
- Non-self, large, complex, easily degradable particulate substances tend to be more immunogenic.

The genetic factors of the host, its health status and age also determine the nature and magnitude of the immune responses. BALB/c mice used in mAb production tend to produce mAbs mostly of IgG_1 subclass to any immunogen due to genetic reasons.

The dose, route of administration and delivery with adjuvants tend to alter the nature and magnitude of the immune responses. For example, anti-rabies vaccine was given intra dermal around the navel in earlier days. This is because the magnitude of immune responses was higher due to the antigen presenting Langerhans cells being abundant in the skin. However since the injection is difficult as if it crosses the skin it would become subcutaneous this has been discontinued.

The epitopes can be either linear or conformational. Linear epitopes are created by primary linear sequence of amino acids while conformational epitopes could be created by the coming together of amino acids that are spatially apart in their linear sequence. An antibody recognizing a conformational epitope may not be able to react with the denatured protein.

Theoretically any sequence of 8–10 amino acid residues of a polypeptide chain can act as an antigen. Just like any sequence stretch of bases can act as a primer in a polymerase chain reaction (PCR). However there are certain design criteria for a good PCR primer. Similarly, certain stretches of amino acids are better epitopic determinants than others. Mostly amino acids that are exposed on the surface (made up of hydrophilic amino acids) are better epitopes for B-cells and those bind to the major histocompatability complex (MHC) are better T cell epitopes.

Immunoglobulins and antibodies are interchangeably used. However the term antibody can be used in the context of an antigen while immunoglobulins are used to denote general antibodies, although this difference is not absolute. For example, it is antibodies to rota virus while it is the immunoglobulins that are passively transferred from dam to calf.

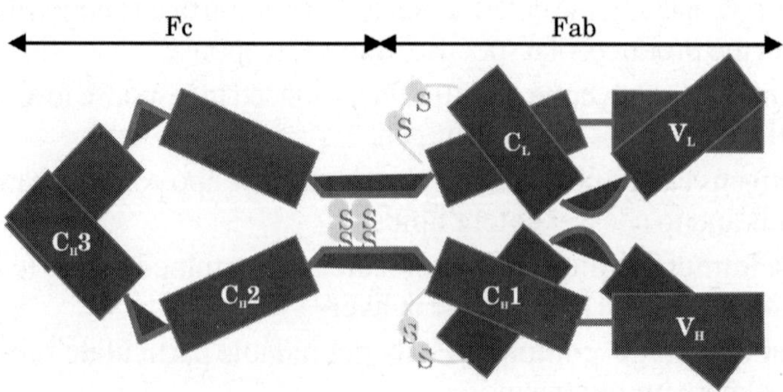

Fig. 1.16: Schematic representation of immunoglobulin molecule

All immunoglobulins have 4 polypeptide chains, two identical light chains (23–25 kDa) and 2 identical heavy chains (50–70 kDa).

The heavy and light chains and two heavy chains are held together by inter chain disulphide bonds.The immunoglobulin structure is designed on the basis of domains of 110 amino acids long that offer structural conservation and a capacity for infinite variability in a single molecule. Ig domains are derived from a single ancestral gene that has duplicated, diversified and modified.

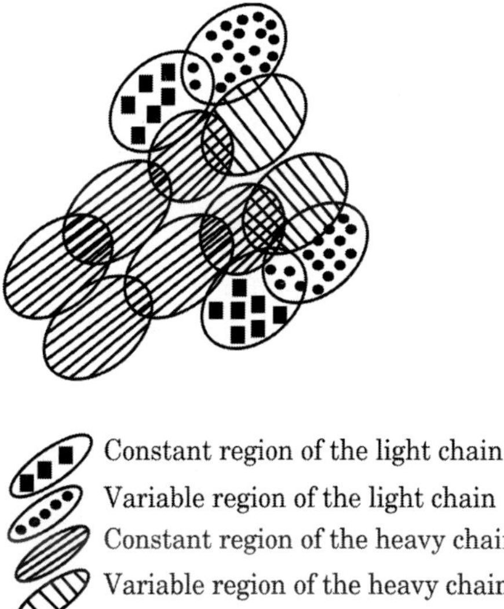

Fig. 1.17: Another representation of immunoglobullin molecule.

So how many hands would an immunoglobulin molecule give on denaturing poly acrylamide gel elecrophoresis?

Two bands

All the disulphide bonds would be broken down by denaturation and by the action of mercaptoethanol or dithiothreitol. This would result into 4 polypeptide chains but 2 bands since the two light and the two heavy chains would bend at the same position as their molecular weights are same. In case of IgG, there would be 2 bands around 50 and 25 kDa. In case of IgM there would be two bands at about 70 kDa and 24 kDa, since the heavy chain of IgM has one more domain in its constant region. If the immunoglobulin molecule is not denatured, there would be only one band.

The heavy and light chains are divided into constant and variable regions based on the extent of amino acid variability. There are sequences in these regions divided into domains. The light chain domains are V_L and C_L. The heavy chain domains are V_H and C_{H1-3} or $_4$. There is a hinge region in the antibody molecule between the C_{H1} and C_{H2} regions that permit flexibility to the molecule. Carbohydrates are attached to the C_{H2} domain in most immunoglobulins. Within the variable region of the light and heavy chains, there are each three distinct hyper variable regions (HVR) or comlementarity determining regions (CDR) that actually participate in bond formation with the epitope on the antigen molecule.

The amino acids between the CDRs are called as framework regions (FR). Although these amino acids do not participate directly in interaction with the epitope on the antigen, they do contribute indirectly by determining the conformation of the amino acids in the CDRs. The amino acid sequences of the six CDRs determine the specificity of the antibody molecule. Different combinations of CDRs in V_H and V_L chains result in antibodies that can bind to different antigenic determinants.

Digestion of the immunoglobulin molecule with papain breaks it into two fragments, one that contains the light chain and V_H and C_{H1} domain of the heavy chain (F_{ab}) and the other fragment containing two heavy chains each consisting of the C_{H2} and C_{H3} domains (F_C) since it is crystallisable. Each F_{ab} is monovalent while the original immunoglobulin is divalent. While the F_{ab} is involved in antigen binding, the F_C mediates the effector functions. Digestion of the immunoglobulin molecule with pepsin, cleaves it into $(F_{ab'})_2$ while the F_C region is digested into small peptides.

Papain cleavage sites –2 × Fab and 1 × Fc
Pepsin cleavage sites –1 × $(Fab)_2$ and small peptides
$(F_{ab'})_2$ can bind to the antigen but can not mediate effector functions.

The effector functions of antibody are triggered only when the antigen binds to the corresponding antibody. Hence the immunoglobulins in the serum are waiting for the corresponding antigen to bind and make use of them. The main effector function of the antibodies is neutralization, which is brought about by binding to the epitope on the antigen and preventing it from exerting its inimical effects on the host. The other functions mediated by F_C are complement fixation, opsonization, placental transfer, mast cell degranulation, antibody dependent cellular cytotoxicity (ADCC), secretory immunoglobulin etc.

The antibody tries to fight off the 'enemy' on its own and when it fails, it tries to garner the help of other mechanisms to help in its ultimate aim of ridding the host of its 'enemy'. Hence immunoglobulin molecule is also of several classes each specializing in a particular function so that their services can be utilized in the process of immune response. There are five different classes of immunoglobulins based on differences in the amino acid sequences in the constant regions of the heavy chains that can be detected by serological methods using antibodies directed against these differences.

IgG – Gamma heavy chain
IgM – Mu heavy chain
IgA – Alpha heavy chain
IgD – Delta heavy chain
IgE – Epsilon heavy chain

All the immunoglobulins within a particular class will have similar heavy chain. Each class of immunoglobulins further classified into subclasses based on small differences in the amino acid sequences in the constant regions of the heavy chains belonging to a particular class.

Subclasses of IgG

IgG_1	–	Gamma 1 heavy chains
IgG_2	–	Gamma 2 heavy chains
IgG_3	–	Gamma 3 heavy chains
IgG_4	–	Gamma 4 heavy chains

Subclasses of IgA

IgA_1 Alpha 1 heavy chains and IgA_2 Alpha 2 heavy chains

The subclasses vary depending on the species of animals. Like heavy chain classes, amino acid differences in the constant region of the light chain also result in immunoglobulin types, kappa and lambda light chains. The light chain also can be divided in to subtypes based on differences in the amino acid sequences in the constant regions of the light chains belonging to a particular type.

Lambda 1	Lambda 2
Lambda 3	Lambda 4

Immunoglobulins are designated based on class and sub-class of the heavy chain and type and sub-type of the light chains. Immunoglobulin molecules are a very heterogeneous mixture of molecules. In addition to the above classes and subclasses, types and sub-types, they would also have different antigen binding characteristics based on the differences in their V_H and V_L region sequences.

1.7.1 Antigenic determinants on the immunoglobulins

Since antibody is also a protein and fulfills all the criteria for immunogens, they can also act as an antigen when the criterion of foreignness is fulfilled by giving this protein in a different species of animal. When an immunoglobulin molecule is inoculated into another species, certain regions of the immunoglobulin molecules acts as epitopes and induces the formation of antibodies to these regions. These epitopes can be classified as isotypic, allotypic and idiotypic determinants.

Isotypic determinants are antigenic determinants that characterize classes and sub-classes of heavy chains and types and sub-types of light chains. They are present in all members of a species and anti-isotypic antibodies are useful for quantification of immunoglobulin classes and sub-classes

Allotypic determinants are those specified by the allelic forms of the immunoglobulin genes. Although by and large the amino acid sequences of each isotypes are same, there could be slight individual differences in the constant region sequences of the heavy and light chains between individuals which give rise to allotypes.

Idiotypic determinants are those created by the HVRs unique to each antibody molecule. And antibodies to these determinants are called as anti-idiotypic antibodies. The structure of the anti-idiotypic antibody molecule would mimic the antigen. Thus it is possible to use these anti-idiotypic antibodies, in place of antigens, for use as vaccines or as diagnostic reagents. However, since the frequency of these anti-idiotypic molecules are so low, that it was not practicable to adopt it in normal practice.

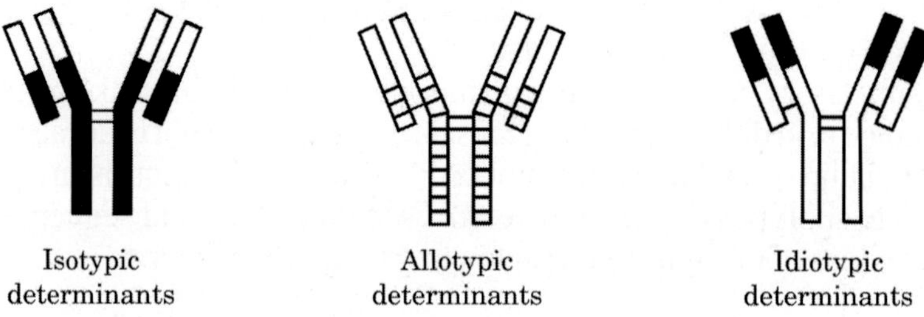

Fig. 1.18: Antigenic determinants on the immunoglobulin molecule

Polyclonal antibodies

When we inject a foreign protein into another species and we bleed the animal after 2–3 weeks and antibodies to this protein are present in the serum. How?

When the foreign protein is injected it is carried either by the blood stream to the spleen or by the lymph to the nearest lymph nodes. Spleen and lymph nodes are secondary lymphoid organs. These proteins are classified as T-cell dependent or T-cell independent antigens. These proteins are taken up by antigen–presenting cells which are dendritic cells, macrophages and B-cells.

These cells engulf the antigen, process them and present them in relation to major histocompatability complex II. The peptide-MHC complex are recognized by the T-helper cells ($CD4^+$), which secrete cytokines that in turn help the B-cells to produce antibodies. Such antigens are called T-cell dependent antigens.

T-cell independent antigens can directly bind to immunoglobulin receptors on the B cells causing it to proliferate and differentiate into plasma cells and secrete antibodies of the same specificity.

In the secondary lymphoid organs, B cells with immunoglobulin receptors of different specificities are present, pre-existent in the body without any prior knowledge on the type of the epitopes that would be encountered by them.

The epitope simply has to select the immunoglobulin receptor on a particular B-cell with which it can facilitate bond formation with the amino acids in its HVRs, which means that it is specific to it.

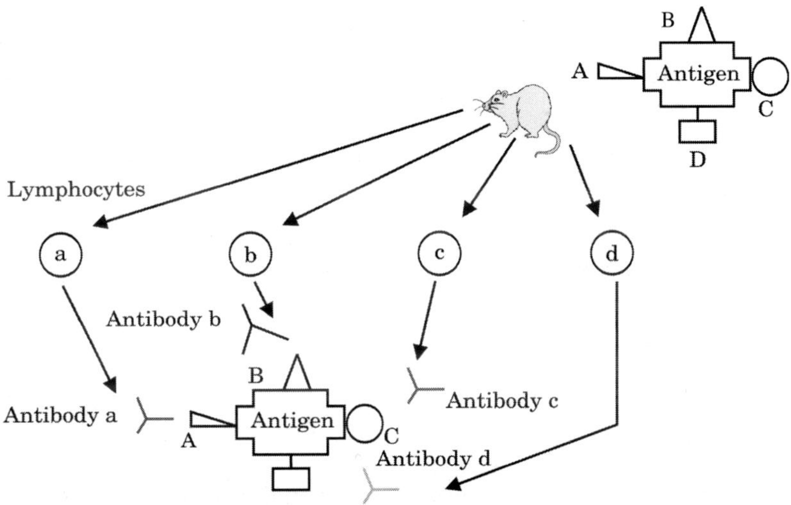

Fig. 1.19: Genertion of a polyclonal response to a multi-epitopic antigen.

This binding send signals to the DNA of that particular B-cell to divide into a clone of cells and differentiate into plasma cells (acquire the paraphernalia such as rough endoplasmic reticulum to secrete more protein in the form of immunoglobulins). These cells secrete immunoglobulins of the same specificity so that there are enough immunoglobulin molecules that can act with the same epitope on the antigen. This is called as clonal selection theory.

The antibodies that are secreted by the B-cell are what we detect in the serum. Most of the antigens have many epitopes. Imagine this situation happening for each epitope separately. The result is each epitope binds to an appropriate B-cell receptor, stimulates and causes secretion of many different antibodies of differing specificities for each immunogenic epitope. Hence such a response is called polyclonal *i.e.* many different lymphocytes are activated resulting in different clones producing antibodies of differing specificities to each epitope.

Two more events occur, affinity maturation and isotype switching.

Affinity maturation is the increase in the affinity of immunoglobulins with time. This happens by a process of somatic mutation. So serum bled later in the course of an immune response would have more high affinity antibodies than early serum.

The affinity constant of anti-dinitro phenyl antibodies prepared in rabbits following immunization of 5 mg per animal after 2, 5 and 8 weeks post immunization was determined to be 0.86, 14 and 120 L/mol × 10^6. The affinity of the anti-DNP antibodies increase with time post-immunization.

The initial isotype of the antibody is IgM. Then it can switch to other isotypes while retaining the antigen binding specificity as same, the Fab is retained while the Fc is changed to the other class. This is enabled by the switching of the expression of the genes coding for the constant region.

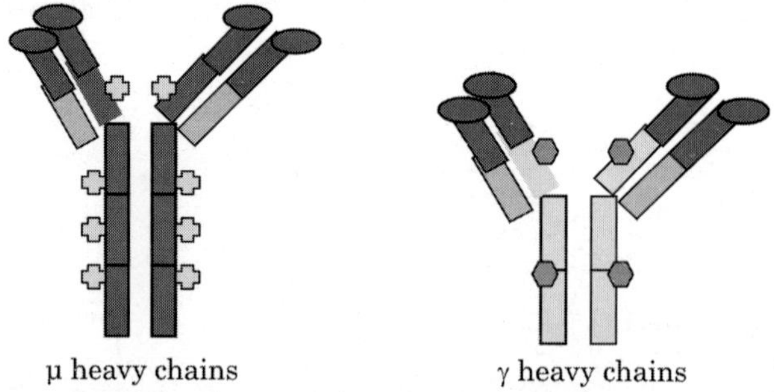

Fig. 1.20: Isotype switching from IgM to IgG-Note the antigen specificity is retained while the heavy chain has changed

This is done in a bid to enhance the removal of the antigen by making use of the 'specialized skills' of each class and subclass of antibodies. For example, IgG_3 is better at fixing complement than other IgG sub-classes and a switch to IgG_3 would help to fight the antigen better through complement mediated lysis. IgA would be better mucosal antibody and IgE for mast cell degranulation. In case of parasitic infestations, a switch to IgE would be useful to mediate mast cell degranulation and removal of the parasites.

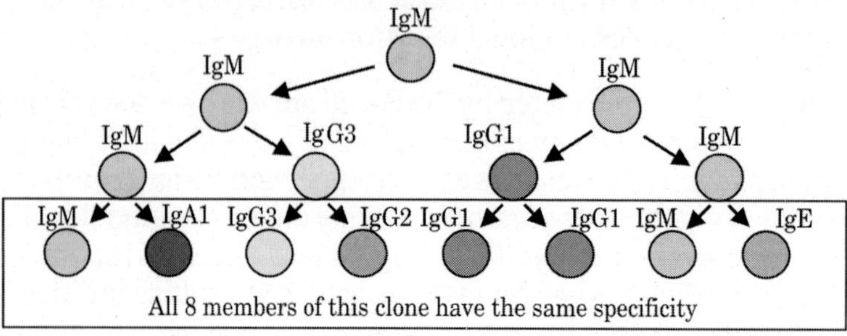

Fig. 1.21: Isotype switching of immunoglobulins during the course of an immune response.

Thus a polyclonal response would be on the following lines

Antigen

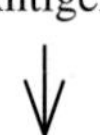

Taken by the blood/lymph to secondary lymphoid organs

Processed and presented by antigen-presenting cells

T-helper cells secrete cytokines

Antigen binding to the immunoglobulin receptor on the B-cells

Clonal expansion, proliferation and differentiation in to plasma cells

Secretion of more antibodies of the same specificity

Same occurs for each epitope resulting in antibodies to different epitopes

Isotype switching occurs resulting in antibodies of different class and subclasses

Affinity maturation resulting in differing affinities of the antibodies

Thus for example, if an antigen has 3 different epitopes, A, B and C, a polyclonal response would result in antibodies to epitopes A, B and C in varied proportions depending on the immunogenicity of each epitope.

There would be IgM class of antibodies to all three epitopes and then for example, a shift to IgG1 to epitope A, shift to IgA to epitope B, shift to IgE to epitope C, then a further shift to IgG3 to epitope B and so on.

These antibodies of differing classes and subclasses would further vary in their affinities, the antibody formed early, say IgG1 would have an affinity of say, 10–12 kd while those formed later say IgG3 would be of higher affinity say 10–15 kd etc.

Thus polyclonal responses are characterized by presence of antibodies to different epitopes, antibodies of different classes and sub-classes and antibodies of different affinities.

1.8 Antigen–Antibody Interactions

Basically, this is a protein–protein interaction which means that the side chains of the amino acids constituting the epitope and those comprising the paratope could be involved in bond formation. When the side chains of the amino acids comprising the epitope and paratope are in correct positions facilitating different kinds of bond formation, then we say that they are specific. This is what we mean by specificity of antigen–antibody interactions in biochemical terms.

One point of difference between nucleic acids and proteins in their interactions with themselves is that nucleic acids are involved in weaker hydrogen bond formation but all the bases are involved in bond formation thereby adding to the strength of interactions. However with proteins only particular regions of the molecules are involved in bond formation (epitope and paratope) but the bonds involved are slightly stronger interactions.

Antigen–antibody interactions are reversible and hence they are not bonded by stronger covalent bonds.

All the four levels of protein structure determine and drive the antigen antibody interactions. The tertiary structure brings the CDRs of heavy and light chains close together and forms the antigen combining site. The quaternary structure brings the CDRs of the heavy and light chains of the antibody molecule together.

1.8.1 *Affinity and avidity*

Antibody affinity is the strength of the reaction between a single antigenic determinant and a single combining site on the antibody.

It is the sum of the attractive and repulsive forces operating between the antigenic determinant and the combining site of the antibody.

It is measured in terms of the ease of association or dissociation.

The higher the affinity of the antibody means it binds to the hapten very efficiently and greater the energy required to dissociate it from it. This is measured for individual epitope binding by a mAb.

The affinity constant is the reciprocal of the concentration of free hapten when half the total antibody is free. This means that the smaller the hapten concentration that saturates half of the total antibody the greater the affinity of the antibody for the hapten. The association constant (K) is determined using the method of equilibrium dialysis.

A dialysis chamber separated by a semi-permeable membrane permitting the hapten to pass across but not the antibody is used with the addition of a known amount of radio labeled hapten on one side and the antibody on the other side. The hapten will start diffusing across the membrane and would attain equilibrium with the hapten concentrations being the same in both sides. However this would not happen since antibody molecule is on one side and some of the hapten would bind to the antibody. Thus the difference in the hapten concentrations between both sides represents the hapten bound to the antibody. The higher the hapten bound the higher the affinity of the antibody.

A high affinity mAb used in a diagnostic assay means that the time required for the interaction between the antigen and conventionally a 45 minutes to one hour incubation are given between each step for antigen antibody interaction to occur of for antibody-anti species antibody interactions to occur. When a high affinity antibody is used this time interval can be reduced and the antigen-antibody complex is more stable.

Diagnostic tests such as lateral flow based assays require the use of high affinity antibodies since there is no time given for the antigen-antibody interactions to occur, the immobilized antibody needs to bind to the antigen as it traverses the antibody line on the membrane. This is only possible only when the affinity of the mAbs used is high so that it can bind very fast and only to the specific antigen in the heterogeneous mixture of proteins that could be present in the sample being tested.

Avidity is a measure of the overall strength of binding of an antigen with many antigenic determinants and multivalent antibodies. Antibody avidity is the tendency for multiple antibodies and multivalent antigens to combine, which is the cumulative binding strength of all individual epitope-antibody pairs. Avidity is influenced by both the valence of the antibody and the valence of the antigen. Avidity is more than the sum of the individual affinities.

For dissociating multivalent antigen antibody interactions, multiple bonds must be broken simultaneously. The reactions between multivalent antigen and multivalent antibodies are more stable because of the cumulative strength of all the individual interactions and hence they are easier to detect.

IgM antibodies have higher avidity than IgG despite that fact that the binding of each Fab in the IgM antibody with the epitope may be similar to the affinity of the Fab from IgG..

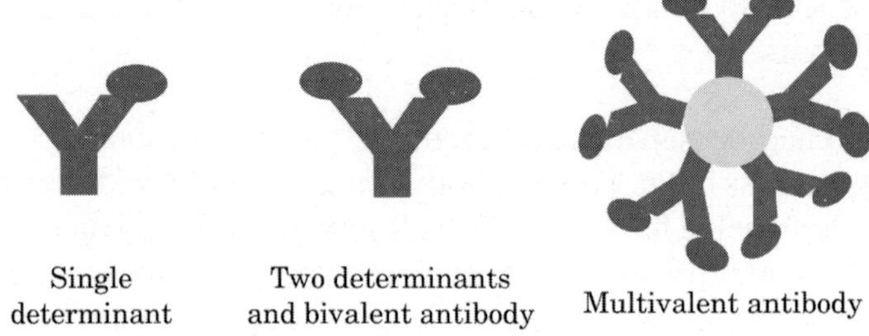

Fig. 1.22: Affinity and avidity of antibodies

1.8.2 Specificity and cross-reactivity

Specificity refers to the ability of an individual antibody combining site to react with only one antigenic determinant or the ability of a population of antibody molecules to react with only one antigen.

Antigen-antibody interactions are highly specific.Cross reactivity refers to the ability of an individual antibody combining site to react with more than one antigenic determinant or the ability of a population of antibody molecules to react with more than one antigen.

Cross reactions arise either because

- the cross reacting antigen naturally shares an epitope in common with the immunizing antigen or
- it has an epitope which is structurally similar to one on the immunizing antigen (multi specificity)

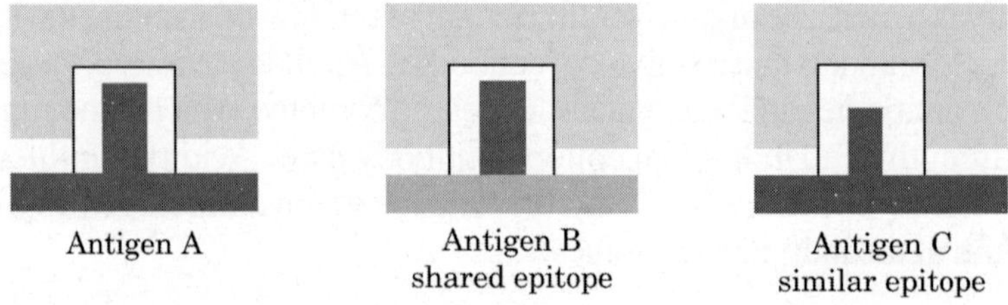

Fig. 1.23: Antigen specificity and cross reactivity between shared and similar epitopes

CHAPTER 2

REQUIREMENTS OF A HYBRIDOMA LABORATORY

2.1 Introduction

A hybridoma laboratory is a sophisticated cell culture laboratory. All the requirements of good cell culture laboratory are needed for hybridoma work in addition, a special animal facility is also a requirement.

2.2 What is Cell Culture?

Cells of a tissue (or individual cells that are prepared as cell suspensions) that are made to grow uniformly *in vitro* by undergoing continuous multiplications without maintaining the original tissue architecture.

Contrast it to organ cultures where pieces of organs or tissues are maintained *in vitro* by providing its requirements in terms of media and sera. In this type of culture, growth is not important as is the maintenance of organization of the tissue. For example, chicken tracheal organ cultures are prepared to support the growth and assay of a variety of avian respiratory viruses such as infectious bronchitis virus. The trachea is collected from 19–20 day-old embryonated chicken eggs and made into slices of 600–700 microns and placed in suitable culture tubes with medium. When observed under an inverted microscope, ciliary beating can be observed indicative of the maintenance of the organ culture. In case of virus infections the movement of cilia ceases and is indicative of virus replication.

Contrast it with tissue culture wherein small pieces of tissues are explanted into suitable culture vessels and maintained with medium and serum. The constituent cells of the tissue may emerge from the tissues as outgrowths.

There are two main types of cell cultures, primary and continuous cultures. Primary cultures are derived from excised tissues and are dissociated into a singe cell suspension by enzyme digestion. Such cultures are heterogeneous but later become dominated mainly by fibroblasts. They have a limited life span and during that time they retain many of the differentiated characteristics of the cells *in vivo*.

Continuous cultures comprised a single cell type propagated for a limited number of cell divisions or indefinitely. Cell lines of finite life span are diploid and maintain their differentiated state. Continuous cell lines can be propagated indefinitely since they have been transformed into tumour cells. They are heteroploid and retain very little of their original *in vivo* characteristics.

Morphologically cell cultures can be classified as growing in suspension or as mono layers that are attached to a culture vessel surface. Normally cells derived from blood (lymphoma, leukemia) tend to grow in suspension while cells derived from solid tissues like kidneys, thyroid etc tend to grow as mono layers.

2.2.1 Cell culture laboratory requirements

The building housing the laboratory should have facilities for decontamination, washing, sterilization, distilled water production, instrumentation and culture room with ante room wherein access should be restricted. A unidirectional flow of work is preferred.

The design of the laboratory should be in compliance with good manufacturing practice (GMP) or good laboratory practice (GLP) requirement as prescribed by regulatory agencies of the country. Laboratories are designated as biosafety levels 1–4 based on their design features, containment facilities and GMP procedures followed. When mAbs are prepared for pathogenic organisms the biosafety levels of the lab required for handling that particular organism is needed. Very low risk organisms can be handled in biosafety level 1 labs simply by adhering to good microbiological techniques (GMT).

Moderate individual risk organism and low community risk organisms require biosafety level 2 labs by adhering to GMT with protective clothing and biosafety cabinets. High individual risk organisms and low community risk organisms require biosafety level 3 labs, with the above features and directional air flow and controlled access. Biosafety level 4 labs are needed for high individual and community risk organisms with provision for airlock entry, special waste disposal, positive pressure suits etc.

In India with the threat of avian and swine influenza, biosafety labs are needed for handling these organisms and making mAbs. Presently, the High Security Animal Disease Laboratory at Bhopal has bio safety level 3 features and can handle avian influenza related work. The air cleanliness of the labs is denoted in terms of the maximum number of particles of size 0.5 μm or larger present per unit volume of air. For example, class 100 space means that only 100 particles of 0.5 μm or larger should be present per cubic foot while class 10000 means that 10000 particles of 0.5 μm or larger can be present per cubic feet. A model plan for a hybridoma laboratory is given in Fig. 2.1.

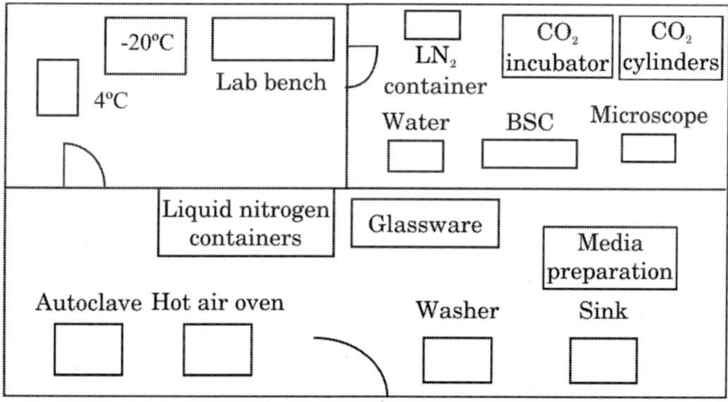

Fig. 2.1: Model plan for a hybridoma laboratory

Specifically for a hybridoma lab, the CO_2 incubator, inverted microscope, liquid nitrogen containers and water bath should be arranged around the biological safety cabinet. The cultures should be taken out of the incubator, examined under the microscope and dealt with appropriately under the biological safety cabinet (BSC). Water bath would be needed for thawing and fusion and LN_2 containers for storage of clones. Entry should be restricted into the culture room. This can also be ensured by having an anteroom wherein other laboratory requirements such as deep freeze storage, balances etc are kept. The equipments should be so arranged so as it is convenient to the user.

2.2.2 Biological safety cabinets

Laminar airflows are clean benches that discharge high efficiency particulate air (HEPA) filtered air across the work surface toward the user. They provide protection only for product inside the bench. They are commonly used for sterile assembly or dust free electronic production.

Biological safety cabinets are containment and protection devices used in laboratories working with biological agents to provide protection, from the potential hazards of handling infectious materials, for the working personnel, products or both. They are fitted with HEPA filters which can remove microorganisms or particles of the size of 0.3 microns or larger at an efficiency of 99.97% from air.

The components of HEPA filters include filter media that consists of folded cellulose/borosilicate media, epoxy or polyurethane sealant, metal or wooden frames and an edge sealant (gasket with clamp or gel seal with knife edge). Biological safety cabinets (BSC) are categorized in to 3 classes, I, II and III based on the method of operation and level of protection offered to personnel or product. Class I and II BSC are used for working with low or moderate risk biological agents while class III cabinets are essential for high risk agents.

Class I BSC is open fronted negative pressure cabinets which offer personnel and environmental protection but not product protection. There is no recirculation of air and there is an HEPA filter in the exhaust outlet. Class II BSC (Fig. 2.2) has an inward air flow for personnel protection and 2 HEPA filters one for affording product protection and the other in the exhaust line for environmental protection. About 70% of the air is re-circulated.

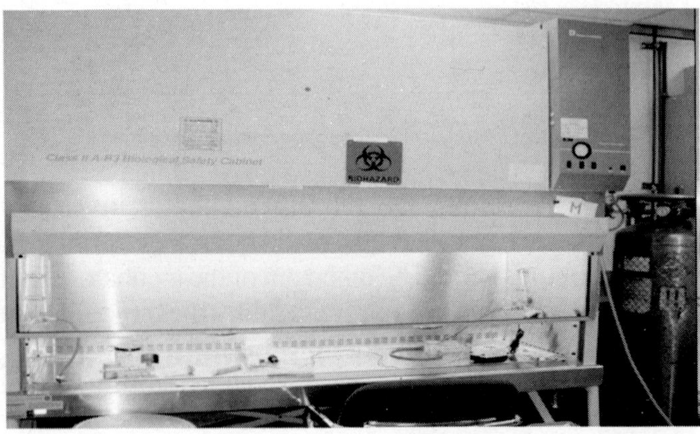

Fig. 2.2: Biosafety cabinets class-II (BSC class-II)

Class III (Fig.2.3) cabinets are totally gas-tight units wherein the operations are conducted through glove ports. The supply air is also HEPA filtered and the exhaust air is passed through two HEPA filters. These cabinets are useful for working with agents that requires biosafety levels III and IV. The protection afforded by the cabinets to personnel, product and environment is given in Table 2.1.

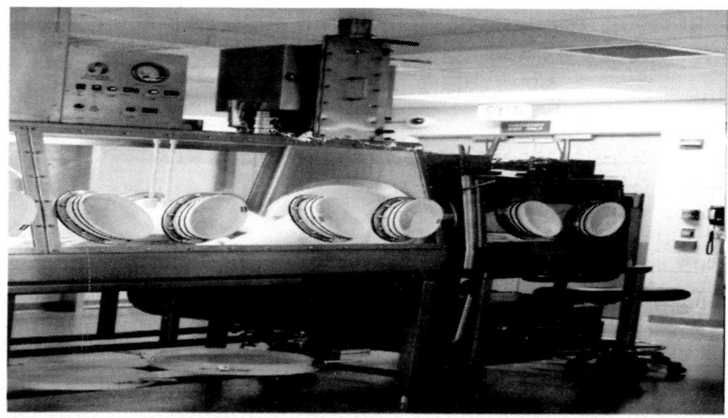

Fig. 2.3: Biological safety unit (Class-III)

Table 2.1: Protection Afforded by the Cabinets to Personnel, Product and Environment

Equipment	*Personnel*	*Product*	*Environment*
Chemical fume hoods	+	–	–
Laminar flow clean bench	–	+	–
Class I BSC	+	–	+
Class II BSC	+	+	+
Class III BSC	+	+	+
Isolator	+	+	+

The performance of these BSC is to be constantly monitored and standards are available. The industry standard (NSF-49) specifies the personnel, product and cross-contamination tests. *Bacillus subtilis* var *niger* spores are used as the marker organisms for these performance criteria.

The HEPA filters are also to be checked for any leakages. This is done with an aerosol of dioctyl phthalate and the down stream of the HEPA filters are to be scanned with a photometer probe. The filter is said to have failed if the downstream reading exceeds 0.1%.

In fluid mechanics, a criterion of whether fluid (liquid or gas) flow is absolutely steady (streamlined, or laminar) or on the average steady with small unsteady fluctuations (turbulent) is defined by the Reynolds number. Whenever the Reynolds number is less than 2000, flow is considered laminar, whereas, at values greater than 2000, flow is turbulent. This mathematical quantity is also applied to other types of flow that are completely enclosed such as in a BSC. Thus a good BSC is required to have a Reynolds number of less than 2000.

2.2.3 Prevention and detection of contamination

Prevention of contamination is half the battle won in case of preparation of hybridomas. It should start from washing and sterilization of all materials used in cell culture. Although most of the labs use pre-sterilized disposable plastic ware such as culture vessels or plates it is better for the worker to have a clear understanding of the sterilization requirements.

Sterilization is defined as any process, physical or chemical which will destroy all forms of life, applied specially to microorganisms including bacterial and fungal spores and inactivation of viruses.

Biological indicators are used for validation of any sterilization process. The D value (Decimal Reduction Value) is the time in minutes required to reduce the microbial population by 90% or one log cycle (to a surviving fraction of $^1/_{10}$) at a specific temperature. When the D value of a biological indicator, *Bacillus stearothermophilus* is 1.5 min. at 121 ºC, if it is treated for 12 minutes under the same conditions, the lethality input is 8D. The main purpose of sterilization is to attain a microbial survivor possibility of 10^{-6}, less than one chance in a million that viable organisms are present.

For example, if the microbial burden in a material is 100, lethality input of 3D yields a microbial burden of 100, *i.e.* 1. A further 5D yields a survivor probability of only 10^{-5}, less than the required 10^{-6}. Hence, the time of sterilization may be increased. But this works on the assumption that the biological indicator organism has the same resistance characteristics as the microorganisms under question in the product or material.

2.2.3.1 *Steam sterilization*

This process involves heating in an autoclave with saturated steam under pressure. The following combinations of time and temperature are normally employed.

Holding temperature (°C)	*Minimum holding time (min)*
115–118	30
121–124	15
126–129	10
134–138	3

The F_0 value of a saturated steam sterilization process is the lethality expressed in terms of the equivalent time in minutes at a temperature of 121°C delivered by that process to the product in its final containers. An F_0 value of not less than 8 to every container in the load is considered satisfactory.

2.2.3.2 *Dry heat sterilization*

This process is suitable for heat-stable non-aqueous products and is done in a hot air oven. Cycles of 180°C for 30 min., 170°C for 1 hr or 160°C for 2 hr are commonly used. A microbial survival probability of 10^{-12} is possible by dry heat sterilization.

2.2.3.3 *Filtration*

This involves physical removal of microorganisms by retention in membranes of pore sizes 0.4 microns, 0.22 microns or less. This method is suitable for certain ingredients that are not stable to heat to permit sterilization by autoclaving. Most of the media and serum are sterilized by filtration. Earlier Seitz filters were used, but they are now obsolete since they contain asbestos and shed fibres during the filtration process. Membrane filters retain particles and micro-organisms that exceed their pore sizes by acting as a physical barrier. Routine laboratory sterilization of most media, buffers, biological fluids is usually done with 0.22 μ pore filter membranes. Clarification and prefiltration of solutions and solvents is best accomplished with 0.45 μ or larger filter membranes.

While filtering materials likely to contain viruses (as used for virus isolation from field samples) ensure that the size of the viruses is lower than the pore size used.

The choice of your membranes depends on:

- Filter membrane characteristics
- Filter housing characteristics
- Chemical compatibility.

***Cellulose acetate*:** Membranes have a very low binding affinity for most macromolecules especially proteins and are especially recommended for applications such as filtering culture media containing sera. However, filtering a small amount of warm purified water through the membrane or filter unit is recommended to remove non-toxic wetting agents that are normally added during manufacture to ensure proper wetting of the membrane since these membranes are hydrophobic.

***Cellulose nitrate*:** Membranes are recommended for filtering solutions where protein binding is not a concern. They are recommended for use in general laboratory applications such as buffer filtration.

***Nylon*:** membranes are naturally hydrophilic and are recommended for applications requiring very low extractables, since they do not contain any wetting agents, detergents or surfactants. They are recommended for filtering solutions such as alcohols and DMSO as they are more chemically resistant and for filtering protein-free culture media.

***Polyethersulfone (PES)*:** membranes are highly recommended for filtering cell culture media. PES has both very low protein binding and extractables. PES also demonstrates faster flow rates than cellulose or nylon membranes.

***Teflon®*:** (PTFE; polytetrafluorethylene) membranes are hydrophobic and hence are ideal for filtering gases, including humidified air. Because of their hydrophobicity, Teflon membranes must be prewetted with a solvent, such as ethanol, before aqueous solutions can be filtered. High chemical resistance of Teflon membranes make them very useful for filtering solvents or other aggressive chemicals for which other membranes are unsuitable.

***Glass fiber*:** filters have high particle loading capacity and are ideal for prefiltering solutions that are difficult to filter such as sera. The filters are available in various sizes depending on the manufacturer. Some the commonly used sizes are 4 mm, 13 mm, 25 mm, 47 mm, 90 mm.

Some commercial companies make filters with 0.1 microns cutoff. This is preferable for exclusion of mycoplasmas. This filtration is possible only if the media is pre-filtered with either 0.4 or 0.22 micron filters earlier.

2.2.3.4 *Gas sterilization*

This process involves exposure to a sterilizing gas. The common gas used is ethylene oxide alone or in combination with an inert gas. After sterilization, adequate time should be given for the residual ethylene oxide or its volatile residues to disperse. This may be confirmed by gas chromatography for the presence of ethylene oxide, ethylene glycol and ethylene chlorhydrin. It is difficult for the gas to reach inner most areas of the products that require sterilization.

2.2.3.5 *Sterilization by ionizing radiation*

This form of sterilization involves exposure of the materials to gamma radiation from a radio isotope source such as cobalt 60 or cesium 137 or electrons from an electron accelerator.

2.2.4 Sterilization of laboratory atmosphere

This is normally achieved by the use of ultraviolet radiation with a wavelength of 254 nm. The UV light is effective only in the absence of any organic matter protecting the microbial cell. The susceptibility of microorganisms to UV light varies depending on the energy emitted from the UV tubes.

Bacteria	–	0.5 to 200 mW sec/cm^2
Mostly	–	10–12 mW sec/cm^2
Yeast	–	4.3–2 mW sec/cm^2
Fungi	–	100–1000 mW sec/cm^2
Viruses	–	Comparable to bacteria

Radiation intensity in mW sec/cm^2 is related to the distance between the lamp and the surface. A 30W UV lamp, at 20 cm distance has a radiation intensity of 745 mW seconds/cm^2 while at 500 cm distance it reduces to 3.9 mW sec/cm^2.

Fumigation may also be used for sterilization of laboratory atmosphere using either formaldehyde spray @ 0.5 to 1 ml per cubic foot. Following overnight action, the formaldehyde may be neutralized with equal amount of ammonia solution spray.

A combination of potassium permanganate (30G and formaldehyde 45 ml) may be used for 100 cubic feet of laboratory space.

2.2.5 Cleaning of glassware

For cleaning glass one of the most useful acids is nitric acid. An effective cleaning fluid for removal of organic matter is by treatment of a chromic acid mixture prepared by dissolving 200 g of sodium dichromate in 100 ml of water, cooling in an ice bath and adding slowly to it, with stirring 1500 ml of sulphuric acid by following adequate safety precautions. Glassware treated with chromic acid mixture should be subjected to prolonged rinsing as glass tends to absorb chromic acid. For general cleaning of glassware, synthetic detergent solutions or alkaline cleansing agents such as trisodium phosphate may be used. All glassware should be finally rinsed thoroughly in distilled water before use.

2.2.6 Media and supplements

Originally, the components of culture media required for cell growth was determined based on the analysis of the composition of the plasma and hence led to formulations with more than 60 ingredients. Later, the number of components was reduced to the bare minimum that was essential for cell growth and called minimum essential media (MEM). Cell culture medium is a complete mixture of salts, carbohydrates, amino acids, fatty acids and lipids, vitamins, growth factors, metabolic precursor, hormones and trace elements.

The inorganic salts in media retain the osmotic balance of cell, provide calcium, sodium and potassium and thus regulate membrane potential. These salts are required for cell attachment and as enzyme co-factors.

The carbohydrates are the main source of energy with the major sugars being glucose and galactose. Some media also contains maltose or fructose. The concentration of sugar varies from 1 g per litre to 4.5 g per litre. The presence of higher concentration of sugars is able to support more diverse cell types. Other carbon sources include amino acids particularly L-glutamine and pyruvate. Glutamine, a heat labile amino acid, is added at high concentrations of 2–4 mM. Normally glutamine is prepared separately, stored at –20°C and added to the culture media. But nowadays heat stable glutamine mixed with the media is also available.

Other proteins/peptides are important in serum-free media and they include albumin, transferrin, fibronectin etc.

Fatty acids and lipids are more important in serum free media and cholesterol and steroids are essential for specialized cells.

Vitamins commonly used in media include riboflavin, thiamine and biotin. They are precursors for many co-factors. Some media have increased levels of vitamins A and E. Vitamin B_{12} is also essential for some cells.

Trace elements such as copper, selenium, tricarboxylic acid intermediates, zinc are needed in the media. Selenium is a detoxifier and helps to remove oxygen free radicals.

2.2.7 Serum supplementation

Serum is a complex mix of albumins, growth factors and is the most important component of cell culture medium. The most commonly used serum is foetal calf serum (FCS). Serum also increases the buffering capacity of cultures and is important when the growth of cells is slow or when the seeding density is low as during cloning of hybridomas. It can also protect cells against mechanical damage when the cells are stirred or scrapped. It can bind and neutralize toxins. It also increases the risk of contamination. A 10% FCS supplement contributes 4.8 mg protein per ml of culture fluid.

Foetal source of serum is preferred because of its high content of embryonic growth factors. One of the disadvantages of the use of serum is that it is not a chemically defined mixture. Hence batches of serum need to be tested for its cytotoxicity and growth promoting effects especially while cloning hybridoma cells when cell densities are low.

Serum is filtered and tested for various microbial and chemical contaminations. It is tested for contamination with bacteria, fungi, mycoplasma and certain viruses such as bovine viral diarrhea virus.

Some of the treatments given to serum are discussed here.

Heat inactivation involves exposure of the serum to 56 °C for 30 minutes to inactivate complement. Gamma radiation wherein the serum is treated to radiation from ^{60}Co source. Ethanol fractionation or polyethylene glycol treatment of serum to reduce the content of gamma globulins. Dialysis against normal saline to reduce the level of glucose to less than 5% mg.

Most cells require pH in the range of 7.2 to 7.4. Regulation of pH is more important immediately following seeding when the culture is establishing itself. The two buffering systems include (*i*) CO_2 balances with the CO_3/HCO_3 content of the culture medium or (*ii*) chemical buffering using a zwitter ion, HEPES (N-(2-hydroxyethyl)-piperazine-N'-2-ethane sulfonic acid). Cultures using bicarbonate/ CO_2 buffering systems should be maintained in an atmosphere of 5–10% CO_2 while HEPES has a superior buffering capacity in the pH range 7.2 to 7.4 and may not require a controlled gaseous atmosphere.

Most of the media have phenol red as an indicator so that the pH status of the media can be constantly monitored by the colour. The media turns yellow when acidic and pink when alkaline.

The osmolality of cell culture media should be in the range of 260–320 mOsm/ kg even though established cell lines can tolerate wide variations in osmotic pressure unlike embryo cultures.

An Osmometer is used for the measurement of the osmotic strength of a solution; thereby the particle number and/or the molecular mass of the dissolved substance can be determined. There are three major types of osmometers commercially available, each measuring a particular colligative property to achieve their analytical results:

Freezing point osmometer: Determines the osmotic strength of solution by utilizing freezing point depression.

Vapor pressure osmometer: Determines the concentration of osmotically active particles that reduce the vapor pressure of the solution.

***Membrane osmometer*:** Measures the osmotic pressure of a solution separated by a semi-permeable membrane.

Measurements of osmolar concentrations are often expressed in osmolarity and osmolality. Osmolarity is a measure of the osmoles of solute per liter of solution. Since the volume of solution changes with the amount of solute added as well as with changes in temperature and pressure, osmolarity is difficult to determine. Osmolality is a measure of the osmoles of solute per kilogram of solvent. Since the amount of solvent will remain constant regardless of changes in temperature and pressure, osmolality is easier to evaluate and is more commonly used, and often preferred, in practical osmometry. Most osmometers give results using osmolality units mOsm/kg. The common antibiotics and anti-fungals used in media and composition of media commonly used in hybridoma cultures are given in Table 2.2 and 2.3 respectively.

Table 2.2: Common Antibiotics and Anti-fungals used in Media

Penicillin	100 U/ml	Gram positive bacteria
Di hydro streptomycin	100 µg/ml	Gram positive and negative bacteria
Gentamycin sulphate	50 µg/ml	Gram positive and negative bacteria and mycoplasma
Kanamycin sulphate	100 µg/ml	Gram positive and negative bacteria and mycoplasma
Amphotericin B	2.5 µg/ml	Fungi and yeasts
Nystatin	50 µg/ml	Fungi and yeasts
Tylosin	100 µg/ml	Gram positive and negative bacteria and mycoplasma

Table 2.3: Composition of Media Commonly used in Hybridoma Cultures

Components	***EMEM***	***DMEM***	***IMDM***	***RPMI 1640***
Inorganic salts (mg/l)				
NaCl	6800	6400	4505	6000
KCl	400	400	330	400
KNO_3	–	–	0.076	–
$CaCl_2$	200	–	–	–
$Ca(NO_3)_2.4.H_2O$	–	–	–	100
$CaCl_2.2H_2O$	–	264.90	218.60	–
$MgCl_2.6H_2O$	–	–	–	–
$MgSO_4.7H_2O$	200	200	200	100
$NaH_2PO_4.2H_2O$	150	140	141.30	1512.00
$NaHCO_3$	2200	3700	2520	2000
L-Amino acids				
Alanine	–	–	25	–
Arginine HCl	126.40	84	84	200
Asparagine. $2H_2O$	–	–	28.40	50
Aspartic acid	–	–	30	20
Cysteine $HCl.2H_2O$	–	–	–	–
Cystine	24.02	–	–	50

Table 2.3: (*Contd...*)

Table 2.3: *(Contd...)*

Components	*EMEM*	*DMEM*	*IMDM*	*RPMI 1640*
Cystine. DiNa	–	56.78	88.05	–
Glutamic acid	–	–	75	20
Glutamine	292.30	584.60	584.00	300
Glycine	–	30	30	10
Histidine HCl.H_2O	41.90	42	42	15
Isoleucine	52.50	104.80	105	50
Leucine	52.50	104.80	105	50
Lysine HCl	73.06	146.20	146	40
Methionine	14.90	30	30	15
Phenyl alanine	33.02	66	66	15
Hydroxy proline	–	–	40	20
Serine	–	–	42	30
Threonine	47.64	95.20	95	20
Tryptophan	10.20	16	16	5
Tyrosine	36.22	–	–	20
Tyrosine. diNa	–	89.46	104.20	
Valine	46.90	93.60	94	20
Trace elements				
$Fe(NO_3)_3.9H_2O$	–	0.10	17.3	
Vitamins				
p-amino bezoic acid	–	–	–	1.00
Ascorbic acid	–	–	–	
Biotin	–	–	0.013	0.2
Choline Cl	1.00	4.00	4.00	3.00
Folic acid	1.00	4.00	4.00	1.00
Inositol	2.00	7.00	7.20	35.00
Nicotinamide	1.00	4.00	4.00	1.00
Pantothenate.Ca	1.00	4.00	4.00	0.25
Pyridoxal. HCl	1.00	4.00	4.00	1.00
Riboflavin	0.10	0.40	0.40	0.20
Thiamine.HCl	1.00	4.00	4.00	1.00
Vitamin B_{12}	–	–	0.013	0.005
Other components				
Glutathione	–	–	–	1.00
Phenol red	10.00	10.00	15.00	5.00
Glucose	1000.00	4500.00	4500.00	2000.00
Pyruvate Na	–	110	110	–
CO_2 gas phase (%)	5	10	10	5

Source: Cell culture, LabFax, Edited by M. Butler and M. Dawson

DMEM has higher concentration of amino acids and vitamins than Eagle's minimum essential medium (EMEM) along with additional non essential amino acids and ferric nitrate. It has 4500 mg per litre of glucose. RPMI 1640 and IMDM have also been widely used for culture of lymphocytes and hybridomas.

2.2.8 Contamination of cultures

The major threats to cell culture include:

- Contamination with other cell lines
- Mycoplasma
- Yeast
- Fungi
- Viruses
- Bacteria

The main areas of quality control in cell culture are:

- Provenance of the cell lines
- Reagents and other inputs used in culture
- The avoidance of microbial contamination.

Bovine serum is a potential source of bovine viral diarrhoea virus (BVDV). Porcine trypsin is also a potential source of *Mycoplasma hyorhinis*. Cell lines are a major source of contamination. Obtaining cell lines from a reputed source ensures that it is fully characterized and is contaminant free.

Potential major sources of contamination include:

- Other cell lines
- Laboratory conditions, and
- Staff.

Bacterial contamination is generally visible to the naked eye and is detected by increase in turbidity and color change of the culture medium due to change in pH. Daily microscopic observation of cultures will ensure early detection of contamination and enable appropriate action. It is always recommended to freeze cultures in liquid nitrogen and thaw when required.

Fungal contamination is common in old building especially when the air conditioners are inefficient. Fungizone (amphotericin B 2.5µg/ml of medium) can be used as a preventive measure but this is stable only for 3–4 days in water and to be effective regular medium changes are required.

Some cell lines contain endogenous viruses and secrete virus particles or express viral antigens on their surface (*e.g.* EBV transformed lines). These cell lines are not considered contaminated. Contamination of cell lines with BVDV causes changes in growth rate. However since the virus is non-cytopathic macroscopic or microscopic changes in the cells will not be noticed.

Mycoplasmas are the smallest free-living self-replicating prokaryotes. They lack a cell wall and lack the ability to synthesize one. They can be observed as filamentous or coccal forms. There are 5 major species that are tissue culture contaminants, namely *M. hyorhinis*, *M. arginini*, *M. orale*, *M. fermentans* and *Acholeplasma laidlawii*. They grow mostly associated with the mammalian cell membranes. The absence of a cell wall gives them the ability to resist beta lactam antibiotics and to pass through 0.2 μm filters.

The effects of mycoplasma infection include:

- Reduced growth rate
- Morphological changes
- Chromosome aberrations
- Alterations in amino acid, and nucleic acid metabolism.

Detection of a potential contaminant is the first line of defense.

2.2.8.1 *Mycoplasma detection methods*

The mycoplasmal infection of cell cultures might often persist for long periods of time without apparent cell damage hence, it is important to use efficient detection methods.

Widely practiced inter laboratory exchange of cell cultures which may have been contaminated, can also lead to transmission and wide spread of mycoplasma contaminations.

Some of the tests used for mycoplasma detection include:

- Microbiological broth-agar colony assay
- DAPI DNA fluorescence staining
- RNA/DNA hybridization
- ELISA with specific polyclonal antisera (*e.g.*, Mycoplasma Detection Kit, Boehringer Mannheim, Germany), immunofluorescence
- Monoclonal antibody CCM-2 (R-Biopharm, Darmstadt, Germany)
- Polymerase chain reaction (16S-23S rR-NA intergenic region, 16srRNA genes)

- PCR ELISA (Boehringer Mannheim, Germany)
- Histochemical staining, electron microscopy, infrared spectroscopy etc.

Identification of mycoplasma species can be done using an immunobinding assay on agar colonies and/or an ELISA (Boehringer Mannheim) using specific antimycoplasma antisera. Mycoplasma contamination can be detected either by agar or medium inoculation.

The recommended procedure is to take 0.2 ml of product sample and spread over two agar plates and incubated for at least 14 days at 36 ± 1 °C at an anaerobic atmosphere. A >10 ml sample is inoculated into 50 ml of medium (Hayflick) and incubated. The minimum time to determine contamination is 28 days. This procedure is very time consuming and cumbersome and may cause delayed cell culture media approvals.

An indicator cell line of Vero or 3T6 cells are used, which are inoculated with 1 ml sample and incubated for 3–5 days at 36 ± 1°C in a 5% carbon dioxide atmosphere. The cells are fixated and stained utilizing Hoechst stain, which is DNA binding. The identification of contaminating mycoplasma is done by fluorescent microscopy.

Staining of infected cultures with DAPI (4, 6 diamidino-2-phenylindole) show typical starry sky appearance due to mycoplasma cells sitting on the cell membrane showing an irregular distribution but uniform in size. In mycoplasma-free cultures, only the fluorescent cell nuclei can be seen. Hoechst 33258 (0.05 μg/ml) or DAPI (0.1 μg/ml) are used. Hoechst 33258 staining is used on fixed cells and DAPI is used on unfixed cells.

The excitation wavelength of DAPI is around 345 nm and fluorescent microscope capable of detecting only FITC (490 nm) may not be useful unless this wavelength of filter is available.

PCR represents the fastest and, probably, the most reliable rapid detection method available. Depending on the PCR method, sensitivity and speed vary; Touchdown PCR provides results within 5–8 hr with a sensitivity of 1 cfu/ml. A major disadvantage of any PCR method is the fact that it does not distinguish between living or dead cells. On the other hand, the speed, accuracy and broad detectability represent advantages so that decisions can be made before the particular component of the media is used.

One of the targets for PCR is the region between 16S and 23S rRNA that differs among each species of mycoplasmas. Some parts of this spacer region vary while some parts are well conserved. Hence an initial PCR is performed to amplify the spacer region using DNA encoding rRNA of 16S and 23S followed by a nested PCR based on a conserved region with in the spacer and another on the 23S rRNA (PCR Mycoplasma detection kit, TaKaRa, Japan).

This system does not allow the amplification of DNA originated from other sources, such as cultured cells, which affect the detection result. Amplification of gene sequence with PCR using primer set enhances not only the sensitivity but also the specificity of detection.

A commercially available test for detection of mycoplasma in cell cultures is the PlasmoTest™ from Invivogen, USA. This test is based on the ability of toll like receptor 2 to recognize the mycoplasma and induce a signaling cascade leading to activation of NF-κB and other transcription factors. These indicator cells also stably express an optimized alkaline phosphatase gene engineered to be secreted (sAP), placed under the control of a promoter inducible by transcription factors such NF-κB and AP-1. The secreted alkaline phosphatase is detectable by the purple/blue coloration of the HEK-Blue™ Detection medium.

Inactivation of the contaminant is the next preventive measure.

2.2.8.2 *Mycoplasma decontamination methods*

Methods of mycoplasma decontamination should be simple, have minimal effect on cell growth, and not lead to loss of special cellular characteristics such as mAb production. Typical inactivation steps for mycoplasma contaminants can be the use of appropriate antibiotics, heat treatment at 45°C for 30 min or 60°C for 10 min, radiation or pH shift.

Heat, pH, and radiation can also alter media components. Heat is mainly introduced by the use of 80°C water for injection, into which the powdered media is mixed and solubilized. Contact time and uniformity of the mixing process are essential for the heat inactivation step. The use of radiation produces a reduction of viable mycoplasma > log 8 at a radiation dose of 25–35 kGy. Application of these methods for mycoplasma inactivation requires prior validation to verify the inactivation robustness versus the media product stability and efficacy.

The other most promising and still relatively simple technique appears to be antibiotic treatment. The most ideal approach would be to identify the contaminating mycoplasma species and determine the antibiotic sensitivity of the contaminant and then to treat the cell culture with such an antibiotic cocktail.

The common antibiotics used for mycoplasma eradication include ciprofloxacin (fluoroquinolone), BM-cyclin which contains a pleuromutilin and a tetracycline derivative, mycoplasma removal agent (MRA) (fluoroquinolone) etc. In a study comparing the efficacy of these treatments, it was found that the efficiency of permanent cure was 64% for MRA, 77% for ciprofloxacin and 84% for BM-Cyclin. Resistance to mycoplasma eradication was observed in few cultures that belonged to the species *Mycoplasma arginini* and *M. orale.* Overall, antibiotic decontamination of mycoplasmas is an efficient, inexpensive, reliable and simple method wherein 75% of the treated cultures can be cured. A combination of two antibiotics, Tiamutin and Minocycline (BIOMYC1 and BIOMYC2) to be added sequentially are also commercially available for mycoplasma treatment.

Antibiotics with medium activity include ciprofloxacin and doxycyclin, those with low activity: include plasmocin, chloramphenicol, azithromycin, clarithromycin, tetracycline and tiamulin. Antibiotics that are not effective against mycoplasma include penicillin, streptomycin, polymyxin, erythromycin (only active against some species), cephalosporin, G418 and bacitracin.

Several methods have been employed with mixed results. These include use of complement and heterologous antisera; passage in nude mice; exposure to mouse macrophages; treatment with trypsin, S-bromouracil, and Hoechst 33258 and so on. If antibiotic treatment fails, co-cultivation with macrophages can be used. This method is based on the ability of the macrophages to phagocytose the mycoplasma and remove them by intra cellular digestion. The infected hybridoma cells can also be injected in to pristine-primed syngenic mice where in the mycoplasmas would be digested by the peritoneal macrophages. For cells from other species nude mice is preferred.

2.2.8.3 *Mycoplasma prevention methods*

Mycoplasma can be removed by filtration with 0.1 μm membrane filters. The ability of these filters to retain mycoplamas depends on factors such as viscosity of the medium, differential pressure, contact time, volume of media filtered and the species of contaminating mycoplasma species. Hence this method requires prior validation as reliance on filter manufacturer's data will not suffice.

2.2.8.3.1 *Bubble point*

Bubble point is a test method used for estimating the pore size of membrane filters and confirming the integrity of sterilizing membrane filters and filter systems. It is a non-destructive integrity test.

The liquid used for filtration is held inside the pores of the filter by surface tension and capillary forces. The minimum pressure required to force liquid out of the pores is a measure of the pore diameter. For measurement of the bubble point, wet the filter with water for hydrophilic membranes or an alcohol for hydrophobic membranes. Then place the filter into the holder and cover the membrane with the wetting fluid. Pressurize the system and slowly increase the pressure until a single, continuous stream of bubbles at the outlet. At this time note the bubble point pressure from the pressure gauge.

Antibiotics such as plasmocin (Invivogen) can be added to the cell culture medium as a preventive measure against mycoplasma. To remove mycoplasma, a multi step approach is necessary. While such an approach must be used by the end-user, the raw material supplier must also enhance assurance.

Current detection, inactivation, and removal methods, in conjunction with appropriate process validation are the best options to prevent mycoplasma contamination. Hybridoma cells contaminated with mycoplasmas can make them sensitive to HAT medium by cleaving the thymidine in the HAT medium. Azaserine selection can be used for overcoming this problem. But do not look for alternatives to mycoplasma contamination but try to avoid, detect and treat them to ensure problem-free mAb production.

2.2.9 Environmental monitoring

The laboratory environment where mAb production is done has to be monitored every 6 months. This can easily be done by periodically placing open blood agar bacteriological culture plates on the cabinet work surfaces or at selected points around the laboratory. After leaving the plates open for 4 hr they are incubated at 32 °C and 22 °C for up to 7 days. At the end of this period the plates are examined for the presence of microbial growth. The position of each plate in the cabinet should be recorded and results used for trend analysis.

Limit of contamination are graded in terms of "alert" levels and "action" levels, the actual values being dependent on the criticality of the work and the levels of cleanness that is needed for the particular operational condition.

Continuous use of antibiotics is not recommended as this could lead to:

- Development of resistant strains
- Require the use of more exotic antibiotics
- Mask low levels of contamination.

Once a contamination has been detected, it is generally recommended to discard the culture and continue the work with earlier stocks that are known to be free of contaminants or obtain fresh stocks from a recognized source. However, if this is not possible eradication of the contaminant, may be attempted appropriately. Viral infections are virtually impossible to remove from cultures since they do not respond to antibiotic treatment nor can be removed by centrifugation or other separation techniques.

In case a few wells of a multi well plate is infected, and the cultures can not be totally destroyed then the contamination can be limited by the addition of copper sulphate (> 20 μg/ml) followed by isolation of the well with a layer of liquid paraffin. Methanol is not useful since the fumes would affect the neighboring cultures while ethanol would evaporate very fast that it may be ineffective especially against spores.

2.3 Mice facility

A closed mice facility is required for a hybridoma laboratory which can be at a distance from the cell culture facility. Animal rooms and maintenance should be in conformity to the regulatory requirement practiced in the respective institutions. Standard mice room should have a floor area of 200 square feet with 8–9 feet high walls. The floor should be smooth and free of cracks. Ceramic surface is preferred since they can be cleaned with detergents or disinfectants.

Windows are not required in the animal room. The area required for mouse weighing 10–25 g varies from 40–100 cm^2 with a height of 12.7 cm. The temperature in the animal room should be between 18–26°C with a relative humidity of 40–70%. The ventilation in the animal room should replenish the air 15–20 times per hour. The light in the room may also be regulated, for mice a 12 hr cycle of light and darkness is suitable.

Noise also should be avoided with care taken on the noise produced by air conditioners. An adult mouse takes about 3–4 g of feed per day. Usually pelleted feed is provided. The feed storage rooms must be dry, cool and well ventilated with low humidity. It should be protected against insects and stray rodents.

The animal must have unlimited access to water. The water could be chlorinated by the addition of sodium hypochlorite at a concentration of 10 ppm, *i.e.* with a stock solution of 6% add 0.16 ml per litre of water. The bedding should be able to absorb dampness and softwood shavings are preferred. The requirement is about 2 kg per 100 mice per week.

For disinfection of the animal room, 0.1% sodium hypochlorite, 25% ethanol, 30 mM sodium hydroxide or 0.01% glutaraldehyde solutions are useful. Alternatively, the room (not with animals) can be fumigated with 20% formaldehyde and sealed for 24 hr. When needed it can be neutralized with 25% ammonia.

During the production of mAbs, the mice used may be screened for mouse hepatitis virus, pneumonia virus, Sendai virus, minute virus and mycoplasmas. Mice may be identified by colour coding using 4% picric acid in 70% ethanol or through punching of the ears. Mice used for immunization may be around 10 weeks old. Subcutaneous, intra venous or intra peritoneal injections are used.

The collection of blood is done from the tail vein (about 0.3 ml), retro orbital plexus (0.7 ml) or about 1.5 ml from the heart. Normally heart bleeding is done terminally. Haematological parameters and floor area requirement of mice and rats are given in Tables 2.4 and 2.5.

Table 2.4: Haematological Parameters of Mice and Rats

Parameter	*Mice*	*Rat*
RBC ($\times 10^6$/mm^3)	7–12.5	7–10
PCV (%)	39–49	36–48
Hb (g/dl)	10.2–16.6	11–18
WBC ($\times 10^3$/mm^3)	6–15	6–17
Neutrophils (%)	10–40	9–34
Lymphocytes (%)	55–95	65–85
Eosinophils (%)	0–4	0–6
Monocytes (%)	0.1–3.5	0–5
Basophils (%)	0–0.3	0–1.5
Platlets ($\times 10^3$/mm^3)	16–410	500–1300

Table 2.5: Floor Area Requirement of Mice and Rats

Animal	*Weight (g)*	*Floor area/animal (cm^2)*
Mice	< 10	38.7
	11–15	51.6
	16–25	77.4
	>25	96.7
Rats	<100	109.6
	101–200	148.3
	201–300	187.0
	301–400	258.0
	401–500	387.0
	>500	>451.5

Thus, the number of animal which can be housed in a particular cage (of different dimensions) can be calculated based on the floor area of the cage, recommended floor area per animal and the weight of animal.

A nude mouse is a mutated mouse (disruption of the FOXN1 gene) that does not have a thymus resulting in a greatly reduced number of T-cells. The nude mouse does not have hair; hence it is called "nude". The absence of functioning T cells prevents nude mice from rejecting not only allografts but also xenografts; that is, grafts of tissue from another species. They are unable to mount most types of immune responses such as antibbody formation, cell mediated immune responses, delayed type hypersensitivity responses, killing of virus-infected or malignant cells and graft rejection. Most strains of nude mice do have a few T cells, especially as they age. For this reason, knockout mice with more complete defects in the immune system have been constructed.

A knockout mouse is a genetically engineered mouse in which one or more genes have been switched off by a gene knock out. By inactivating the gene and observing any differences in phenotypic behaviour, the function of the gene deleted can be identified. The first knockout mouse was created by Mario R. Capecchi, Martin Evans and Oliver Smithies in 1989 for which they were awarded the Nobel Prize for Medicine in 2007.

To generate a gene knockout mouse, first a vector consisting of two homologous regions which have complementary strands of DNA on either side of the targeted gene in the genome is constructed. The vector binds to the genome at these two points of homology. Then by a process of recombination the disrupted gene is swapped for the real one. The disrupted gene along with a gene coding for neomycin resistance are included between the homologous regions. A thymidine kinase gene is included outside the homologous region.

Once the vector is introduced into the host cell:

- It can either be incorporated into the genome by homologous recombination (the desired result),
- Undergo complete insertion into the genome at an undesirable point or
- Not be taken up by the cell at all.

If there is no insertion cell get killed by neomycin.

- If there is a random gene insertion cells are resistant to neomycin but killed by gancyclovir.
- If there is a targeted gene insertion, cells are resistant to both neomycin and gancyclovir.

Neomycin resistance is used to select for cells in which the vector has been taken up. If the vector has not been inserted, all cells will die when the cells are grown in neomycin.

If recombination has taken place, the TK gene will not be in the genome and so cells will be insensitive to gancyclovir. However if the vector has been inserted into the genome completely, the cell will die when grown in gancyclovir. Thus through positive and negative selection, cells with the correct insert can be isolated.

Once a vector has been incorporated correctly into the genome of the embryonic stem cells, the cells are expanded in culture and injected into 3.5 day old mouse blastocysts. The blastocysts are injected into the uterus of a pregnant female and the embryos are allowed to come to term.

Often, embryonic stem cells which give rise to mice with a brown coat colour are injected into blastocysts which give rise to mice with a white coat colour. In a completely white mouse, no injected cells was grafted with the blastocyst. On the other hand the mouse with both brown and white markings on its coat, was successfully injected with knockout embryonic stem cells. Mice with brown coat colour are selected and bred to make pure knockout mice.

Gene knockout mice offer one of the most powerful means now available for studying gene function in a living animal.

A transgenic mouse is one that has a foreign gene introduced into their cells. This allows studies of gene expression and protein function within live animals.

Essentially the steps necessary for the production of transgenic mice are:

- Construction of a transgenic vector containing a suitable promoter, a genomic clone or DNA and intron fragment and polyadenylation addition sequences.
- Microinjection of the transgenic into the pronuclei of fertilized ova or injection of embryonic stem cells into blastocysts to generate mice containing copies of that transgenic integrated randomly in their genome.

CHAPTER 3

PRODUCTION OF MONOCLONAL ANTIBODIES

3.1 Introduction

While producing monoclonal antibodies, three things need to be considered. (i) Choice of animal for hybridoma production, (ii) Choice of cell lines, and (iii) Choice of immunogenies, needed and each choice depends upon the final product.

3.1.1 Choice of animal for hybridoma production

Mouse, rats, humans and rabbits have been used to make mAbs. The mouse system was historically the first to be developed. The choice of the animal largely depends on the immunizing antigen. For example, rats can be used for preparation of mAbs against mouse antigens.

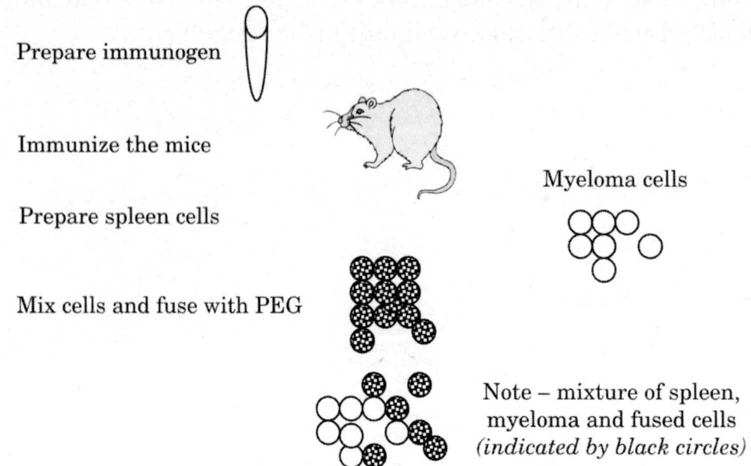

Seed cells into wells and select in selection medium

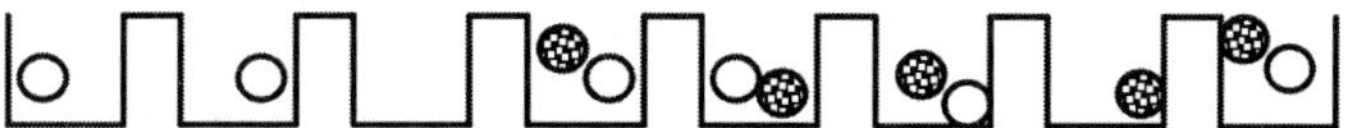

Screen clones and expand positive hybridomas

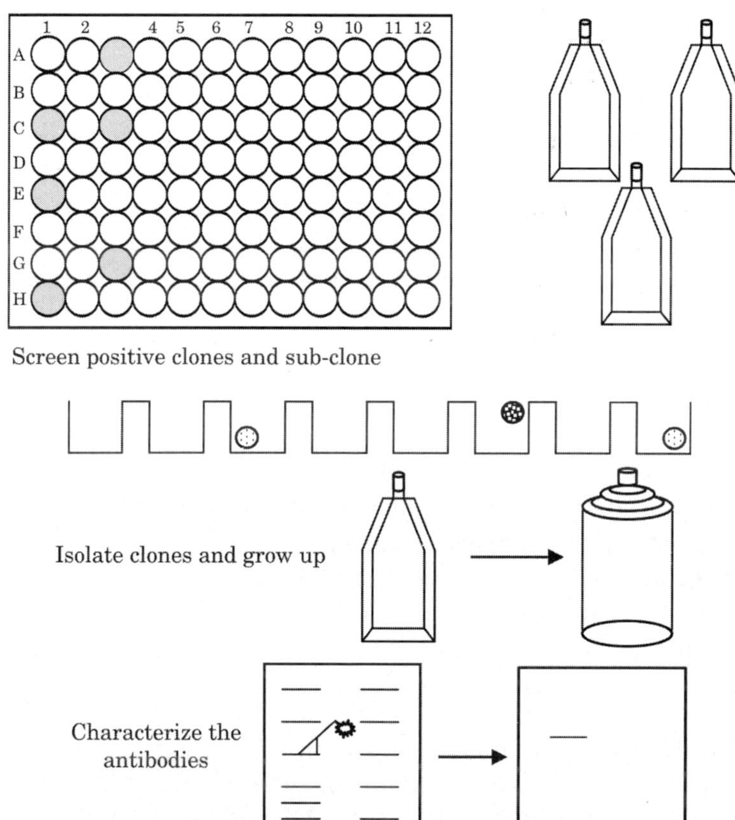

Freeze; Grow *in vitro* or *in vivo*

Fig. 3.1: Schematic representation of the production of mAbs

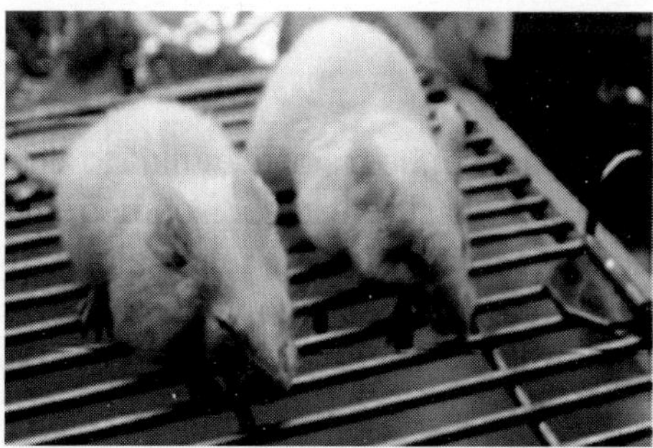

Fig. 3.2: BALB/c mice

The advantages of the rat system include:

- Lower reversion of the parent cell line to non-secreting forms
- Higher number of fusion hybrids expressing spleen immunoglobulins
- Larger volumes of ascitic fluid.

One of the disadvantages of the rat system is the inability of the rat immunoglobulins to bind to protein A.

The application of human mAbs include:

- Passive immunotherapy
- Diagnosis
- Analysis of B cell repertoire
- Antibodies to polymorphic determinants.

However the problems of human mAbs include:

- Unavailability of suitable human myeloma cells
- Source of lymphocytes: peripheral blood lymphocytes
- Dependence on "immunized humans"
- Auto immune patients.

Cross species fusions or hetero hybridomas have been prepared between say mouse × bovine or human × mouse etc.

The ideal choice of the mouse strain for immunization is BALB/c (B albino) since it is compatible with the available parent myeloma cell lines and hence hybridomas can be grown as ascites without the problem of immune rejection. Most hybridomas have origins in BALB/c plasmacytomas and spleen cells and hybridoma recipient mice must also be BALB/c strain or alternatively immunodeficient animals have to be used.

Although many different mouse strains can be used for immunization, there are strain differences in responses. Hence if another strain such as SJL or NZB mouse is found to be better in eliciting an immune response, it can be used for immunization with subsequent use of an F_1 hybrid between BALB/c and SJL/NZB mouse for ascites production. Generally, female retired breeder mice are preferred because of availability, large size and tendency not to fight. Lou/C and Lou/M rats have also been used. Ileo caecal tumours in these animals have the features of plasmacytomas from which myeloma cell lines have been developed.

3.1.2 Choice of cell lines

The basic characteristics of the myeloma cell line used as a fusion partner are:

- The cell line by itself should not make and secrete any immunoglobulin
- Lack of defects in the ability to make or secrete immunoglobulin
- Should have good fusion efficiency
- Low reversion frequency.

If the parent myeloma cell line also produces immunoglobulin, immunoglobulins produced by the hybridomas would be a mixture of heavy and light chains against the target antigen, and the 'basal' immunoglobulin of the myeloma would lead to lowering of overall affinity and specificity. If only the light chains are secreted by the myeloma partner, the problem is less since the irrelevant immunoglobulins would be limited but not completely eliminated.

Although it should not produce immunoglobulins on its own, it should be capable of producing immunoglobulins after fusion with the spleen lymphocytes. The fusion efficiency of the myeloma cell line should be high leading to a high numbers of fused cells. Although it depends on the ratio of myeloma and lymphocytes, fusing agent, the method of fusion, etc. in general mouse myelomas should yield hybridization frequencies of 1–100 clones per 10^7 lymphocytes. The fused cells should not lose their secretion potential of mAbs following continuous culture. A measure of this characteristic can be assessed from the number of wells that are positive for antibody secretion in the first screening, and should continue to remain so thereafter.

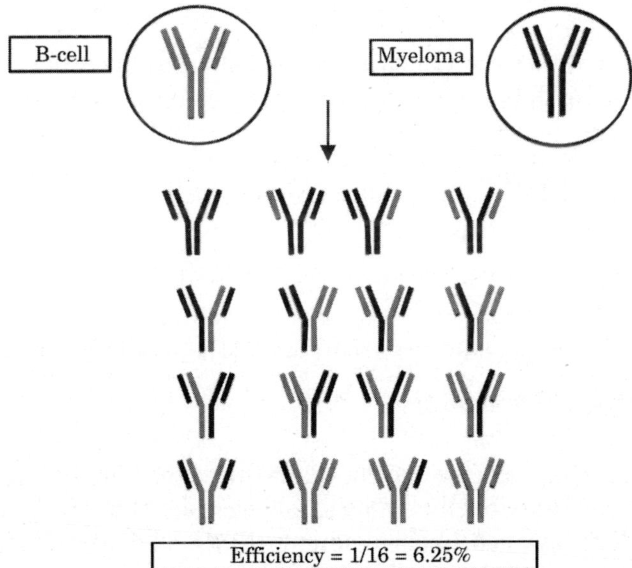

Fig. 3.3: Effect of myeloma cells also synthesizing immunoglobulins

Table 3.1: Commonly used Mouse cell-lines

Cell line	*Ig secretion*	*Derived from*
X63–Ag8	IgG1, k	MOPC–21
NS1–Ag4/1	k, intra cellular	X63
X63–Ag8.653	None	X63–Ag8
SP2/0–Ag14	None	X63–Ag8 × BALB/c
NSO/1	None	NS1–Ag4/1
FO	None	Clone of SP2/0
FOX-NY	None	NS1

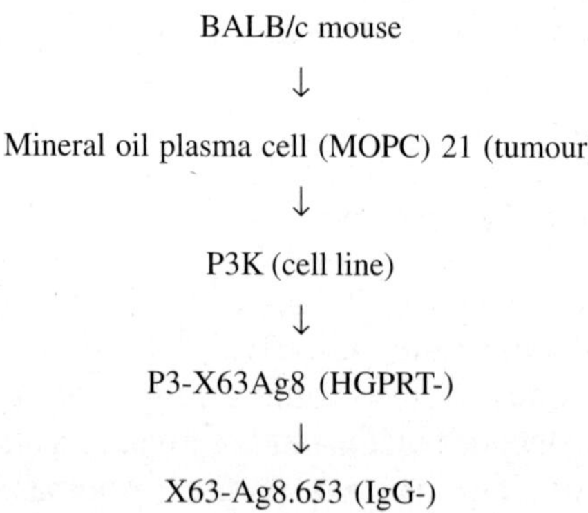

The rat cell lines include:

- Y3-Ag1, 2, 3 cell line that secretes a light chain and
- YB$^{2}/_{3}$ Ag20 that makes no immunoglobulins.

Some of the human cell lines available and used in earlier trials includes SKO–007 (U–266ART)–azaguanine resistant, secretes epsilon heavy chain and lambda light chain.

- GM1500–6TG–2–thioguanine resistant, secretes gamma-2b heavy chain and kappa light chain
- LICR–LON–HMy2–azaguanine resistant, secretes gamma one heavy chain and kappa light chain
- UC729–6–thioguanine resistant, secretes IgM and kappa light chain.

3.1.2.1 *Selective drug markers*

The metabolic requirements of nucleotides are met either through dietary intake or synthesis *de novo*. However, the ability to salvage nucleotides from sources within the body precludes any nutritional requirement for nucleotides. Hence purine and pyrimidine bases are not required in the diet. The salvage pathways are a major source of nucleotides for synthesis of DNA, RNA and enzyme co-factors.

In *de novo* pathways, the nucleotide bases are assembled from simpler compounds using ATP hydrolysis. The framework for a pyrimidine (thymine and cytosine or uracil) base is assembled first and then attached to ribose. While a purine (adenine and guanine) base is synthesized directly onto a ribose-based structure the salvage pathways recycle already used bases by reattaching them to a ribose. Synthesis of the purine nucleotides begins with 5-phosphoribosyl-1-pyrophosphate (PRPP) and leads to the first fully formed nucleotide, inosine 5'-monophosphate (IMP). The synthesis of IMP requires five moles of ATP, two moles of glutamine, one mole of glycine, one mole of CO_2, one mole of aspartate and two moles of formate. The formyl moieties are carried on tetrahydrofolate (THF) in the form of N^5, N^{10}-methenyl-THF and N^{10}-formyl-THF.

IMP represents a branch point for purine biosynthesis, because it can be converted into either AMP or GMP through two distinct reaction pathways. The pathway leading to AMP requires energy in the form of GTP; that leading to GMP requires energy in the form of ATP. The accumulation of excess GTP will lead to accelerated AMP synthesis from IMP. Conversely, since the conversion of IMP to GMP requires ATP, the accumulation of excess ATP leads to accelerated synthesis of GMP over that of AMP.

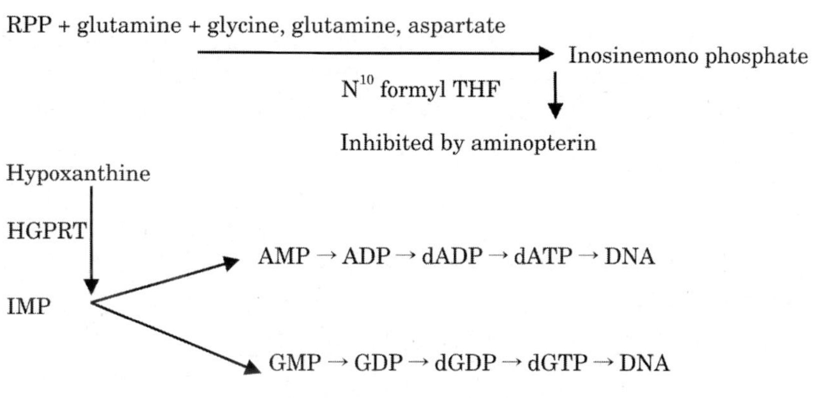

Fig. 3.4: Synthesis of purines

The synthesis of pyrimidines differs in two significant ways from that of purines. First, the ring structure is assembled as a free base, not built upon PRPP. PRPP is added to the first fully formed pyrimidine base (orotic acid), forming orotate monophosphate (OMP), which is subsequently decarboxylated to UMP. Second, there is no branch in the pyrimidine synthesis pathway. UMP is phosphorylated twice to yield UTP (ATP is the phosphate donor). The first phosphorylation is catalyzed by uridylate kinase and the second by ubiquitous nucleoside diphosphate kinase. Finally UTP is aminated by the action of CTP synthase, generating CTP. The thymine nucleotides are in turn derived by *de novo* synthesis from dUMP or by salvage pathways from deoxyuridine or deoxythymidine.

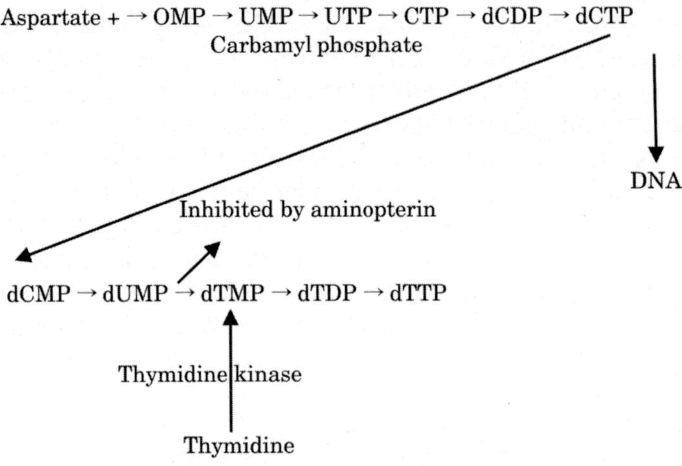

Fig. 3.5: Synthesis of pyrimidines

Both the salvage and *de novo* synthesis pathways of purine and pyrimidine biosynthesis lead to production of nucleoside-5'-phosphates through the utilization of an activated sugar intermediate, 5-phosphoribosyl-1-pyrophosphate (PRPP) and a class of enzymes called phospho ribosyl transferases.

The free purine bases, adenine, guanine, and hypoxanthine, can be reconverted to their corresponding nucleotides by phosphoribosylation. Two key transferase enzymes are involved in the salvage of purines: adenosine phosphoribosyltransferase (APRT), which catalyzes the following reaction:

$$\text{adenine} + \text{PRPP} \leftrightarrow \text{AMP} + \text{PP}_i$$

and hypoxanthine-guanine phosphoribosyltransferase (HGPRT), which catalyzes the following reactions:

$$\text{hypoxanthine} + \text{PRPP} \leftrightarrow \text{IMP} + \text{PP}_i$$
$$\text{guanine} + \text{PRPP} \leftrightarrow \text{GMP} + \text{PP}_i$$

The thymine nucleotides are in turn derived by *de novo* synthesis from dUMP or by salvage pathways from deoxyuridine or deoxythymidine.

The salvage pathway to dTTP synthesis involves the enzyme thymidine kinase which can use either thymidine or deoxyuridine as substrate:

$$\text{thymidine} + \text{ATP} \leftrightarrow \text{TMP} + \text{ADP}$$
$$\text{deoxyuridine} + \text{ATP} \leftrightarrow \text{dUMP} + \text{ADP}$$

Aminopterin blocks the main biosynthetic pathway for purine and pyrimidine biosynthesis mainly by the inhibition of the enzyme dihydrofolate reductase.

The salvage pathway of purines involves the enzyme HGPRT with exogenous hypoxanthine. The salvage pathway of pyrimidines involves the enzyme TK with exogenous thymidine. Cell lines can be made deficient in either one of these two enzymes by growth and selection in either azaguanine or thioguanine (for TK^-) and bromodeoxy uridine (for $HGPRT^-$).

In normal cells these analogues are incorporated into the DNA and it becomes cytotoxic. Hence only enzyme negative cells survive in the presence of these compounds. It is easier to select for HGPRT than TK negative cells since the HGPRT locus is on the X-sex chromosome. Only one X chromosome is transcriptionally active, hence, mutation in one chromosome is sufficient for a cell to become HGPRT negative.

6-thioguanine is better a 8-azaguanine for selection of HGPRT negative mutants because 8-azaguanine is incorporated into both DNA and RNA hence the cell is better protected from the mutagenic effect.

The cells can be mutagenised by irradiation or exposure to ethyl methane sulphonate. Then the cells can be exposed to 8-azaguanine or bromodeoxy uridine at increasing concentrations from around 1 μg/ml to about 30–100 μg/ml in 6–8 weeks. Then the surviving cells (resistant) is cloned by limiting dilution and chosen for high growth rate and low reversion frequency.

Oubain resistance is another marker where human cell lines are used. Rodent cell lines can grow in the presence of 10^{-3}M oubain while human cell die at levels of even at 10^{-7}M oubain.

Instead of aminopterin that blocks purine and pyrimidine biosynthesis, another inhibitor, azaserine blocks only purine biosynthesis. Hence thymidine need not be added as in HAT medium, only hypoxanthine is enough. Thymidine inhibits DNA synthesis at milli molar concentrations in most mammalian cells; hence sometimes it is better avoided.

Another selection medium is AAT (Adenine-Hypoxanthine-Thymidine) instead of HAT. This is based on adenosine phosphoribosyltransferase (APRT) mutants (in place of HGPRT) and hence is supplemented with adenine (instead of hypoxanthine). The FOX NY cell line is APRT and HGPRT negative. Selection is done in the presence of 2, 6, di amino purine which is the toxic analogue of adenine.

3.1.3 Immunization

According to the clonal selection theory, B-cells of different specificities pre-exist in the body. The immunizing antigen binds to the specific membrane immunoglobulin receptor on the B-cell causing it to proliferate and differentiate so that more of the specific antibodies produced by that particular B-cell are secreted to neutralize the antigen.

In mAb production, the purpose of immunization is to increase the number of B-lymphocytes capable of producing antibodies of the desired specificity in the spleen of the mouse so that more such B-cells would be involved in fusion with the myeloma cells.

However, rodents, and especially mice, are almost always the animal of choice. This is primarily due to the availability of mouse myeloma cell lines, but other methods are available for production of human or rabbit mAbs.

If production of ascites tumors is envisaged, the mouse strain used for the immunization should match the mouse strain from which the myeloma cells were derived so that the injected cells are histocompatible and are not rejected.

The mice are immunized, boosted and tested until an antibody response of the desired specificity is elicited. It is critical that the mouse exhibits antibodies of the desired specificity before proceeding with the fusion which ensures adequate number of stimulated B-cells that can participate in fusion.

Immunization strategies include alterations in the:

- Inoculation routes
- Dosage
- Timing
- Use of adjuvants

The same basic factors (*i.e.,* immunogen preparation, dose, adjuvants, etc.) for the generation of polyclonal sera also apply to the production of mAbs.

3.1.3.1 *Factors influencing immunogenicity*

3.1.3.1.1 *Contribution of the immunogen*

- ***Foreignness*:** The immune system discriminates between self and non-self and hence only foreign molecules are immunogenic. More distant the phylogeny the better would be the immune responses. For example, mouse proteins may not stimulate a good immune response in rats as that in chickens.

- ***Size*:** The larger the molecule the more immunogenic it is likely to be.
- ***Chemical composition*:** Chemically more complex molecules tend to be more immunogenic.
- ***Physical form*:** Particulate antigens are more immunogenic than soluble ones and denatured antigens more immunogenic than the native form.
- ***Degradability*:** Antigens that are easily phagocytosed are generally more immunogenic since development of an immune response requires antigen processing and presentation by the antigen presenting cells (APC). Dendritic cells, macrophages and B-cells are the professional APCs.

3.1.3.1.2 Contribution of the host

- ***Genetic factors*:** The genetic background of the mice used for mAb production affects the magnitude and type of immune responses generated.
- ***Age*:** Usually the very young and the very old have a diminished ability to mount a good immune response. Use 8–12 week-old mice.

3.3.1.3 *Method of administration*

- ***Dose*:** The dose of the immunogen is critical and needs to be optimal. Higher doses may lead to tolerance while lower doses may not elicit a good immune response
- ***Route*:** The route of antigen administration can also alter the nature of the response
- ***Adjuvants*:** Substances that can enhance the immune response to an immunogen are called adjuvants. Adjuvants can be used to potentate and also direct the immune responses generated.

So, for better success in mAb production, the course and magnitude of immune responses of individual mouse must be assessed before fusion.

3.1.3.2 *Immunization procedures*

The site of injection should be clipped thoroughly and prepared aseptically. A disinfection solution is suitable for disinfection of the skin, followed by wiping the area with 70% ethanol.

3.1.3.2.1 *Routes of inoculation*

- ***Intra dermal route*:** The intra dermal route is inappropriate in the mouse or for other rodents

- ***Subcutaneous route***: In rabbits, the site of choice is the inter-scapular region (between the shoulder blades skin on the dorsum, avoiding the neck where the rabbit is restrained, administering up to 0.25 ml of inoculum per site in a maximum of four sites. In the mouse, up to 0.1 ml may be given in the neck region.
- ***Intramuscular route***: In rabbits, intramuscular injections of FCA may be administered in the thigh muscle; up to 0.5 ml preferably in one site. Intramuscular injection of FCA is not recommended for small laboratory animals such as rats, mice etc.
- ***Intra peritoneal route***: The intra peritoneal route for injection of FCA is permitted in mice and rats only. FCA should be administered only once, and be limited to minimal volumes of up to 0.1 ml.
- ***Intravenous route***: FCA should not be used for intravenous injections.
- ***Footpad injection***: FCA should not be injected in the feet of rabbits or rodents unless there is scientific evidence indicating this route is essential as a specific requirement for the production of immune response. In rats and mice, only one footpad may be used with the volume of to be injected into the footpad must not exceed 0.05 ml for a mouse and 0.1 ml for a rat.
- ***Intra spleenic route***: Technically demanding, preferred for IgM type of mAbs and also for injection of plasmid DNA or haptens.

Immunization schedules vary depending upon the nature of the antigen. There is no universal immunization schedule for the production of mAbs. A good immunization needs at least 3–4 months. Regardless of the method or antigen mixture used, all antigen preparations should be prepared aseptically and final mixtures should be cultured for presence of contaminating bacteria. The first injection of the antigen normally given with FCA stimulates primary antibody response that greatly expands number of B-lymphocytes specific for the immunizing antigen.

Intravenous (tail vein) inoculations (0.1–0.5 ml) are routinely used for particulate antigens and subcutaneous (0.05–0.2 ml) and intra peritoneal (up to 0.5 ml) routes are generally used for antigen/adjuvant mixtures. Although the first injection may utilize FCA, subsequent (booster) injections must be only of incomplete Freund's adjuvant (IFA) or saline.

The second injections of the antigen should be given when the serum titres tend to fall. If secondary boosters are given when the serum titres are high, it may result in neutralization of the antigen by the anti sera resulting in the absence of booster effect and simultaneous fall in antibody titres as well.

The antibody titers are generally determined in blood samples taken at 10 to 24 days after the boost and, when peak titers are reached, animals are rested for 3–4 weeks. Mice are then given a final intravenous aqueous antigen boost and euthanatized by cervical dislocation or CO_2 narcosis 3 days later. Animals failing to achieve high antibody titers may be boosted multiple times.

A 'thumb rule' immunization schedule could be:

- Day 1–priming with antigen (100 μg/100 μl/mouse) + FCA (100 μl) intra peritoneal
- Day 14–Boost with antigen (50 μg/100 ul/mouse) + IFA (100 μl) intra peritoneal
- Day 21–Boost with antigen (50 μg/100 μl/mouse) + IFA (100 μl) intra peritoneal
- Day 28–Boost with antigen (50 μg/100 μl/mouse) intra venous
- Day 31–Fusion.

The time between two immunizations can be extended to 3–4 weeks and a total of 4–5 immunizations may also be tried.

Since more number of antigen-specific lymphocyte fusions are achieved from the spleen collected from mouse whose serum has high titre of antibodies, this should be the benchmark for selection of the mouse spleen for fusion. The time interval between intra venous injections and fusion should be always three days. This interval is critical.

The resting B-cell that has more of membrane immunoglobulins is not a good fusion candidate as also differentiated plasma cells which have more cytoplasmic immunoglobulins. The intermediary stage of lymphoblasts is the ideal fusion candidate cell since their membrane has more fluidity which also expresses higher amounts of membrane immunoglobulins.

The interval of three days after the last injection and fusion is critical to produce more antigen-specific lymphoblasts. Some schedules recommend intra venous injections on all the three days prior to fusion.

3.1.3.3 *Adjuvants*

Adjuvants are substances that enhance the overall immune response. The advantage of using a smaller antigen dose is that only the higher affinity clones of B cells are stimulated, thus improving the quality of the antibody produced. Most adjuvants contain two components. One component will form a 'depot' that prevents the rapid breakdown of the antigen and promotes its slow release.

The second component non-specifically stimulates the immune system. For example, killed bacteria especially mycobacteria, or bacterial components such as lipopolysaccharide (LPS) or muramyl didpeptide (MDP), a synthetic analogue of the adjuvant-active component from the cell walls of mycobacteria. These substances stimulate macrophages and other immune effector cells to release cytokines which then enhances the antibody response. The immunomodulatory component may also influence the class of immunoglobin produced.

A second way an adjuvant can work is to serve as a vehicle to help deliver the Ag to the spleen and/or lymph nodes where Ag is trapped by the follicular dendritic cells and where most of the cell to cell interactions take place to generate plasma cells.

For example, microdroplets of oil containing Ag, such as those formed in an oil-in-water adjuvant emulsion, are readily ingested by macrophage and taken to draining lymph nodes or spleen. Emulsions aid tissue dendritic cells in their capture of Ag.

A third way an adjuvant can work is by activating the various cells involved in the immune response, either directly or indirectly. Surfactants may serve this function as well as helping to stabilize oil-water emulsions.

3.1.3.3.1 Freund's complete adjuvant (FCA)

FCA is a mixture of non metabolizable oil (mineral oil), a surfactant (Arlacel A), and mycobacteria (*Mycoplasma tuberculosis* or *M. butyricum*). It is prepared as a water-in-oil emulsion by combining one volume FCA with one volume aqueous antigen solution.

In the emulsion, antigen is distributed over a large surface area thereby increasing the potential for interaction with relevant cells. To check whether the water-in oil emulsion has been prepared properly, drop the emulsion on the surface of cold water in a beaker. The first drop may spread over the surface but subsequent drops should float as white drops just below the surface of water. This confirms that the antigen-containing aqueous phase is totally enclosed in the oil phase.

3.1.3.3.2 Incomplete freund's adjuvant (IFA)

IFA contains the ame oil/surfactant mixture as FCA but does not contain any mycobacteria. It is frequently used to boost animals that received a primary antigen injection in CFA, but it can be used as the adjuvant for the primary injection as well.

3.1.3.3.3 Other adjuvants

Montanide ISA (Incomplete Seppic Adjuvant) [Seppic, Paris, France] is a group of oil/surfactant based adjuvants in which different surfactants are combined with non-metabolizable mineral oil, metabolizable oil, or a mixture of the two. They are prepared for use as an emulsion with aqueous Ag solution. The surfactant for montanide ISA 50 is mannide oleate, a major component of the surfactant in Freund's adjuvant. The performance of these adjuvants is similar to IFA with lesser inflammatory responses.

Ribi's Adjuvants are a mixture of oil, detergent, and immunostimulator to which an aqueous antigen solution should be added and mixed to form a stable oil-in-water emulsion. The adjuvant utilizes a metabolizable oil (squalene) and a mycobacterial component, trehalose dimycolate (TDM), serves as a surfactant and an immunostimulator as well as an adherence factor in binding protein Ag to the oil droplets. Ribi's adjuvants provide different detoxified bacterial products as immunostimulators for different species. Hence the name Ribi's Adjuvant System (RAS) is used.

Hunter's TiterMax is an oil/surfactant-based adjuvant prepared as a water-in-oil emulsion in a manner similar to that used for Freund's adjuvants. It uses squalene as the metabolizable oil and synthetic nonionic copolymers of polyoxyethylene and polyoxypropylene as a nonionic surfactant.

Other commercial adjuvants such as Titermax Gold™ (Sigma Immuno-chemicals) can be used in lieu of FCA with relatively similar levels of induction of a productive humoral immune response. This adjuvant provides for a stable immunization emulsion as this adjuvant has the following constituents a block copolymer, CRL–8300 (a patent pending product) and squalene (a metablolizable oil) and a microparticle stabilizer. The components facilitate increased emulsification of the antigen compared to FCA. This reduces the viscosity of the immunogen and facilitates delivery via narrow bore needles resulting in less pain to the animals used in the immunization protocol.

Aluminum salt adjuvants are used with protein antigens either as alum-precipitated vaccines or as alum-adsorbed vaccines. Aluminum salts are generally weaker adjuvants than emulsion adjuvants but because of milder inflammatory reactions, safety, and efficacy for generating memory, they are the primary adjuvants utilized in humans. Adsorption of protein is dependent on the pI of the protein and the pH of the medium. A protein with a lower pI adsorbs to the positively charged aluminum ion more strongly than a protein with a higher pI. The mineral adjuvants work by establishing a depot of Ag, which is released slowly over a period of 2-3 weeks, nonspecific activation of macrophages and complement activation. The effectiveness of aluminum salt adjuvants has been increased by the addition of gamma-inulin, detergents or *Bordetella pertussis*.

3.1.3.4 *Immunogen preparation*

Typically a purified protein is used as an immunogen. Partially purified preparations can be used. For example, virus purified from infected cell cultures could be pelleted and used. However, in such preparations the presence of cellular proteins can not be ruled out. This can result in a strong immune response against the cellular contaminants. Under such circumstances, if the same partially purified protein is to be used for hybridoma screening, there is no way to eliminate the possibility of hybridoma clones secreting mAbs to the cellular protein contamination present in the immunogen preparation.

If in the case of hapten the carrier used in the immunogen and that used for screening are made different the antibodies produced against the carrier do not interfere with the screening. For example, if progesterone coupled to bovine serum albumin is used for immunization, progesterone coupled to keyhole limpet haemocyanin can be used for screening.

Immunization with non denatured (*i.e.*, native) proteins tends to produce antibodies against conformation epitopes, whereas immunization with denatured proteins tends to produce antibodies against linear determinants. It is easier to obtain a higher degree of purity under denaturing conditions.

Other immunization antigens include:

- Synthetic peptides coupled to carrier proteins
- Recombinant proteins expressed in *Escherichia coli*, yeast, baculo virus or mammalian vectors
- DNA vaccination using plasmid encoded immunogenic gene
- Denatured antigens or fixative treated antigens especially for use in immuno histochemistry (IHC).

3.1.3.5 *In vitro* immunization

Exposure of the spleen cell suspension of host animal to the antigen *in vitro* is followed by use in fusion with myeloma cells. The spleen cells are suspended at a density of 5×10^6 cells/ml, to which an antigen concentration of 0.05 to 5 μg/ml are exposed for 3–4 days and then used in fusion. The cultures can be supplemented with thymocyte conditioned medium and with polyclonal activators such as lipo polysaccharide (LPS) or poke weed mitogen (PWM).

The advantages of *in vitro* immunization are:

- Shortened immunization time (days instead of weeks)
- mAbs against antigens suppressed in the normal response
- Preferable if IgM isotype of mAbs is required
- Very small and defined quantities of antigen are required and
- Wider library of antibodies produced because of lack of *in vivo* phenomena such as suppression or tolerance.

3.1.3.5.1 Intra spleenic immunization

Intra spleenic immunization involves direct injection of antigen into the spleen through surgery. Intraspleenic injection is recommended:

- When there is limited supply of antigen
- Other routes of immunization did not elicit a strong response.

Three days after injection is completed the mouse is killed and the spleen is removed for fusion.

3.2 Collection of Spleen

The immunized mouse spleen serves as the source of lymphocytes to be fused with mouse myeloma cells to form hybridoma cells. The spleen is the preferred source as it is easily obtainable. Lymph nodes and peripheral blood are also occasionally used as lymphocyte sources. In humans, peripheral blood is often the only source used, unless the spleen or some lymph nodes were being surgically removed and are made available. Identify the mouse to be used for fusion which is based on high serum titres to the antigen of interest.

Bleed the mouse either through the tail vein or retro orbital plexus. This serum can be used as the positive control serum in the ELISA based screening assays. Set up a sterile glass Petri-dish containing about 5–10 ml of cold, sterile Hank's Balanced Salt Solution (HBSS) for placing the spleen after removal from the mouse. Sacrifice the mouse humanely by cervical dislocation. Place the dead mouse on its back or right side on a clean surface and wipe the abdomen and left side thoroughly with 70% alcohol. Trim back the fur and skin using gloved hands and scissors and forceps. Using another set of sterile forceps and scissors cut a slit into the abdomen. Enlarge the slit with the scissors. Locate the spleen by gently pushing the stomach to the animal's right side. The spleen will appear as a dark red, thin, flat organ about one inch in length by one-quarter inch width. Collect the spleen and place it in a sterile, glass Petri-dish containing cold, sterile HBSS. Trim the excess fatty or connective tissue.

3.2.1 Preparation of spleen cell suspension

Various methods have been proposed for spleen dissociation and collection of splenocytes. One method is to take some medium and pump it into the stroma of the spleen tissue half way (and not through and through). Due to the pressure build up inside the tissue, the medium would come out of the tissue thereby bringing with it the cells of the spleen.

After collection of the medium containing the spleen cells, the spleen tissue is placed on a fine wire mesh. A few drops of the medium are added and using the plunger of the 5 ml syringe, the spleen is crushed and the dissociated cells are made to pass through the wire mesh. Gentle grinding of the spleen across the mesh with the plunger will help hasten the dissociation.

If cell clumps are seen, it is recommended to split the clumps using gentle pipetting or passing through a 20 gauge needle.

If clumps are not removed at this stage, it will continue to be present in the pellet.

Another way to remove the pellet is to allow the clumps to settle by gravity (leave for 1–2 minutes) and then collect the supernatant.

After complete dissociation of the spleen cells, only the connective tissue and fatty tissue would remain on the wire mesh

The spleen cell suspension can be centrifuged at 200 × g for 10 minutes.

Discard the supernatant carefully with out dislodging the cell pellet which would remain in the bottom of the tube.

Add 5–10 ml of cold, sterile HBSS/RPMI 1640 medium and resuspend the cells using a sterile pipette and wash the cells thrice.

3.2.1.1 *Cell count and cell viability*

Using a haemocytometer, sterile 0.4% trypan blue, and medium as a diluents, the total number of viable lymphocytes/ml of the suspension can be estimated as follows:

Using separate, sterile pipettes for each addition, mix 0.1 ml of the resuspended spleen cell suspension + 0.1 ml of 0.4% trypan blue + 0.8 ml of sterile HBSS in a small, microfuge tube. Allow this mixture to stand at room temperature for about 1 minute. Cells would begin to die if held too long in trypan blue mixture. Using a microtip, carefully fill one chamber of the hemocytometer under coverslip. Using a light microscope, number of viable lymphocytes in all the 4 large corner squares is counted.

The viable cells exclude the trypan blue stain while the dead cells would appear blue. If stained for a long time, even the viable cells would appear blue. Live cells have an intact membrane and hence the trypan blue which is negatively charged cannot enter the cells. Other cells that may be present that should not be included in the count include erythrocytes (light reddish brown round cells), monocytes (that would appear larger than lymphocytes) and polymorphonuclear neutrophils (multinucleated cells).

Optimum dilution of the cell suspension is essential for correct counting. Too many cells or too few cells counted may lead to erroneous results. Optimum dilution should result in 50–70 cells in each large square that can be counted properly.

The number of viable lymphocytes/ml

Average cells per large square × 10^4 × dilution factor

Based on the estimated cell counts of viable cells (cells that excluded trypan blue) and dead cells (cells stained with trypan blue) that percentage of viability can be assessed.

The percent viability should be always greater than 95%. If it is lower, the collection procedure needs to re-evaluated. It is possible that the cells are being handled roughly; centrifugation is at higher speeds or for longer duration and so on. Based on the cell count, determine the volume of cells needed for fusion.

3.3 Myeloma Cell Preparation

Several different mouse and human myeloma cell lines are available for use in hybridoma formation. However, only a very few are used frequently. One of which is the P3 × 63, Ag 8.653. This cell line is a non-secretor (*i.e.*, does not produce antibodies on its own), is 8-azaguanine resistant (important during selection of hybridoma cells), is derived from the BALB/c strain of mice (the same strain that was used for immunization), is very easy to culture, and is not dangerous to use (it is a mouse tumor, but is harmless to humans). Myeloma cells would be almost perfectly round or oval, in small to large clumps, in suspension or loosely attached to the bottom surface of the flask.

Look for any cells with an unusual morphology and any signs of contamination. The myeloma cells are non-adherent cells and hence sub culturing can be done either by simple dislodging the cells from inside the flask, or using a pipette to force cell culture fluid over the cell layer several times coupled with giving the tightly closed cell culture flask a strong tap on the palm of your hand.

Dulbecco's Modified Eagle's Medium (DMEM) with 4.5 g of glucose/liter to which has been added L-glutamine, antibiotics and antimycotics and 10–15% FBS is most often used. Cultures are most often maintained in 25 cm^2 cell culture flasks at 37ºC in 5% CO_2. The flask cap should not be tightly closed since this would prevent exchange of CO_2 that acts as a buffer by dissolving in the medium. The position of the flasks should at right angles to the direction of the shelf movement. The split ratio can be 1:2 or 1:3 depending on the growth of the cell line. The cells may be sub cultured once every 4–5 days to maintain them in the log phase.

3.3.1 Ensuring 8-azaguanine resistance

The myeloma cells are HGPRT negative and thus are not capable of converting hypoxanthine to GTP. Given the rapid cell division and long-term culture of myeloma cells, it is not unusual for a few of the myeloma cells to mutate and acquire the ability to produce HGPRT. In such cases the myeloma cells will be able to use hypoxanthine to make GTP will not be killed in the HAT medium. 8-azaguanine is an "analog" of hypoxanthine, but will kill the cell if it is incorporated into DNA.

When the myeloma cells become HGPRT positive, 8-azaguanine gets incorporated into the DNA and kills the cells. If a cell survives in 8-azaguanine, it implies that it is HGPRT negative. These cells are known as 8-azaguanine-resistant (Ag8). The myeloma cells used for fusion should be resistant to 8-azaguanine. Such HGPRT positive cells should be eliminated by culturing the myeloma cell line in 8-azaguanine once or twice a year leaving only 8-azaguanine resistant cells.

Another simpler way to find out whether the unfused myeloma cell line is susceptible to HAT is to grow them in HAT medium. All the cells should be killed in 4–5 days without any cells being left alive. If you suspect that some cells are not being killed in the HAT medium, it is better to passage the myeloma cell line in 8-azaguanine to ensure that all the cells are HGPRT negative.

3.3.2 Counting myeloma cells

Using the method described above, the number of viable myeloma cells/ml in the culture can be estimated. Based on this, the volume of the culture needed to obtain a total of 2×10^7 viable myeloma cells for the cell fusion technique can be calculated made ready for the fusion day.

3.4 Fusing Agents

The earliest fusion agent used by Kohler and Milstein in 1975 was inactivated Sendai virus. Some of the viruses belonging to the *Paramyxo* virus group have the property of causing fusion of the infected cells as a means of intra cellular spread of the virus and consequent production of syncytium or multi nucleated giant cells.

It has been largely replaced by polyethylene glycol (PEG). The molecular structure of PEG is $HO\ (CH_2CH_2O)_n\ CH_2CH_2OH$. PEG is obtained in the molecular weight range of 200–20000. Most fusions are performed with PEG in the range of 600–6000.

High molecular weight PEG is used for concentration across a dialysis membrane through which water and other solutes are pulled out based on the molecular weight cut-off of the membrane. PEG 6000 is also used for protein precipitation such as virus precipitation from the tissue culture fluids or immunoglobulins from serum collected from adult animals.

The exact mechanism of fusion is not well understood but it is thought to be due to the removal of the physical free water leading to agglutination of cells which occurs in the concentrations of 40–50%. PEG acts simply by volume exclusion, resulting in an osmotic force driving membranes into close contact in a dehydrated region.

An efficient alternative is electric field-mediated cell fusion, which offers several advantages over conventional biological (virus-induced), and chemical (PEG-induced) fusion methods:

- Higher fusion efficiencies
- Better reproducibility
- Fewer antigen–stimulated B-cells required
- Better growth properties in the early stage following fusion
- Possibility of tailor-made fusion protocols for specific cells
- Better control of fusion-results.

3.4.1 Basics of electro fusion

Applying an electrical field to cells in the form of short, intense pulses increases the permeability of the membrane as well as the membrane flow. The resulting local perforation of the cell membrane allows cell fusion to form a new cell with the properties of the fusion partners. The prerequisite for successful electro fusion is the direct membrane contact between the individual cells before the electrical pulse is applied. The process of electro fusion comprises three steps:

- ***Alignment of the cells*:** The cells to be fused must be aligned in chains between the electrodes. Fusion will occur at the flattened areas of the cell membranes, where the cells are in close contact with one another forming long strings ("pearl chains"). For alignment to occur 4–6 V for 20–30 sec is sufficient.
- ***Membrane fusion*:** Very short field pulses with high intensity leads to a reversible electrical breakthrough of the cell membranes. This results in the formation of temporary pores in the contact zone of two cells, which may then become fused. The pulse voltage for fusion is 20–60 V, 15–20 μ sec with 1–3 pulses.
- ***Post-alignment*:** Rounding off the fusion products is carried out by expanding the primary fused membrane sections, resulting in a so called plasmogamy. For post-alignment 4–6 V at 20–30 sec can be used.

3.5 Components of HAT Medium

Hypoxanthine is not toxic to cells hence concentrations of 0.1 mM are used. Thymidine is toxic even at millimolar levels due to feed back inhibition leading to reduced dCTP, for which the concentrations of thymidine is used at 0.016 mM. Sometimes, thymidine inhibition is reversed by the use of deoxy cytidine.

100 × HT

Dissolve 136 mg hypoxanthine and 38.75 mg thymidine in 100 ml of 0.02 M NaOH pre-warmed to 60ºC. Cool, filter sterilize, and store in aliquots at –20ºC.

100 × A

Dissolve 1.9 mg aminopterin in 100 ml of 0.01 M NaOH, filter sterilize and store in aliquots at –20ºC.

HAT medium

Add 1% (v/v) 100 × HT and 100 × A to the cell culture medium.

Readymade HAT and HT media are commercially available.

3.6 Fusion of spleen lymphocytes and myeloma cells

Lymphocytes-produces antibodies, but cannot survive in tissue culture beyond 7–10 days. Myeloma cell line-does not produce antibodies, but can survive in tissue culture indefinitely. Fusion combines these two characteristics into one hybrid cell. In the presence of the fusion agent such as 50% polyethylene glycol (PEG) the cell membranes of the 2 cells are fused, that is the two separate nuclei are enclosed in one cell membrane. After a temporary phase of tetraploidy, the two nuclei will join and the chromosomes will mix together. Following subsequent cell divisions, the fused cells would contain a diploid nucleus. A few of such hybrids would contain the desired combination of antibody production, antigen specificity and immortality in tissue culture that is dependent on the right 'mix' of the chromosomes. The fusion procedure should have high fusion efficiency so that the favouable 'mix' of chromosomes is achieved in more numbers of hybrid cells. The optimum cell ratio for fusion is 2 parts lymphocytes with 1 part of myeloma cells. For example, 4×10^7 lymphocytes mixed with 2×10^7 myeloma cells (2:1 ratio).

Various concentrations (25%–65%) and molecular weights (1500–6000) and preparations of PEG have been used but 50% PEG 1500 is optimal. The exposure of the lymphocyte and myeloma cell mix to PEG and the recovery following exposure to the fusion agent are very critical for good fusion. 50% PEG is added very slowly with very gentle mixing to the lymphocytes and myeloma cells mixture, followed by 1 minute incubation. PEG is concentration would become 25%. Then, the PEG is diluted out slowly to approximately 12% concentration with very gentle mixing and 1 minute incubation. Finally, the PEG is diluted slowly to nearly 0% with very gentle mixing. More than the counts of lymhocytes and myeloma cells the ratio is important. The volume of HAT needed based on the cell counts are given in Table 3.2.

Table 3.2: The ratio of splenocytes and myeloma cells to be used for fusion

Total number of lymphocytes	*Total number of myeloma cells*	*Volume of HAT medium required*
1×10^8	5×10^7	50 ml
9×10^7	4.5×10^7	45 ml
8×10^7	4×10^7	40 ml
7×10^7	3.5×10^7	35 ml
6×10^7	3×10^7	30 ml
5×10^7	2.5×10^7	25 ml
4×10^7	2×10^7	20 ml
3×10^7	1.5×10^7	15 ml

The addition of 200 µl of medium per well would require about 20 ml per 96 well plate. Use control wells for each plate, two wells each containing unfused spleen lymphocytes and myeloma cells with added HAT, so that the time required for their complete death can be checked out every time the plate is being screened. Some protocols also suggest adding normal medium with FCS (not HAT) on the day of fusion and shifting to HAT medium from the next day to reduce the 'insult' (blocking of the *de novo* pathway of DNA synthesis) for the fused cells. The medium has to be replaced every 3–4 days to prevent nutrient depletion, maintain pH (along with CO_2) and remove the waste products. The step wise fusion protocol is given below.

- The total numbers of lymphocytes and myeloma cells available after collection from the immunized mouse and sub culturing the myeloma cells is determined by multiplying the cells/ml × total volume of the cell suspension available in the centrifuge tube. Then decide how many cells of each type (lymhocytes and myeloma cells) has to be used. Then calculate the volumes of each suspension needed that would contain this number of cells.

$$\text{ml of cell suspension needed} = \frac{\text{total number od cells needed}}{\text{number of viable cells / ml}}$$

- Thoroughly resuspend the cells in the two suspensions. Then, using separate, sterile pipettes, mix together in a new, sterile 50 ml centrifuge tube the calculated volume of the spleen cell suspension and the calculated volume of the myeloma cell suspension to obtain a cell mixture with a 2:1ratio of lymphocytes/myeloma cells.
- Use the extra cells available for control wells.
- The HAT will need to be pre warmed to 37°C before use, so the HAT medium can be placed into a 37°C water bath at this stage.
- Add cold, sterile medium to this mixture to bring the total volume in the tube to 20 ml and centrifuge the mixture of cells at 200 × g for 5 minutes.
- Very carefully (without disturbing the cell pellet) as much of the supernatant as possible is removed by gentle tilting of the tube. Then vigorously "flick" the bottom tip of the centrifuge tube against the palm of your hand to break up the flat cell pellet and distribute the cell mixture evenly over the bottom of the tube. Now the cell mixture would flow when the tube is tilted.
- Now add 0.8 ml of sterile, pre-warmed (37°C) 50% PEG prepared in DMEM without FBS very slowly and evenly over a period of one minute while very gently and continuously mixing the cell suspension and PEG.
- Now place the tube in a 37°C water bath for one minute. It is recommended to have a small water bath paled inside the laminar flow hood for this purpose.
- Then add 1 ml pre-warmed (37°C) DMEM (without FBS) very slowly and evenly over a period of one minute with continuous mixing to ensure that the PEG is diluted properly. Place the tube back into the water bath for another minute.

- Then add 10 ml of the pre-warmed (37°C) DMEM (without FBS) very slowly and evenly over a period of two minutes with continuous mixing to ensure that the PEG is diluted properly. Replace the tube cap, and place the tube back into the water bath for one minute.
- Centrifuge the cells at 200 × g for 5 minutes. Then discard the supernatant and add 15–50 ml of pre-warmed (37°C) DMEM + FBS + antibiotics containing HAT supplement (this medium is called HAT medium). The amount of HAT medium to be used will depend on the total number of cells you mixed together before fusion (see the Table 3.2 above). Gently resuspend the cells making sure to break apart cell clumps to ensure a uniform cell suspension. Then add 200 microliters of this suspension to each well of one to four 96 well culture plates depending on the final volume of cells/HAT medium available.
- Gently agitate the suspension in the tube every minute or two, or tightly replace the cap on the tube and then invert the tube a couple of times to re suspend any cells that may have settled to the bottom of the tube. Replace the lids on the culture plates and label them. Small pieces of tapes can be sued to keep the lid in place. Incubate the cells at 37°C in 5% CO_2. It is recommended not to open the incubator doors during the most critical phase after cell fusion.
- After 4–7 days, very carefully aspirate off a portion the medium in each well of the 96 well plates, leaving approximately 100 microliters with out disturbing the cells that are at the bottom of the well. Add 100 microliters of fresh HT medium (not HAT) to each well to bring the volume of medium to near the top of the well. Monitor the control wells. If the myeloma cells have died under the HAT medium then the medium can be replaced with HT medium. Or else, continue couple of more changes in the HAT medium itself. Once hybrids are well established and other un-fused cells have died, then aminopterin is no longer needed. Aminopterin is toxic in high concentrations (used to make HAT medium), hence it should not be used any longer than necessary.
- Hypoxanthine (H) and thymidine (T) are still included in medium because hybrids are accustomed to using these readily available sources of nucleotide precursors. Continue to change the HT medium when necessary in the 96-well plates, observing the wells each time using an inverted microscope to determine when hybrid cells are growing. Depending on the growth of the hybrid, the medium may be changed more often move the cells into a larger volume (*i.e.*, into a 24-well plate) and go for screening assays.

The positive clones have to be cloned to prevent outgrowth by non-antibody secreting fused cells.

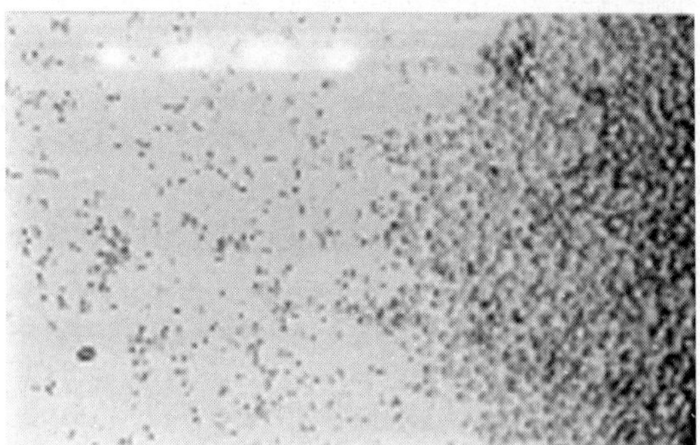

Fig 3.6: A hybrid clone growing in he edge of a 96 well plate

3.7 Cloning by Limiting Dilution

A clone is a cluster of cells resulting from cell division of a single isolated cell and mAbs are antibodies produced by an isolated clone that originated from an isolated hybridoma cell.

After fusion by PEG and culturing in HAT medium, hybridoma cells would produce antibodies of several different specificities that are not separated from each other. It is possible that many clones arising from individual fused myeloma and antibody producing lymphocytes are present in the same well producing antibodies of same or different specificities to the target antigen. It is also possible that clones have arisen from fused myeloma and non-antibody or 'not the desired' antibody producing lymphocyte. To separate the antibody producing clones from one another, the process of cloning the antibody positive hybrids is needed.

Limiting dilution is one method to isolate individual hybridoma cells from each other and culture these isolated hybridoma cells individually to produce isolated clones.

Cloning by limiting dilution is a procedure for separating cells based on the dilution of the hybrid cells surviving in HAT medium, to a concentration that would result in dropping of a single cell per well of the tissue culture plate used, normally a 96-well plate. If this cell remains viable and proliferates an isolated clone of cells would have been established in the well. Now if the supernatant of this well is shown to produce antibodies against the desired antigen, it is likely to be a mAb, antibodies secreted from a single clone of cells. Such antibodies would be against a single epitope.

Since this is done on the basis of numerical probability of landing a single cell per well, it is recommended that the cloning by limiting dilution is repeated thrice so that the chances of a clone of antibody producing cells arising from a single parent antibody producing cell is totally ensured.

The number of times that the cloning by limiting dilution has to be done to achieve monoclonality is based on the number of wells in the first cloning where growth is seen. If growth is seen in about 37% of the wells cloning needs to be done thrice. If fewer wells show growth in the first cloning it can be limited to twice but if more wells show growth it may have to be done more than thrice. A better indicator is the microscopic observation that only a single cluster of cells are seen in one well.

3.7.1 Feeder cells

Cell density is crucial for cell survival in tissue culture. While cloning hybridomas, hybrid cells have to be cultured at a very low density. These low-density seeded hybrid cells need to be grown in the 'vicinity' of other cells called feeder cells, until the hybrids divide enough to create their own density.

The feeder cells:

- Will provide the necessary cell density until hybrids divide
- Will "condition" the medium by providing a cocktail of growth factors
- Will die off after a few days.

Feeder cells commonly used include:

- Lymphocytes from the spleen
- Macrophages from the peritoneal cavity
- T-lymphocytes from the thymus.

Spleen cells are convenient to be used as feeders but the macrophages are probably the best feeders. Cells should be used from the same strain of mice as that used for fusion to avoid histo-incompatibility.

Cells that can be washed from the peritoneal cavity consist of a mixture of resting and activated macrophages, lymphocytes, polymorpho nuclear cells, mast cells and eosinophils. About 2–3 ml of medium is injected at the midline with a 25 G needle, the abdomen massaged gently and the fluid collected using a 22G needle. Activated macrophages are obtained by intra peritoneal injection of 1 ml of 10% sodium thioglycollate 4 days prior to collection. Such activated macrophages are useful for elimination of mycoplasma from infected hybridomas. The thymus is a bilobed grayish soft tissue which is ventral and anterior to the heart at the top of the thoracic cavity.

Normally 2×10^6 viable feeder cells/ml are needed. To obtain this cell number from the available lymphocyte cell suspension, the calculation is as follows.

$$\frac{2\times106\,\text{cells / ml}}{(\text{undiluted lymphocyte cell suspension})} = \frac{1}{X}$$

Mix 1 volume of undiluted lymphocyte cell suspension with (X-1) volumes of diluent to obtain a suspension of cells that contains 2×10^6 viable lymphocytes/ml.

Then add 0.1 ml of this suspension to each well of a 96-well plate and incubate at 37°C 5% CO_2 incubator.

It is best to prepare the feeder layer 24 hours prior to seeding the wells with the isolated hybridoma cells. A variety of enriched media containing defined amounts of growth promoting properties of the feeder cells are commercially available and can be used if cell culture contamination issues are a problem in the sustenance of the hybridomas.

3.8 Hybridoma cells

Step-wise dilutions are made to avoid or lessen errors. Ultimately the cell concentration needed is 1×10^1 cells/ml *i.e.* 10 cells per ml that is 1 cell in 0.1 ml that is added per well. Suppose the original cell concentration, for instance was 5.3×10^6 cells/ml. By adding 0.1ml of hybridoma cell suspension with 9.9 ml diluent (100 fold dilution), the cell concentration would become 5.3×10^4 (first step dilution). By further diluting 0.1ml of the first step dilution with 9.9 ml diluent (again 100 fold dilution), the cell concentration would become 5.3×10^2 (second step dilution).

Now to obtain a concentration of 1×10^2 cells/ml, 1 ml of the second step dilution, has to be diluted 5.3 folds, *i.e.* 1 ml of this dilution with 4.3 ml of diluent. For a final concentration of 1×10^1 cells/ml, 0.1 ml of the second-step dilution, has to be diluted 53 folds, *i.e.* 0.1 ml of this dilution with 5.2 ml of diluent. These two concentrations, 10 cells per well (0.1 ml) and 1 cell per well (0.1 ml) can be added to one half of a 96 well plate.

Thus, some wells would receive 10 cells/well, some would get any number between 1–10 cells/well, some would have 1 cell/well, and some may receive no cells at all. However, if the procedure of counting and dilution is done *carefully*, several wells will actually be seeded with a single cell. During the process of dilution and seeding, the cells should be agitated gently to keep the diluted hybridoma cells uniformly suspended in the medium.

Always ensure that the final volume of these diluted cells is more than 5 ml to add to 48 wells of a 96 well plate. Exact volumes of 4.8 ml would not be enough for the calculated numbers of wells due to pipette and pipetting errors and some frothing due to presence of at least 15–20% of FCS.

The suspension of hybridoma cells is prepared in HT medium. The dilutions prepared with higher concentration of hybridoma cells may also be seeded in tissue culture flasks or 48-well plates for back up. Incubate the plate at 37 °C in 5% CO_2 for 4–7 days without changing the medium.

Observe for growth of isolated clones of hybridoma cells (an isolated true clone of hybridoma cells that resulted from cell division of one isolated cell will usually have a very uniform, almost circular, border).The supernatants from all wells that contain one hybridoma clone/well can be assayed for production of the desired antibody specificity by the screening assay used. Positive clones can then be transferred into larger volumes of medium (24 well plates, 25 cm^2 flasks, etc.).

Often, a second cloning by limiting dilution of what appears to be an isolated clone is performed to totally ensure that it is a clone from a single parent. Cloning by multiple rounds of limiting dilution is an extremely labor-intensive and time-consuming technique to single-cell clone a hybridoma clone. Thus it is very difficult to isolate a large number of hybridoma clones from each cell fusion, since such cloning needs to be done for each and every positive antibody-secreting well.

For example if 10 such positive clones are chosen, each clone needs to be diluted in to one 96 well plate, that is, 10 plates that needs to be prepared with feeder cells, screened visually for the occurrence of clones and screened for antibody production. Each of these clones also needs back up in larger volume plates or flasks to ensure against loss of such antibody-positive clones during the process of cloning.

Some hybridoma clones overgrow others prior to cloning. Often, these faster growing cell lines do not synthesize antibodies, resulting in a failure to obtain the best antibody-producing hybridoma clones.

Hence alternate methods for cloning are available:

- Cloning in soft agar
- Flow cytometry.

The cells are diluted and spread over a dish containing low concentration of agar and left for 7–14 days. When cells are visible, they are collected using a sterile pipette under a microscope and transferred into a 96 well plate. After sufficient growth, the supernatant can be assayed for production of the desired antibody.

Some of the advantages of cloning in soft agar include

- Slower growing and faster growing clones are physically separated thus eliminating the risk of overgrowth
- Selection of duplicate clones producing the same antibody is unlikely and thus the amount of screening required is reduced
- Fewer manipulations are necessary there is no need for medium exchanges, HAT feeding
- Lower risk of contamination.

Agar, agarose, and methylcellulose have been used as semi-solid media for the growth of monoclonal antibody-producing hybridomas. Methylcellulose has been shown to be superior to other semi-solid media because it is inert and has greater optical clarity.

The fluorescence activated cell sorter (FACS) can be used for separating specific antibody producing hybridomas from the mixture of cells after fusion. It uses the antigen coupled to a fluorescence dye and is allowed to react with the fused cells. The reacting fused cell can be 'sorted' that is, directed into a separate tube or well wherein it can be cultured and then screened for antibodies of desired specificity and also of the desired isotypes.

3.8.1 Flow cytometry-a technology to count and sort cells

Flow cytometry literally means measurement of certain characteristics of particles including cells when they are in liquid stream (flow-in liquid stream, cyto-cells/and metry–measurement). Instruments built to utilize this technology can gather information on the physical, biochemical and antigenic traits of cells by measuring visible and fluorescent light emissions and also permit separation of cells based on the above characters (cell sorting).

The two major advantages of a flow cytometer is multi parametric measurement and the speed. By multi parametric measurement we mean that several parameters can be measured from the same cell at the same time. For example if a lymphocyte fraction of the blood is labeled with CD3, CD4 and CD8 mAbs at the same time, each mAb being coupled to a different fluorescent dyes, such that all these dyes get excited at more or less the same wavelength but emit at different wavelengths then it is possible to analyze the number of lymphocytes bearing CD3, CD4 and CD8 on its surface. In addition it can also analyze the number of CD3 cells bearing CD4 or CD8 and number of CD4 cells bearing CD8 and number of cells bearing neither CD4 nor CD8.

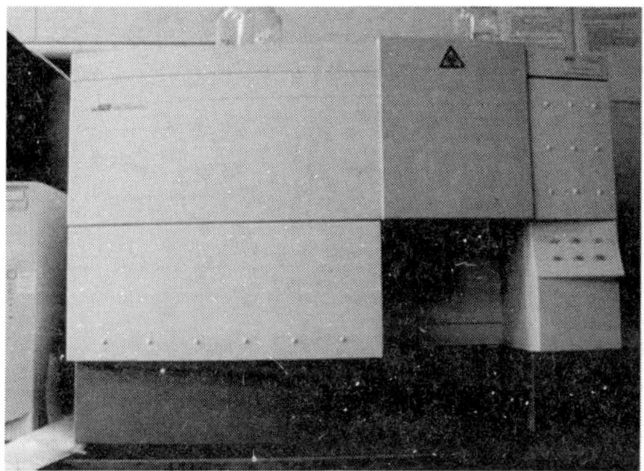

Fig. 3.7: A flow cytometer. Front of desktop flow cytometer-the Becton-Dickinson FACSCalibur. *Source*: http://en.wikipedia.org/wiki/Flow_cytometry

What are these cells that do not bear either CD4 or CD8?

They must predominantly be B –cells. The instrument can count about half to one million cells every minute that is humanly impossible. The advantages of counting such large numbers are the degree of accuracy of the data is largely enhanced.

3.8.2 Functions of a flow cytometer

- Enumerate particles in suspension
- Separate "live" from "dead" particles
- Evaluate 10^5 to 5×10^6 particles/min
- Measure particle-scatter as well as fluorescence
- Sort single particles for subsequent analysis.

3.8.3 Components of a flow cytometer

A flow cytometer, sometimes called a fluorescence activated cell sorter (FACS), has the following key components:

1. An ***excitation source***, typically a laser (acronym for Light Amplification by Stimulated Emission of Radiation) that emits light at a particular wavelength.

2. A ***liquid flow system*** that moves the suspended cells thought the instrument and past the laser.
3. A ***detector*** (photodiode or photomultiplier tube), which is able to measure the flashes of light emitted as cells flow past the laser beam and convert them into digital signals.

In a flow cytometer, when single cells flow past the excitation laser light source and the light after hitting the cells is either scattered or absorbed and then re-emitted (fluorescence) if the cells are labeled with a fluorescent dye. The extent of scatter depends on physical characteristics such as size, internal complexity, shape and surface topography. The relative size is measured on the basis of the forward scatter (FSC) and the internal complexity on the basis of side scatter (SSC).

If blood cells are analyzed in a flow cytometer, which cells would have the maximum FSC and which cells the maximum SSC? In other words which are the largest cells and which are the granular cells? The neutrophils are large and granular cells while monocytes are large but less granular and lymphocytes are small and very less complex. So based on these preliminary characteristics the cells could be grouped.

However the major application of flow cytometer is based on fluorescence which depends on the absorption of light by the cell and the subsequent re-emission of this light at a different frequency. Flow cytometers uses barrier filters to block the original light source from reaching the detector, while the fluorescence emission is allowed through for detection. Detection of the second wavelength is used as a measure of the presence of the dye on the cell and thus the component it is labeling.

Various fluorescent dyes are commercially available, their emitted colors beaing similar to reds and green colours seen in fireworks. The most common fluorescent dyes are Texas-Red, fluorescein isothiocyanate (FITC) and phycoerythrin (PE). The Table 3.3 shows some of the different fluorochromes, their excitation and emission wavelengths, and their emission color.

Table 3.3: Different Fluochromes used in Flow3 Cytometry

Flurochrome	*Excitation wavelength (nm)*	*Wavelength emission (nm)*
Texas Red	488	615
Phycoerythrin (PE)	488	575
Fluorescein isothyocanae (FITC)	490	514
Tetra methyl rhodamine	540	570

Table 3.3: (*Contd...*)

Table 3.3: (*Contd...*)

Flurochrome	*Excitation wavelength (nm)*	*Wavelength emission (nm)*
Phycocyanin	620	650
Allophycocyanin	650	660
Hoechst 333341 or 33258	343	482
DAPI	345	455
Ethidium bromide	482	616
Propidium iodide	493	630
Acridine orange-DNA	480	510
Acridine orange-RNA	509	533
di-O-C_n(3)-oxycarbocyanines	485	505
Carbody fluorescein-high pH	495	520 (bright)
Carbody fluorescein-low pH	450	520 (weak)

3.8.4 Gating

A subset of data can be defined through a gate. A gate is a numerical or graphical boundary used to define the characteristics of cells to include for further analysis. For example, analysis of lymphocytes only, in a blood sample containing a mixed population of cells, a gate can be set on the FSC vs SSC plot to allow analysis of only the cells of the size of lymphocytes.

3.8.5 Display and interpretation of flow cytometry data

What happens when a single cells passes through the sample injection port and is incident with the laser beam of light is called an EVENT. The amount of light a cell scatters or fluoresces is measured by the detectors and subsequently displayed as a dot. If the X- and Y-axes measure the different emissions, display of a dot is done showing the particular emission for both the dyes for each of the cell analyzed. Then using isotype matched controls quadrants are generated so that each cell (dot) can be placed in the particular quandrant. For example, if X axis is showing green emission and if say green emitting fluorescent dye (FITC) was coupled to CD4 mAbs and if Y axis is showing a red emission and if that dye (Texas Red) was coupled to CD8 mAbs then a cell fluorescing for both red and green light is placed in the upper right quadrant while cells not showing either green or red emission is placed in the lower left quadrant and so on. This can immediately enable to calculate the percentage of cells showing that particular marker with respect to the other. The percentage of cells in the lower right quadrant would be CD4 bearing cells and cells in upper left quadrant CD8 bearing cells.

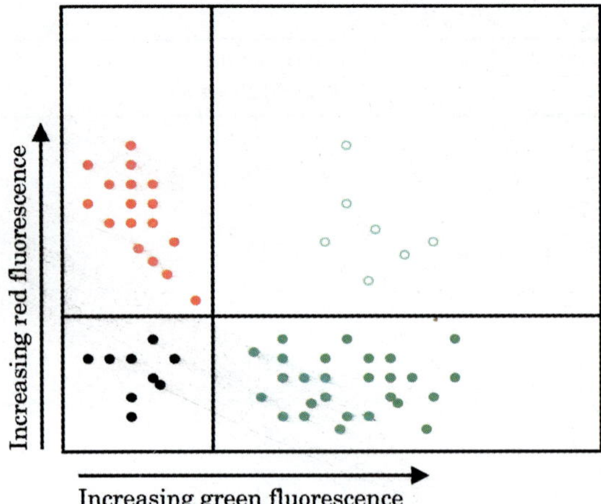

Fig. 3.8: A dot plot of double staining of membrane antigens in a flow cytometer.

Histograms are also used to display data from flow cytometry experiments wherein the X-axis shows the intensity of the detected signal and the Y-axis measures the number of events (cells) counted.

Horizontal axis: Parameter's signal value in channel numbers
Vertical axis: Number of events per channel number

Each event is placed in the channel corresponding to its signal value. Signals with identical intensities accumulate in the same channel. Brighter signals displayed in channels to the right of dimmer signals. An isotype control is used to determine where the markers will be placed. M1 is placed around the (–) peak of the isotype control. M2 is placed to the right of M1 to designate (+) events.

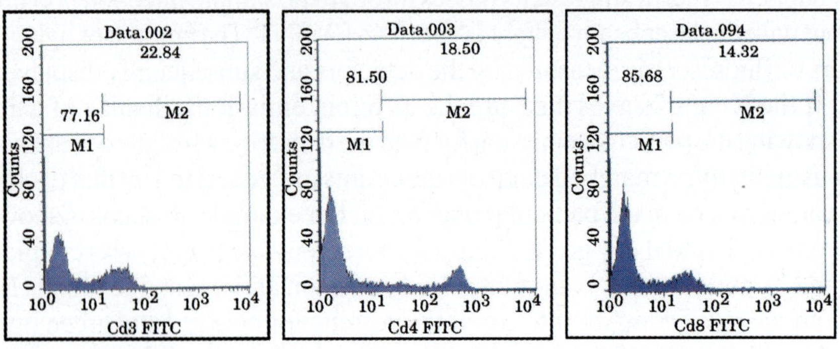

Fig. 3.9: Histogram of single fluorescence in a flow cytometer against membrane antigen

3.8.6 Applications of flow cytometry

Flow cytometry is used for a variety of different applications in fields such as immunology, pathology and medicine. A few of the most common applications are listed below:

3.8.6.1 *DNA content*

Fluorescence staining of DNA followed by flow analysis has been used to determine a cell's DNA content. Stained cells with one copy of their genetic material (a haploid cell) will be half as bright as cells with two copies (a diploid cell). A cell varies between these states during the cell cycle and flow cytometry can be used to determine its position in the cell cycle based on its DNA content.

3.8.6.2 *Evaluation of cell-surface markers*

Immunologists frequently use flow cytometry to determine the types of markers and receptors on the surface of a cell. For these experiments, a fluorescent dye is attached to antibodies or receptor ligands. These cells can then be subjected to flow cytometry and the amount of the receptor of their surface detected as a level of fluorescence.

These experiments can be designed to incorporate more than one fluorescent marker at a time, giving the ability to detect multiple cell-surface markers simultaneously. Building upon the example of staining for particular markers or receptors, staining with more than one fluorescence dye allows researchers to determine whether there are populations of cells that contain multiple receptors.

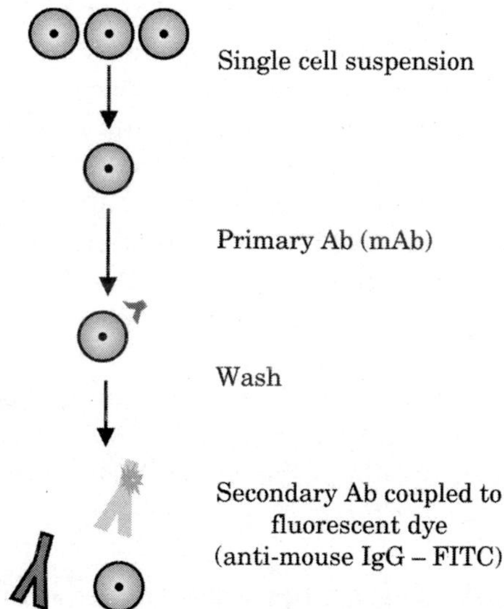

Fig. 3.10: Fluorescent antibody staining of single cell suspension for analysis in a flow cytometer.

Apoptosis is another burgeoning area in which flow cytometers have extensive application.

3.8.7 Cell sorting

Flow cytometry can be used to select and purify a specific subset of cells with a population. This is a popular application with researchers, since you can selects cells expressing a particular receptor, in a phase of the cell cycle, or perhaps expressing a particular transgenic protein, followed by culturing of these cells as a pure population. Amazingly, a FACS can sort cells as fast as 15000 cells/sec to a very high purity (over 98%).

3.8.8 Why use flow cytometry?

As a technology, flow cytometry provides a way to measure the biochemical properties of thousands of individual cells in a liquid suspension. The speed at which a flow cytometer can do this is un-paralleled, counting thousands of cells a second, while still looking at each cell individually. This ability, combined with its flexibility to observe many different cellular characteristics, has made it a core technology of the cell biologist.

3.8.9 Application in cloning of hybridoma cells

Individual hybridoma cells can be distributed into microtiter wells in an automated manner based on their forward angle light scatter properties and their reaction to fluorescein-conjugated anti-mouse-IgG. Then the frequency of immunoglobulin-secreting cells can be determined by automated laser nephelometry. Inclusion of propidium iodide in the hybridoma cell sorting mixtures led to improved cloning efficiency by facilitating enhanced discrimination and elimination of nonviable cells. Flow cytometric-assisted single cell deposition thereby provides a tool for selection of enhanced immunoglobulin producing cultures.

Several new methods for selecting and screening cells using flow cytometry and cell sorting have recently been developed; these include gel microdrop technology, which encapsulates the cells in gelatine beads, and matrix-based secretion assays.

In this method, the cells are first encapsulated in an unique derivatised gel matrix followed by the addition of streptavidin to create a bridge to which a biotinylated "capture" antibody would be subsequently be bound. The gel microdrop with the cells and bound capture antibody are incubated for secretion and capture of the target protein. A fluorescent-labeled "detection" antibody is incubated with the gel microdrops, and the samples are analyzed in a flow cytometer and sorted. The fluorescence intensity of each gel microdrop is quantified and high producers are isolated and recovered based on secretion of the specific target protein.

Using this method, mAbs/antibody producer cells can be identified shortly after transfection or fusion. This method reduces the time required for manual limiting dilution cloning, improving yields and productivity while reducing product development time and costs. Some modifications of the hybridoma technique include fusion and cloning together in a single step. It is possible that after fusion of the myeloma and splenic lymphocytes, the fused cells are directly diluted in large volume of medium and suspended into say twenty numbers of 96 well plates thereby achieving cloning cells also simultaneously.

This method eliminates the possibility of overgrowth of potentially valuable slow-growing clones by fast-growing clones, which normally are 'non-producers'.

The antibody producing clones have the added function of production and secretion of antibodies hence they tend to grow little slowly. However this is not a universal rule.

One such method, an Omni-Hybridoma Platform is designed to select and clone hybridoma cell clones immediately after fusion. HAT selection and cloning of hybridomas are performed simultaneously in a single step. In this platform, newly fused hybridoma cells are sub cloned, grown and selected using an agarose-based semi-solid medium containing growth factors, B-cell stimulators and medium supplements optimized for the growth of single hybridoma cells.

Another example is ClonaCell-HY method where a methylcellulose-based semi-solid selective medium is used to combine the hybridoma selection with HAT and cloning in one step. Selection and cloning is done simultaneously. There is also a reduction in time required to 16–20 days as against 39–42 days in conventional fusion and cloning by limiting dilution.

3.9 Taggert Hybridoma Technology

An alternative to the HAT selection is another method developed by Taggert and Samloff which uses the mouse myeloma cell line FOX-NY that is deficient in both HGPRT and APRT enzymes. Thus FOX-NY is resistant to both 8 azaguanine and 2,6, diamino purine, toxic analogues of hypoxanthine and adenine respectively. APRT enzyme locus is on chromosome 8 and selection medium used is AAT instead of HAT.

The spleen used is from the 5BNR mouse which has the heavy chain immunoglobulin gene on chromosome 12 translocated onto chromosome 8 by Robertsonian fusion.

When the above spleen cells and myeloma cells are placed in AAT medium one is actually selecting for the presence of chromosome 8 containing the ARPT gene but also selecting at the same time retention of the immunoglobulin gene on the chromosome 12 translocated on the chromosome 8. Thus there would be a decreased probability of any non-secretor hybridomas formed. Since the immunoglobulin and APRT loci were linked in this system hybridomas that survived AAT selection also would have immunoglobulin secretion.

3.10 Naming the Hybridoma Clones

Proper labeling of the hybrid clones is needed since several populations of cells are generated through positive clones after fusion, cloning and sub cloning.

The designation should include the number of the primary well and the number of the clone.

- The first number would designate the plate number of a fusion say 2nd plate
- The next number denotes the well number say B2
- The next number could denote the clone number from the cloning of the above clone say clone 5
- The next number could denote the sub clone number from the cloning of the above clone say a
- Thus it would read as 2B2.5a
- Alphabets can also be avoided by using consecutive numbers from 1–96 wells of plate 1 followed by 97 to 192 wells etc
- The mAbs are also designated based on its specificity also.

Whatever the method adopted by individual labs it should be simple and avoid confusion since a mAb production laboratory would be handling several thousands clones against a variety of antigens.

3.11 Immunoassays for Screening of mAbs

The basis of antigen- antibody reaction is their specificity. The amino acids in the epitope of the antigen and CDR of the antibody should be able to form protein-protein interactions through their side chains.

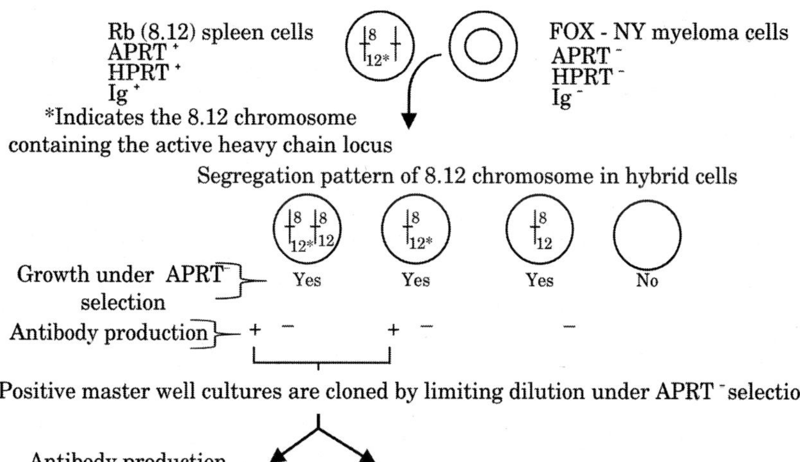

Fig. 3.11: Taggert hybridoma technology

This is equivalent to specific base pairing by hydrogen bonds between the two strands of the DNA molecule. This phenomenon is used in hybridization assays between nucleic acids. The formation of double stranded nucleic acid molecules indicates that their bases are complementary.

The general procedure used in all immunoassays is:

- To allow antibody-antigen complex formation,
- Detection of the antibody-antigen complex.

Antigen antibody complexes are formed by incubating the antibody with an extract containing the antigen. Alternatively, the antigen is absorbed or fixed to a solid support and then antibody binds to the immobilized antigen. The detection of the complex will depend on the assay being performed. One method is to directly label the antibody (or antigen) with a detectable marker (*e.g.,* radioactivity, fluorescence, or enzyme). Alternatively, a labeled secondary antibody (prepared in another species) that recognizes the primary antibody can be used to detect the complex.

Similarly, either protein A or protein G labeled with a marker could be used to detect the antigen-antibody complex. Protein A and protein G are proteins isolated from *Staphylococcus areus* or *Streptococcus*, respectively, that bind to the Fc-region of IgG. Protein G recognizes more immunoglobulin subclasses, as well as a wider range of species, than protein A.

Similarly, due to the highly specific nature of the antigen antibody interactions, if one component is known, the other can be determined as to whether it is specific to the known. If a purified virus is used as an antigen and if a serum sample is added and it has been shown that an antigen (virus) and antibody (from serum) interaction has occurred, this means that antibodies to the virus were present in the serum sample that was used for testing.

However there could be cross reactions occurring between some extra component in the virus preparation and equivalent antibodies that are fortuitously present in the serum (undesirable to us but the interaction is specific). This can be avoided by further purification of the virus and ensuring only the components of the virus is present and no other proteins are present in the antigen preparation that has been used for coating.

A common example is when a prokaryotically expressed protein is used as an antigen. It is likely that some components of the host bacteria, *E. coli*, could be contaminated in the protein prep and it is likely that antibodies to *E. coli* can be present in the serum sample that is used for testing. If we are not aware, this antigen (from *E. coli*) and antibody (present in the serum sample) interaction would be construed as the one between the virus and antibody and given as a positive test.

Another possible cross reaction could occur, when there is epitope sharing between the antigen in question and some other related cross reacting antigen that exists in nature. For example, PPRV and rinderpest virus are closely related and belong to the same family of Paramyxo virus and genus Morbilli virus. They share several epitopes and antibodies to PPRV could cross-react with rinderpest virus. This is not our making and can only be avoided only by using specific epitopes that are not shared among these two viruses.

In the context of application of immunoassays for mAb screening the following considerations are important.

- Screening method should be applicable for analysis of several samples easily and rapidly
- Should be as close to the final application of the mAbs
- The nature of the antigen used for screening should also be as close as in the final use
- The ability to exclude possible cross-reactions
- The sensitivity and specificity of the assays.

Generally the number of plates used for initial fusion with spleen cells from one mouse would be 4 × 96 well plates. So, typically 400 samples need to be screened for the presence of antibodies. Even if the wells are first screened and supernatants only from wells with growing hybridomas are used for screening there should be at least 300 wells, if fusion efficiencies of 80% are obtained.

Then after sub cloning, several thousands of wells need to be screened. So the assay used for screening should facilitate this. It should also be ensured that there is enough antigen available before your fusion. It is also required that the same batch of antigen is used if variability is likely between batches.

The timing of screening is also critical and there should be a via media between the times required for the production of enough amounts of antibodies in the well that falls above the threshold of sensitivity of the assay system while at the same time ensuring that there is no overgrowth by the non-secretors.

Two tier screening may also be practiced. Early screening to detect the high producing and high affinity clones and a later screening to detect low affinity and lower yielding clones.

If the screening assay is far removed from that of the final application of the mAbs, positive samples detected by the first screening assay may be tested in the final application assay. For example, if the mAbs are to be used for neutralization assays, the ELISA positive clones may be screened using virus neutralization tests, since the numbers of clones are much higher than the ELISA positive ones.

The pH optimum of the assay is also critical, since when the clones are rapidly growing the pH would become lower. If these supernatants are directly transferred from the hybridoma plates to the screening plates, the pH may interfere with the antigen-antibody interactions in the test.

The common assays used for primary screening are the solid phase assays, liquid phase assays are less common and biological assays are the least commonly used.

The most common solid phase assay is the ELISA. There has been a logarithmic explosion of assays using ELISA since it was first described by Engvall and Pearlman in 1971. Several modifications of the ELISA are used.

The simplest ELISA uses the antigen is bound to the ELISA plate and incubated with the mAb to be tested. Then a second antibody coupled to an enzyme is used to detect the first reaction.

The point for understanding is that the first reaction that occurs in the above ELISA reaction is between the epitope on the antigen and the CDR of the mAbs. The Fc portion of the mAbs is free.

The second reporter reaction that occurs is between the Fc portion of the mAb and the CDR of the anti-species antibody that is coupled to the enzyme, which is a reaction between two immunoglobulins. How this happens is because the immunoglobulins from one species acts as an antigen (foreign protein) in another species and antibodies are produced in the second species against epitopes that are present on the first immunoglobulin molecule (isotypic, allotypic and idiotypic determinants).

Then substrates and chromogen are added and colour formation is detected spectrophotometrically. The intensity of the colour is directly proportional to the amount of the first antibody bound which determines the amount of the second antibody and in turn the amount of enzyme immobilized with the second antibody.

The solid phase support most commonly used is polystyrene or polyvinyl or membranes such as nitro cellulose or nylon.

The plates are generally coated with some proprietary material which encourages the binding of antigen.

The parameters useful to evaluate the ELISA plates are:

- Signal to noise ratio rather than the strength of the signal alone
- Coefficient of variation (CV) of protein binding should be less than 5%
- High protein binding capacity such as 400 ng/cm^2 (1 cm^2 = 100 μ volume).

Some plates could give high OD values with serum from immunized animals (signal) but also may give a high back ground with negative serum (noise).

The binding of the antigen to the ELISA plate is mostly non-covalent and is mediated by hydrophobic interactions. The amount of binding depends on:

- Diffusion coefficient of the protein
- Surface area to volume ratio
- Time and temperature of adsorption.

When a soluble protein is used then a 100 μl volume of a 1–10 μg/ml solution of protein can be tried initially.

Generally a small percentage of the protein added only is bound to the plate and in some rare cases it is also possible to reuse the antigen solution used for binding to the ELISA plate. The supernatant after incubation can be collected and used to coat another plate after again estimating the antigen concentration.

Cells have also been used for screening by fixing them to the plates. This is performed using 10–50 ug of poly lysine for pre-coating the plate for one hour at room temperature. Then the cells are added at a concentration of 5×10^3 to 5×10^4/ml for 45–60 minutes. The cells may then be fixed with 0.1 to 0.25% glutaraldehyde for 3–5 minutes and then washed thoroughly.

This method of cell-ELISA is particularly useful when the antigen can not be purified to homogeneity, especially in case of viruses. If the virus is not completely pure and is used as an immunizing antigen and the same antigen is also used for screening, it is possible that the clones appear positive due to antigen-antibody reactions occurring between the cellular contaminant proteins present in the antigen preparation and its equivalent antibodies likely to be induced in the mice. This could be avoided by screening the clones with both infected and uninfected cells and choosing the clones that react with the infected cells and not with the uninfected cells. If the clones were secreting mAbs against contaminating cellular proteins, it would be positive to both infected and uninfected cells.

Chemically activated plates are commercially available such as maleimide activated plates than can couple the peptides covalently to the plate surface. In addition the plates may first be bound to molecules such as protein A or G to orient the antibodies by exposing their F_{ab} regions by binding to their F_c regions. Secondary antibodies can also be used with the same purpose. Plates are also available with streptavidin coating to permit binding to biotinylated proteins.

The conventional coating buffer is the carbonate-bicarbonate buffer pH 9.6. At this high pH the antigen tends to be more negatively charged and would bind better to the plates which tend to have a positive charge. When immunoglobulins are sued for coating PBS at neutral pH can also be used. Again conventionally coating is done at 40°C overnight. It can also be done at 37°C for 1–3 hrs with continuous gentle shaking.

All the solid supports used in ELISA are capable of binding to the proteins and if the antigen binding has not completely saturated the well surface then it is possible that the immunoglobulins and other proteins present in the serum can directly bind to the plate surface (irrespective of the antigen). In this case the secondary anti-species antibody would also bind to the immunoglobulins and produce a colour which has no relation to antigen mediated binding of antibody (background). Therefore once the antigen is bound it is imperative to block the unbound sites on the support with blockers that include any one or a combination of the following.

- Bovine serum albumin 1–4%
- Gelatin 0.2 to 0.5%
- Non-specific serum 1%
- Bovine gamma globulin 1%
- Skimmed milk powder 5%
- Casein hydrolysate 1–3%

The use of detergents such as 0.01% Tween 20 or Triton X–100 also reduces the background. If glutaraldehyde has been used wash buffers containing 100 mM glycine should be added to block reactive glutaraldehyde sites.

Sodium azide should not be used or must be washed off when peroxidase labeled secondary antibodies is used as azide inhibits peroxidase.

If alkaline phosphatase conjugates are used, the blocking buffer used should be Tris buffered saline (TBS) and not phosphate buffered saline (PBS) since it interferes with alkaline phosphatase.

The blocking buffer should also not in any way alter or obscure the antigen bound to the plate. The ideal blocking buffer must be determined empirically using the signal to noise ratio which is the signal obtained with a sample containing the target analyte as compared to the sample that does not contain the target analyte.

While inadequate blocker would cause a high background (noise) too much blocker may mask the antigen antibody interaction or inhibit the enzyme.

Washing steps in ELISA are required to remove the unbound reactants. Inadequate washing would cause high background while excessive washing may cause elution of the antigen or antibody and result in decreased sensitivity. The wash buffer commonly used is physiological buffers such as TBS or PBS with detergent such as 0.05% Tween 20 to remove the non-specifically bound material.

To determine the optimal dilutions of the reagents used in the ELISA a checker board titration has to be performed. It is also called two dimensional serial dilutions. In a single experiment the concentrations of two components are varied in each direction.

For example the concentrations of the primary antibody are varied across the plate while the enzyme labeled secondary antibody is serially diluted down the plate. This permits analysis of different concentration of two reagents in each well to obtain the best signal noise ratio.

The choice of secondary antibody depends on the animal where the primary antibody was developed. For example if your primary antibody is raised in a mouse, you will need an anti-mouse secondary antibody. If it was raised in a rabbit, you will need an anti-rabbit secondary antibody.

The choice of the conjugate is also critical. Of course anti-mouse enzyme conjugate has to be used. But it may be available as anti-mouse IgG whole molecule peroxidase conjugate affinity purified prepared in various species such as goat, rabbit and so on, anti-mouse IgG Fc part etc.

For example, anti-mouse IgG 0(whole molecule) peroxidase conjugate developed in goat means that purified mouse IgG was used as an immunogen and inoculated into goats. After production of antibodies in goats (to mouse IgG) the goat serum was used in an affinity column coupled with mouse IgG and only antigen-specific antibodies were isolated. Thereby all the goat serum proteins including immunoglobulins, that do not specifically bind to mouse IgG are removed. Identity and purity of this antibody is established by immunoelectrophoresis prior to conjugation. Electrophoresis of the antibody preparation followed by diffusion against anti-goat IgG and anti-goat whole serum should result in single arcs of precipitation. Then this affinity purified antibody is coupled to HRPO enzyme. The conjugate titre is determined by direct ELISA. Titer is defined as the dilution of conjugate sufficient to give a change in absorbance of 1.0 at the appropriate wavelength after 30 minutes of substrate conversion at 25°C. Microtiter plates are coated with purified mouse IgG and used to determine the titre. However in case of screening assay, the amount of mouse IgG available (mAb) depends up on the amount bound to the antigen and hence this titre does not reflect the actual working dilution that has to be determined through checker board titrations.

Anti-mouse IgG (gamma chain-specific) peroxidase conjugate is also developed similarly except that during affinity purification, antibodies which bind specifically only to the gamma-chain of mouse IgG is separated and used.

The various specificities of secondary antibodies include:

- Polyvalent antibodies–reacts with all classes of immunoglobulins
- Fc and heavy-chain specific–reacts with heavy chains only (*i.e.* gamma chain specific reacts only with IgG; μ chain specific reacts only with IgM, etc.)
- Fab and whole molecule specific–reacts with heavy and light chains. Due to the light chain reactivity, they can react with all classes.

- Light chain (kappa, lambda) specific–reacts with all classes, since all classes contain either kappa or lambda light chains only.

Generally affinity isolated antibodies are preferred due to its limited cross reactions. However when the secondary antibodies are of high affinity to the immunogen, they bind too strongly to the immunogen in the affinity column and may not be eluted. Hence there is a possibility of losing the high affinity antibodies which would be preserved if the IgG fraction of the serum is used.

If working with human tissues, cells or proteins, a secondary antibody adsorbed with human serum or human IgG is preferred since these products will reduce non-specific background. When using cells that Fc receptors (thymus, spleen, blood, leukocytes, B cells etc.), choose an $F(ab')_2$ fragment to eliminate non-specific binding through Fc receptors present on cells. Alternatively, Fc receptors can be blocked by using purified IgG from the host species where the secondary antibody has been produced.

Several substrates (Table 3.4) are available which differs in terms of their sensitivity and the requirement of instrumentation

- Colorimetric
- Chemiluminiscent
- Chemifluorescent.

Chemiluminiscent and chemifluorescent substrates are more sensitive and produce a stronger signal than colorimetric substrates. ELISA conditions need re-optimization when changing the substrates using higher dilutions of the reagents.

Table 3.4: Different Types of Substrates used in Immunoassays

Feature	*Colorimetric substrate*	*Chemi luminiscent substrate*	*Chemi fluorescent substrate*
Sensitivity	Low	High	High
Substrates	Many	Few	Few
Signal generation	Slow	Rapid	Rapid
Linear range	Small	Large	Large
Equipment	Spectrophotometer	Fluorometer	Luminometer

Horse radish peroxidase (HRPO) is a 40kDa protein that catalyses the oxidation of substrates by hydrogen peroxide. HRPO functions optimally at neutral pH and can be inhibited by cyanides, sulfides and azides. The specific activities of both the enzyme and antibodies are higher than alkaline phosphatase conjugates. The characterisation of substrates for HRPO enzyme are given in Table 3.5.

Table 3.5: Characteristics of substrates used in enzyme immunoassays

Enzyme	*Substrate*	*Colour*	*Sensitivity*
HRPO	3, 3', 5, 5'-tetra methyl benzidine (TMB)	450 nm–stopped–Yellow 652 nm–non stop Blue	2–8 pg/well well
HRPO	2,2'-azinobis (3-ethylbenzothi-azoline–6 sulphonic acid (ABTS)	410 nm/650 nm Green	0.25 ng/well
HRPO	o-phenylenediamine dihydro-chlorine (OPD)	490 nm–stopped–Green 450 nm-nonstop–Yellow/Orange	7 pg/well
AP	Para nitro phenyl phosphate (PNPP)	405 nm–Yellow	10 ng/well
Beta-gala-ctosidase	o-nitrophenyl-beta-D-galactopyramoside (OPNG)	420 nm–Yellow	10 ng/well

There are several types of ELISA systems (Table 3.6) in use, each with a distinct advantage over others. The main principle is same but variations exist in the order of reagent addition and complex formation. The main types include:

- Indirect ELISA
- Antigen-capture or sandwich ELISA
- Competitive ELISA or blocking ELISA
- Class capture ELISA.

Table 3.6: Characteristics of different types of ELISAs

Reactants	*Indirect ELISA*	*Antigen capture ELISA*	*Competitive ELISA*	*Class capture ELISA*
Coating	Antigen	Antibody specific to antigen being detected (capture antibody)	Antigen	Antibody against a particular class (isotype) of antibodies detected
Wash	+	+	+	+
Block	+	+	+	+
Wash	+	+	+	+
Reagent added	Serum or mAb being tested	Sample likely to contain antigen to be tested	Serum sample likely to contain antibody against coated antigen + known mAb against antigen	Serum sample being tested
Wash	+	+	+	+
Reagent added	Anti-species antibody conjugated to	Another antibody directed against antigen being	Anti-species (mouse) antibody conjugated to	Known antigen against which

Table 3.6 (*Contd...*)

Table 3.6 (*Contd...*)

Reactants	***Indirect ELISA***	***Antigen capture ELISA***	***Competitive ELISA***	***Class capture ELISA***
	enzyme	detedted (detector antibody)	enzyme (not against the species from which the sample serum is being tested but agaisnt the species from which the known antibody is being used, if mAbs are used anti-mouse enzyme conjugate)	the antibody and its class are being tested
Wash	+	+	+	+
Reagent	–	Anti-species antibody (against the detector antibody) conjugated to enzyme	–	Known antibody against the antigen conjugated to the enzyme
Wash	–	+	–	+
Substrate	+ (substrate specific for the enzyme)	+ (substrate specific for the enzyme)	+ (substrate specific for the enzyme)	+ (substrate specific for the enzyme)
Colour development and positivity	Colour development indicates positivity	Colour development indicates positivity	Colour development indicates negativity that is lack of antibodies in the serum sample being tested	Colour development indicates positivity
Major application	Using known antigen, presence and quantity of antibody/mAbs	Using known capture and detector antibody, the presence of antigen	Using known antigen and mAb against a specific epitope, presence of antibody aginst the specific epitope	Presence of antibody against a specific antigen and its class (isotype)

Some of the features of each ELISA system are discussed here.

In the indirect ELISA, known antigen is coated and antibodies in serum are quantified. It is useful for detection and quantification of vaccinal responses, sero epidemiological surveys etc. It is not highly useful for the detection of antigen using known mAbs or serum. Why?

The antigen that needs to be detected from a suspected sample would be present in a heterogenous mixture of unrelated proteins and other substances. If this sample is directly coated on the ELISA plates, all the proteins would bind to the well surface. Of all the bound proteins only a small proportion would be the antigen that needs to be detected. This would reduce the sensitivity of the indirect ELISA if it is used for antigen detection and also show increased background ODs due to contaminating proteins that are likely to be coated on the ELISA wells.

3.11.1 Antigen-capture ELISA

The antigen-capture or sandwich ELISA is similar to the indirect ELISA except for the addition of the coating antibody on the plate prior to the addition of the ample antigen being tested.

So what is the role of this antibody? It actually purifies the antigen from the heterogenous mixture of proteins likely to be present in the sample and all the unwanted proteins are not bound to the known mAb/serum and hence are washed out. The rest of the assay is like indirect ELISA.

The features of the capture and detector antibodies used in the sandwich ELISA are given here.

- Both these antibodies should be against different epitopes if mAbs are used
- If polyclonal serum is used, these antibodies should be from different species. If they are from the same species, the anti-species antibody enzyme conjugate against the detector antibody can also bind (independently of the antigen) to the coating antibody and produce colour and positivity
- If both the capture and detector antibodies are mAbs, the detector antibody should be labeled with the enzyme. The use of anti-mouse enzyme conjugate would bind to the capture antibody independent of the antigen.
- Alternatively the detector mAb can also be biotinylated followed by the addition of streptavidin peroxidase conjugate
- It is possible to use polyclonal serum as coating antibody and mAb as detection antibody either coupled to enzyme or followed by the use of anti-mouse enzyme conjugate.

3.11.2 Competitive ELISA

This test is also useful for the detection antibodies against the test antigen similar to indirect ELISA. But what other information this gives that is not possible to obtain in indirect ELISA? This test is useful to detect epitope–specific antibodies, the epitope being determined by the mAb used for competition.

Suppose you get bitten by a dog and you are advised anti-rabies vaccination. After the vaccination, you want to check whether you have developed protective antibodies against the virus. Protective antibodies mean antibodies against the surface glycoprotein of the rabies virus, the G protein. Only antibodies against the G protein of rabies virus would prevent the virus entry into the nerve cells, the target cells in the host. Once the virus enters the neurons and starts multiplying there is no escape from its fatality. Hence only the induction of antibodies against the G protein of the virus would correlate with protection. There would be induction of antibodies to other proteins of the virus such as nucleoprotein or matrix protein etc. but they may not be related to protection and hence may not be directly useful. The detection and semi-quantification of antibodies against the G protein is possible in competitive ELISA using known mAbs against the G protein. Only antibodies against the rabies virus G protein present in the serum would only compete and inhibit the binding of the known mAbs and produce a reduction in colour development.

In an indirect ELISA using whole rabies virus as a coating antigen, antibodies against all the proteins of the virus would bind to the whole virus and produce a colour. It is not possible to separately identify antibodies against one component protein of the virus. Alternatively this can be done if a purified rabies virus glycoprotein or a recombinant expressed G protein is used as a coating antigen in indirect ELISA (in place of whole purified virus).

Alternatively, if a high correlation exists between results of ELISA and serum neutralization test, indirect ELISA results also would be a better indicator of protection.

While the mAbs used in sandwich ELISA should be directed against the most abundantly present protein in the target antigen the mAb used in competitive ELISA should be against the protective antigen that would be a better measure of protection.

For example, in PPRV the sandwich ELISA may use mAbs against the nucleoprotein (N) of the virus, the cELISA should use mAb against the haemagglutinin protein of the virus.

Similarly, in case of bluetongue virus, the sandwich ELISA should use mAbs directed against the conserved viral protein 7 (VP7) while the mAbs in cELISA should be directed against the serotype specific viral protein 2 (VP2).

In case of infectious bronchitis virus (IBV) affecting chickens, the conserved N protein of IBV is the ideal target for diagnosis of IBV while antibodies against the spike protein (S) is the ideal target for detection of serotype-specific antibodies.

The other distinctive feature of cELISA is the ability to detect antibodies in the serum from a wide variety of species without the need for specific anti-species conjugates.

This is possible because in cELISA the conjugate used is against the mAb used in competition (anti-mouse enzyme conjugate) and not against the species from which the sera is being tested. For example, if sera of wild birds need to be tested for presence of avian influenza antibodies, we could still use an mAb against the virus and sera from any species of birds or animals (except that from which the mAbs have been prepared).

The critical factor in cELISA is the limiting antigen concentration used for coating. The epitopes on the antigen should be limiting to favour competition between the mAbs and antibodies present in the serum. If excess epitopes are present, the mAbs and antibodies in the serum can bind to them independently of each other and this would not bring any competition and subsequent reduction in OD values.

The difference between competitive ELISA and blocking ELISA is that in competitive ELISA both mAbs and serum to be tested are added simultaneously ensuring competition while in blocking ELISA, the serum to be tested is added first and incubated followed by the addition of the mAb. In this case the antibodies in the sera are allowed to bind to the epitopes first and when mAbs are added they would bind to only epitopes that are free (unbound by the antibodies in the serum). Hence the blocking ELISA would be slightly more sensitive than cELISA.

3.11.3 Class-capture ELISA

This variant of ELISA provided information on both the antigen specificity of the antibody as well as its isotype.

The wells are coated with the anti-isotype antibodies say anti-mouse IgM and then the mAbs are added. In this case only if the mAbs belong to the IgM class it will get bound through its Fc part, but it is not known at this stage whether it is also against the antigen of interest. Then the antigen of interest is added and if the Fab of the trapped IgM binds to the corresponding epitope on the antigen, it means that the antibordy belong to IgM class and is also against the antigen of interest. This reaction is detected using another known enzyme labeled antibody. This assay is valuable when mAb of a desired isotype is alone required.

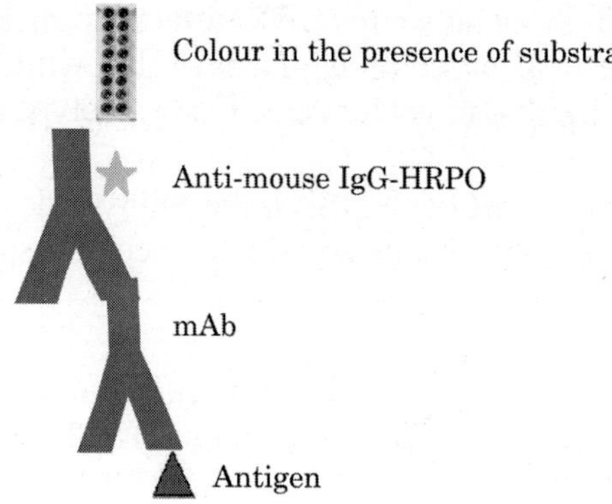

Fig. 3.12: Indurect ELISA

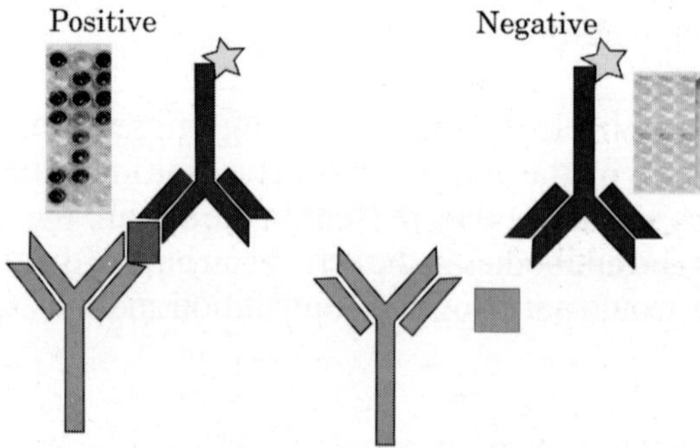

Fig. 3.13: Sandwich ELISA

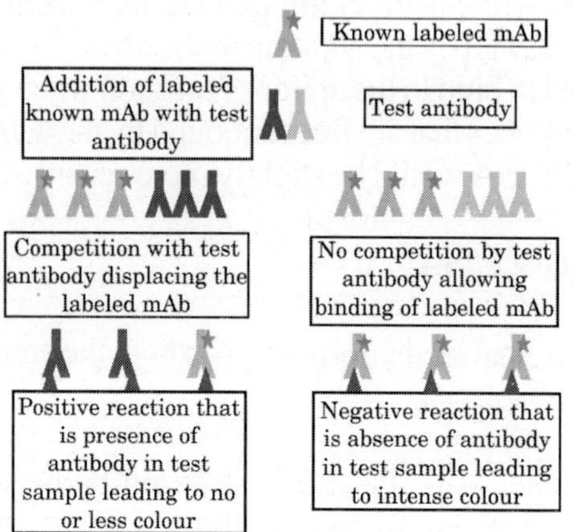

Fig. 3.14: Competitive ELISA.

3.11.4 Additivity index

Once the mAbs is found positive in the initial screening using indirect ELISA and if the application of the mAbs is in the development of an immuno capture ELISA

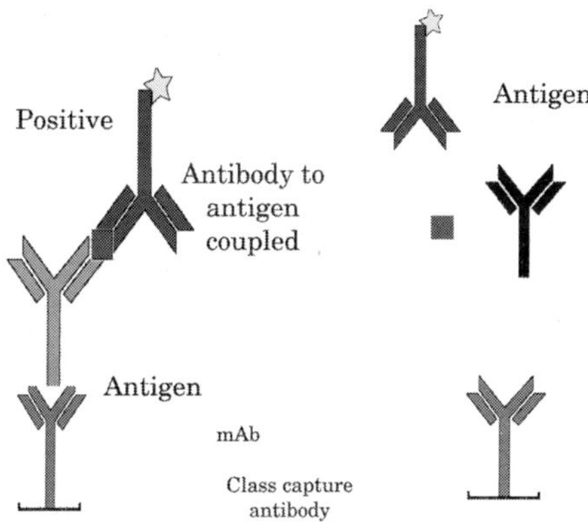

Fig. 3.15: Class capture ELISA.

for antigen detection, an appropriate pair of mAbs has to be identified for use as a coating and detector antibody. As suggested earlier, one of the features of these mAbs is that they bind to different epitopes. A simple preliminary test to assess this is based on the additivity index (AI). This is based on the principle that when two mAbs at the saturating concentrations are placed simultaneously in the same well, and if they bind to spatially different epitopes, the OD value would be significantly higher than either of their individual values. However if they bind to the same epitope and epitopes close together, one mAb binding interferes with the binding of the other mAb, and their OD values tend not to be different from their individual values. Using these OD values an AI can be calculated using the formula

$$AI = [[(2\, A_{1+2})/(A_1 + A_2)] - 1] \times 100$$

where A_1 and A_2 are the ODs obtained when the mAbs are assayed separately, and A_{1+2} is the OD when the same amounts of the two mAbs are pooled in the same well. Provided the concentrations of the mAbs are saturating for the antigen, the AI will tend to be 0 if both the mAbs recognize the same epitope, but close to 100 if the two epitopes are topographically unrelated. The lowest AI for mAbs that recognize different epitopes was 40 and this can be considered the threshold for evaluating epitope relatedness.

3.11.5 Avidin-biotin systems

To generate increased amplification, a two-step biotin/avidin system may be used. Biotin binds with very high affinity to avidin resulting in an essentially irreversible interaction. The association constant of avidin and biotin is the strongest in biological systems. A biotinylated secondary antibody is applied first, then avidin, ExtrAvidin or streptavidin conjugated to an enzyme or fluorochrome binds to multiple sites on the biotinylated secondary antibody, thus amplifying the signal and resulting in greater sensitivity than that achieved with an antibody-enzyme or antibody-fluorochrome conjugate alone.

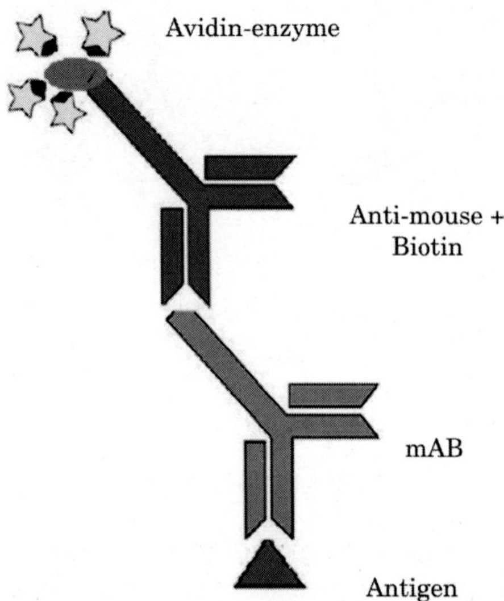

Fig. 3.16: Avidin-biotin ELISA

3.11.6 Fluorescence based assays

- Fluorochrome is a dye or molecule that is capable of exhibiting fluorescence.
- Fluorophore is the region of the molecule capable of exhibiting fluorescence.

A fluorochrome absorbs light energy over a range of wavelengths that is characteristic for that compound. This absorption of light raises an electron in the fluorochrome to a higher energy level. The excited electron quickly decays to its ground state, emitting the excess energy as a photon of light. This transition of energy is called fluorescence.

This process repeats in a cyclical manner unless the fluorophore is destroyed by photobleaching. The energy of the emitted photon is lower than the energy of the excitation photon due to energy dissipation in the excited state. Lower energy means longer wavelength. The difference in energy or wavelength is called the Stokes shift. The Stokes shift allows the emission photons to be detected and isolated away from the excitation photons. A single fluorophore can be repeatedly excited and detected.

Fluorescence has been reinvented recently with a lot of molecular biological techniques such a automatic sequencing, microarray, flow cytometry etc using them.

Immunofluorescence is used to localize antigens to specific cell types or in sub cellular compartments. The assay can also be adapted for the detection and quantification of antibody. The general procedure is to incubate fixed cells or tissue sections or impression smears with the primary antibody and detect the antigen-antibody complex with a secondary antibody conjugated with a fluorochrome. Fluorescein and rhodamine, which fluoresce green and red, respectively, are two most common conjugates. The location of the protein recognized by the primary antibody is determined by examining the sample under UV illumination.

Once the mAbs are found positive in ELISA based assays, fluorescence based assays can also be used, if required. Some viruses that do not produce any cytopathic effects (CPE) when inoculated into cell culture then, fluorescence based assays come in handy, *e.g*., rabies virus, classical swine fever virus etc.

The developed mAbs are added onto infected cell cultures followed by the addition of anti-mouse FITC. After washing the slides are observed under a fluorescent microscope and presence of intra cytoplasmic apple green fluorescence indicates that the mAbs bind to the virus. Appropriate controls of uninfected cells or cells infected with unrelated viruses are required. The infected cells are normally fixed with acetone to permit intra cytoplasmic penetration of the mAb and the conjugate into the cells.

Both direct and indirect fluorescence antibody techniques (FAT) are used similar to the direct and indirect ELISA. In the direct FAT, the primary antibody (mAb) is labeled with the fluorescent dye while in the indirect FAT the secondary antibody (anti-mouse) is labeled with the fluorescent dye.

Direct detection methods are quicker to carry out since an antibody incubation step and the associated washing steps are eliminated. In addition, there is sometimes less background. However, the primary antibody must be first purified and conjugated with the appropriate label. The ready availability of secondary antibodies from commercial sources makes the indirect methods easier to perform. In addition, signal amplification may occur during the secondary antibody step.

The preparation of the cells or tissue for FAT is a crucial step that depends on the type of cells being analyzed and upon the application.

The samples that can be used for FAT include:

- Cryostat sections
- Adherent tissue culture cells grown on cover slips or microscope slides
- Cells grown in suspension cyto centrifuged or dried onto microscope slides
- Cells in suspension.

The fixation procedure should not affect the ability of the antibody to recognize the antigen. Organic solvents, such as ethanol, methanol and acetone, or paraformaldehyde are routinely used. Glutaraldehyde is not a good fixative since the bonds formed by the cross linking of glutaraldehyde exhibit a strong endogenous fluorescence.

Fixation also permeabilizes the cell so that the antibody has access to internal cellular structures. The permeability can be enhanced by treating with a detergent after the fixation. Intact and unfixed cells can be used to demonstrate the surface localization of an antigen.

The sub-cellular structures recognized by the antibodies will appear as a bright image against a dark background. By comparing the epifluorescence with the bright field image the protein of interest can be localized to a particular sub-cellular compartment or to a particular cell type within a tissue.

Fluorescent dyes which bind to particular subcellular compartments or cell types (vimentin or cytokeratin) can also be used to assist in the localization of the protein of interest.

Dual-labeling experiments can also be used to demonstrate the extent of co-localization between two different proteins. The most convenient method is to used antibodies generated in different species (*e.g.*, mice and rabbits) as the primary antibody and then used species specific secondary antibodies conjugated with different fluorochromes.

If only mAbs raised in the same species are available, it will be necessary to purify the two antibodies and conjugate them with different fluorochromes. The two different fluorochromes can be viewed separately through the use of filters specific for each fluorochrome. It is also possible to digitally merge the two images to demonstrate the extent of co-localization between the two proteins.

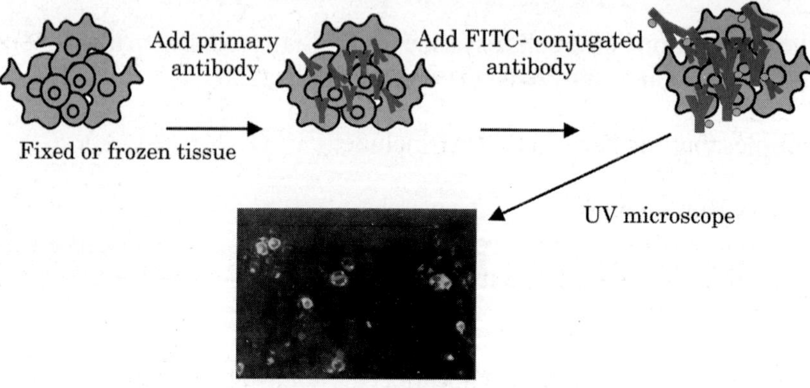

Fig. 3.17: Fluorescence antibody test

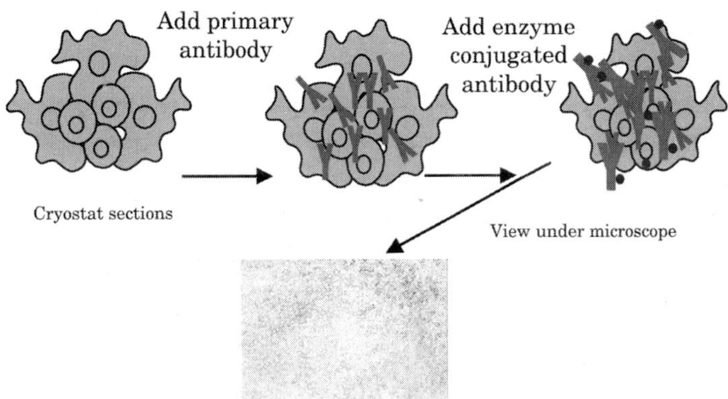

Fig. 3.18: Immunoperoxidase test

If the mAbs belong to two different isotypes, say anti-CD3 marker mAb belongs to IgM and anti-CD4 marker to IgG2, it is possible to use commercially available anti-mouse IgM coupled to FITC and anti-mouse IgG2 coupled to rhodamine and use it in FAT or flow cytometry techniques.

Live FAT, using unfixed live cells in suspension is useful to identify mAbs against surface glycoproteins of virus being expressed in infected cell membranes. For example, mAbs against the N protein of PPRV can be demonstrated by FAT or IPT staining of fixed infected cells while mAbs against the H protein can be stained using live infected cells without fixation.

Similar to FAT immuno peroxidase (IPT) tests are used by replacing the fluorescence label with an enzyme label and adding the appropriate substrates and counter staining with histologial stains to improve contrast. These tests are more applicable with mAbs against cell surface markers primarily to identify the cell types in the tissues that express the surface markers, for example the localization of CD3 cells in spleen sections or B-cells in bursal sections.

3.13.7 Immunochemistry substrates

Table 3.7: Substrates used in Immunochemistry

Enzyme	*Substrate*	*Colour*	*Mounting media*	*Counter stain*
HRPO	3,3' diamino benzidine (DAB)	Brown	Organic or aqueous	Mayer's hematoxylin, methyl blue, methyl green, neutral red
HRPO	3-Amino-9-ethylcarbazole (ACE)	Red	Aqueous	Methyl green, mayer's ematoxylin, methyl blue
AP	5-Bromo-4-chloro-3-indol-ylphosphate (BCIP)/Nitro blue tetrazolium (NBT)	Purple	Organic	Nuclear fast red, light green

3.12 Neutralization Assays

In a neutralization test, antibodies and virus are allowed to interact (neutralize) followed by quantitation of the un-neutralized virus in a suitable host (animal, eggs or cell culture).

- If antibodies are absent, disease, death or lesions may result.
- If antibodies neutralize the virus no such effects would be seen.

There are two methods of performing neutralization tests. In the alpha procedure, equal quantities of a constant amount of serum and increasing dilutions of the virus are incubated together and then inoculated into a suitable indicator system.

In the beta method, virus at a fixed concentration (100 $TCID_{50}$) is incubated with two-fold serial dilutions of serum before inoculation into the indicator system

In the alpha neutralization test (constant serum and varying virus), the neutralization effect of the serum of mAb is expressed in terms of neutralization index.

This is determined by titrating the virus in the presence of diluent and in the presence of mAb or serum and calculating the 50% vendpoints. Then, subtract the exponent of the latter from the former disregarding the negative sign.

For example,

$TCID_{50}$ of virus + diluent = $10^{-6.5}$
$TCID_{50}$ of virus + mAb = $10^{-4.5}$
Neutralization index = $10^{2.0}$ or 100
Log of neutralization index = log 100 = 2.0
when titrations are done in 10-fold dilutions, it varies by a factor of 10 or $\log_{10} = 1.0$

Thus neutralization index of less than 10 (less than log1) is not significant, values between 10 and 50 (log 1.0 to 1.6) are suspect and only indices above 50 (log 1.7 or greater) are considered significant.

For the beta method, 2-fold or 10-fold dilution series of serum or mAb with 100$TCID_{50}$ of virus are used. The highest dilution of serum showing 50% protection is taken as titre.

3.12.1 Calculation of virus titre

The virus titre is calculated from the proportion of hosts observed to become infected when inoculated with a series of virus dilutions into an appropriate host system. The method of calculation is that of Reed and Muench.

As an example,

A	*B*	*C*		*D*		*E*
Virus dilution inoculated	*No. infected / No. inoculated*	*No. infected*	*No.not infected*	*Summing No. inf*	*No. not inf.*	*% infected*
10^{-2}	5/5	5	0	18	0	100
10^{-3}	5/5	5	0	13	0	100
10^{-4}	4/5	4	1	8	1	89
10^{-5}	3/5	3	2	4	3	57
10^{-6}	1/5	1	4	1	7	13
10^{-7}	0/5	0	5	0	12	0

Inoculum volume = 100 ul

In this example, the 50% end point lies between virus dilutions 10^{-5} and $10^{-6.}$ Then we need to calculate the exact proportionate distance between 10^{-5} and 10^{-6} dilutions at which 50% end point lies.

$$\text{Pr oportionated diss tan ce} = \frac{\%\,\text{above}\,50\% - 50\%}{\%\,\text{above}\,50\% - \%\,\text{below}\,50\%} = \frac{57-50}{57-13} = 0.11$$

- The 50% infectivity endpoint is $10^{-5.11}$
- Titre of the original virus suspension is $10^{-5.11}$ in 0.1 ml.
- For running the beta neutralization test, we need 100 $TCID_{50}$ of virus. How to make this dilution?
- As above if the virus titre is $10^{-5.11}$ in 0.1 ml or $10^{-6.11}$ in 1 ml.
- Then 10 $TCID_{50}$ would be in $10^{-4.11}$ in 100 µl
- Then 100 $TCID_{50}$ of virus would be $10^{-3.11}$ in 100 µl
- Make regular dilutions till $10^{-3.0}$
- Find the antilog of 0.11 (which is 1.288)
- 1.00 (virus) = 0.3, therefore take 1 part of $10^{-3.0}$ dilution of virus and add 0.3 parts of diluent.

3.13 Radio Immuno Assay

Radio immuno assay (RIA) uses an immune reaction to estimate a ligand. RIA was developed by Rosalyn Yalow and Solomon Aaron Berson in 1960 and Yallow received the Nobel Prize in 1977 in Medicine for RIA for insulin. It has been largely been replaced by ELISA but still useful for measuring small haptens and pharmaceutical compounds and hormones.

A known labeled antigen and antigen that may be present in the sample are allowed to compete to the binding sites on the known antibody. If specific antigen is present in the sample the binding of the labeled antigen is reduced hence the radioactivity in the bound residue, measured after adequate washing, is also reduced. The ligand concentration is inversely related to radioactivity.

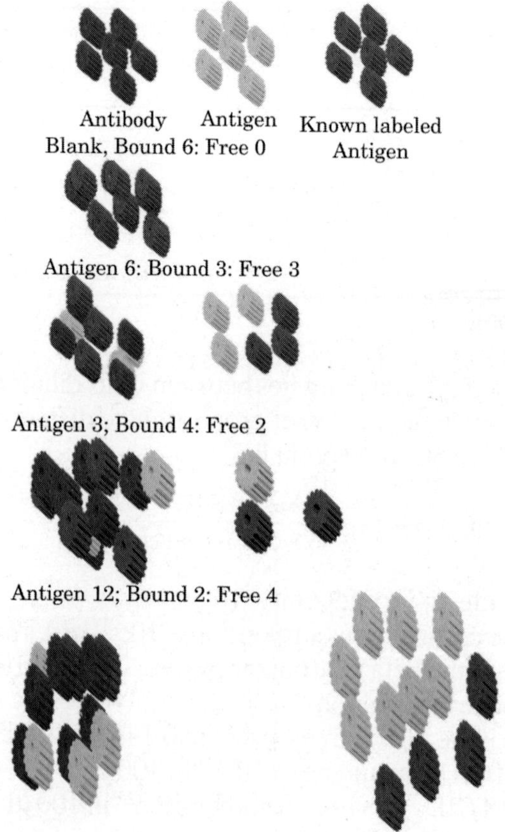

Fig. 3.19: Radio immunoassay procedure

Advantages

- Highly specific
- High sensitivity

Disadvantages

- Radiation hazards
- Requires specially trained persons

- Labs require special license to handle radioactive material
- Requires special arrangements for
    - Requisition, storage of radioactive material
    - Radioactive waste disposal.

^{3}H, ^{14}C, ^{125}I are commonly used as radioactive tags for antigen. The labelling should affect antigenic specificity and antigenic activity. A crucial step is separation of unbound antigens which is achieved by binding the antibodies to the microtitre well surface [Solid phase RIA]. Then add known amounts of the test sample + labelled antigen into the microtitre wells. Incubate →allows the reaction to reach completion →Decant and wash the contents of the well →remove all unbound antigens. Radioactivity remaining in the microtitre wells measured by a Counter [GM counter, Scintillation counter etc].

Intensity of radioactivity is inversely correlated with the concentration of antigens in the test sample.

A standard curve is prepared by measuring the bound radioactivity in the presence of different concentrations of standard known antigen. Then based on the measurement of bound radioactivity in the presence of unknown antigen its concentration can be established from the standard curve (Fig.3.18).

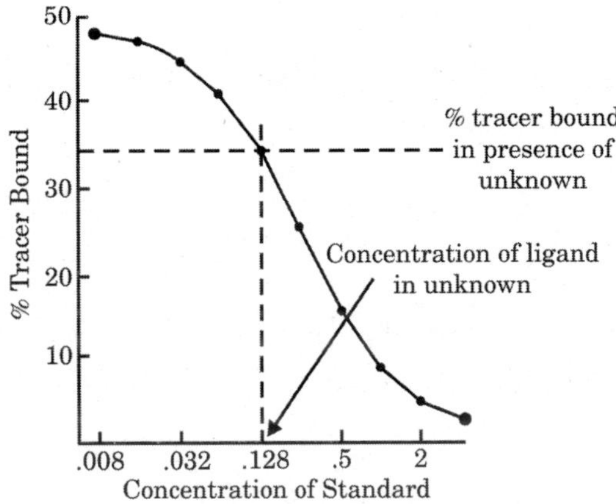

Fig. 3.20: Concentration of standard

Indirect solid phase RIA has also been used for screening hybridomas. For example, in the preparation of mAbs against bovine immunoglobulin subclasses, the particular sub-class has been coated on to flexible polyvinyl chloride 96-well plates followed by the addition of hybridoma supernatants and ^{125}I labelled rabbit antibody to murine immunoglobulins. Washing is done between each step to remove the unbound reactants. Then the wells are cut and transferred into gamma counting tubes and counts per minute (CPM) were measured in a gamma counter. The CPM is proportional to the amount of rabbit antibody bound to the plate, which in turn is proportional to the mouse monoclonal anti-bovine immunoglobulins.

CHAPTER 4

CHARACTERIZATION OF MONOCLONAL ANTIBODIES

Just recap the major features of mAbs

- It is against a single epitope
- It belongs to a single class and subclass
- It has a particular affinity.

So if we need to characterize a particular mAb produced, we should be able to identify the following

- To what epitope on the target antigen it binds
- What is the isotype of the mAb–both heavy chain and light chain
- What is the affinity of the mAb

In addition, mAbs are applied in various diagnostic, therapeutic or research purposes. So as part of the characterization requirement it is also needed to ascertain whether the mAb is applicable for the particular intended use. Before starting characterization, we also need to confirm that we are really dealing with the mAbs. Several techniques are available to obtain there objectives.

4.1 Polyacrylamide Gel Electrophoresis

Polyacrylamide (PA) gels have the following properties making it an ideal matrix for electrophoresis.

- High reproducibility being synthetic
- Stable to wide range of pH and ionic strengths
- Low fixed charge
- Ability to include additives in the gel
- Strong gels permitting easy handling

Agar, another common gel matrix is a natural biological material produced simply by boiling and cooling and hence there is little control on its biological composition. In PA gels, two monomer ingredients are used, monoacrylamide, whose concentration determines the length of the polymer and a cross linking agent, N, N' methylene bis acrylamide (bis) making the gel having a network of pores. The letter 'T' (in G/100 ml) denotes the total monomer concentration (acrylamide and bis acrylamide, and the letter 'C' denotes the percentage of 'T', which is due to the cross linker alone. If 28.94 G of acrylamide and 1.06 G of bis is added in 100 ml of water would mean a gel with 30% T and $^{1.06}/_{30}$ = 3.53% C.

A thumb rule is that C should be nearly 6.5–0.5 × T

Acrylamide monomers are activated in the presence of free radicals forming long chain polymers through a reaction known as vinyl addition polymerization. However these polyacrylamide molecules do not form a gel because they are not cross linked. Polymerization of acrylamide monomers with cross linker bis results in a mesh like structure as shown in Figure 4.1 below.

Structure of acrylamide

$CH_2 = CH–CONH_2$ Acrylamide MW = 71.08

Structure of bis acrylamide

$CH_2 = CH–C–NH–CH_2–NH–C–CH–CH_2$ N, N' methylene bis acrylamide MW = 157.17

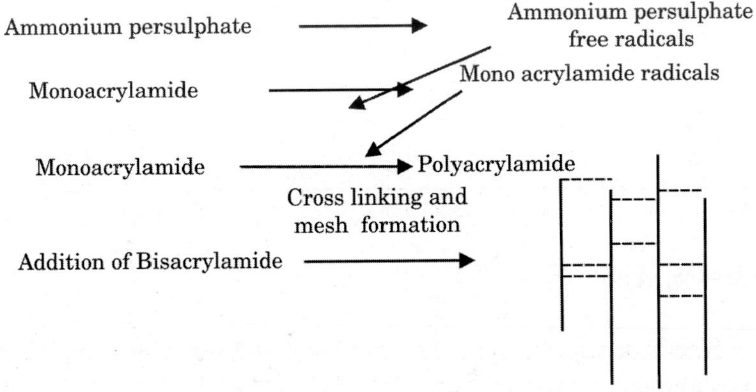

Fig. 4.1: Formation of polyacrylamide from mono acrylamide and free radicals

Polymerization process involves mixing the acrylamide and bis in particular ratio in the presence of catalysts, accelerators and buffer. Oxygen inhibits polymerization. The cross-linking of the acrylamide polymers results in 'pores' of a defined size. The total acrylamide concentration and the ratio of bis-acrylamide to acrylamide will determine the average pore size. Polymerization is catalyzed by free radical production which involves tetra methyl ethylene diamine (TEMED) and ammonium per sulphate (APS).

Another alternative for TEMED is riboflavin or riboflavin phosphate (which is more soluble than riboflavin) which would also provide the necessary free radicals. Oxygen and light are required to convert the riboflavin into another derivative that is the catalytic form. Advantages of riboflavin are better control of the catalytic activity (and intern the polymerization) by switching the light on and off and catalytic function at low concentrations. However the TEMED system is the most commonly used.

Higher percentage of gels will result in smaller average pore sizes. Hence smaller molecules will be able to pass through these gel pores more easily resulting in larger molecules having a lower mobility than smaller molecules. Thus the gel acts like a molecular sieve and retains the larger molecules while letting the smaller ones pass through. This is in contrast to gel filtration where the larger molecules have a higher mobility because they do not enter the gel.

Thus the mobility of a protein during gel electrophoresis is primarily a function of its charge/mass ratio. Protein shape and other factors will still affect mobility, but to a lesser extent. The gel concentration and the molecular weight of proteins which can be separated on PA gels are given in Table 4.1.

Table 4.1: Separation of Proteins on Polyacrylamide Gels

Concentration	*Mw (KDa)*
15%	10–50
10%	15–100
5%	25–250
3.3%	Up to 1000

The cytochrome C protein (12 KDa) is about 3 nm, ribosomes are 25 nm, bacteria is 1500 nm.

4.1.1 SDS–PA gels

The role of SDS in denaturing the proteins and coating them with a uniform negative charge and aiding movement in one direction has already been described earlier. Compared to normal PA gels wherein electrophoresis is dependent on both the size and charge of the protein, in SDS-PA gels it is dependent only on the size of the protein subunits. Thus SDS-PA gels are technically less demanding and have some advantages over non-denaturing gels.

1. The separation in less influenced by pH and ions since charge differences are not important so sample desalting and buffering are not so crucial
2. Electrophoresis is fast since charge density is high
3. Since the proteins are in denatured form, cooling the gel is not very crucial
4. The use of detergents also improves the solubility of the proteins electrophoresed.

Two types of electrophoresis are commonly used – the continuous and discontinuous gel systems.

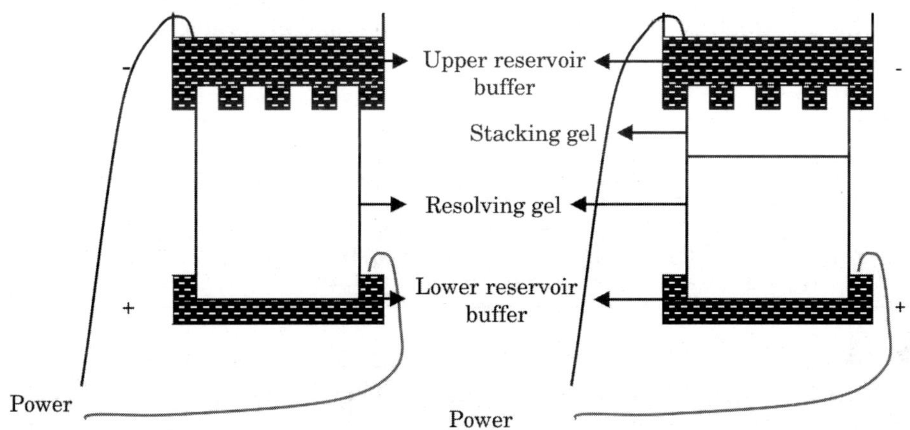

Fig. 4.2: Continuous and discontinuous gel systems

In a continuous gel system, there are certain features which are highlighted below:

1. Wide range of buffers can be used (as compared to discontinuous gel systems in which only certain buffer combinations are suitable).
2. It is quick and easy to set up with high reproducibility.
3. Separation is usually inferior to discontinuous gel separations.
4. Sample needs to be concentrated since there is no concentration step in the electrophoresis (stacking process in discontinuous gel system).

In the discontinuous gel systems, there are 2 different gel mixes and buffer systems. The upper stacking, spacer or top gel and the lower separating, running or resolving gel.

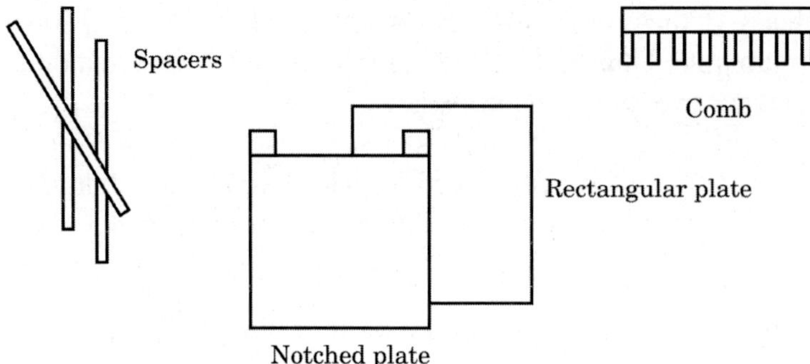

Fig. 4.3: Materials used for preparation of polyacrylamide gels

Three buffers are normally used, one each for the gel systems and one for the electrode compartments. The two gel buffers have the same ions but different pH while the electrode buffer has different buffer ions and pH (Table 4.2).

Table 4.2: Concentration, pH and Ionic Strength of Stacking and Separating Gels

	Stacking gel	***Separating gel***	***Electrode buffer***
Acrylamide	3–4.5%	6–20%	–
pH	6.8	8.8	6.7
Ionic strength	0.125 M Tris	0.375 M Tris	25 mM Tris, 192 mM glycine

The stacking gel has a lower acrylamide concentration (open pores, no sieving effect), a lower pH and a lower ionic strength than the separating gel. The lower ionic strength of the stacking gel results in a greater local electric field strength than in the separating gel. The field strength difference combined with the lower acrylamide concentration results in proteins having a higher mobility in the stacking gel than in the separating gel. No separation occurs in this stacking gel and hence this gel can be discarded following electrophoresis.

The glycine ions in the tank buffer have a lower mobility in the stacking gel than in separating gel because of the pH differences. Therefore, proteins will migrate faster than the glycine in the stacking gel. When proteins reach the separating gel their mobility is decreased because of the increased acrylamide concentration and decreased field strength, whereas the increase in pH results in glycine having a higher mobility. These factors result in the proteins becoming compressed at the interface between the two gels and thus increasing resolution–protein band sharpening. This stacking process does not work well with nucleic acids (probably because of their larger sizes). Hence they are only subjected to continuous gel electrophoresis.

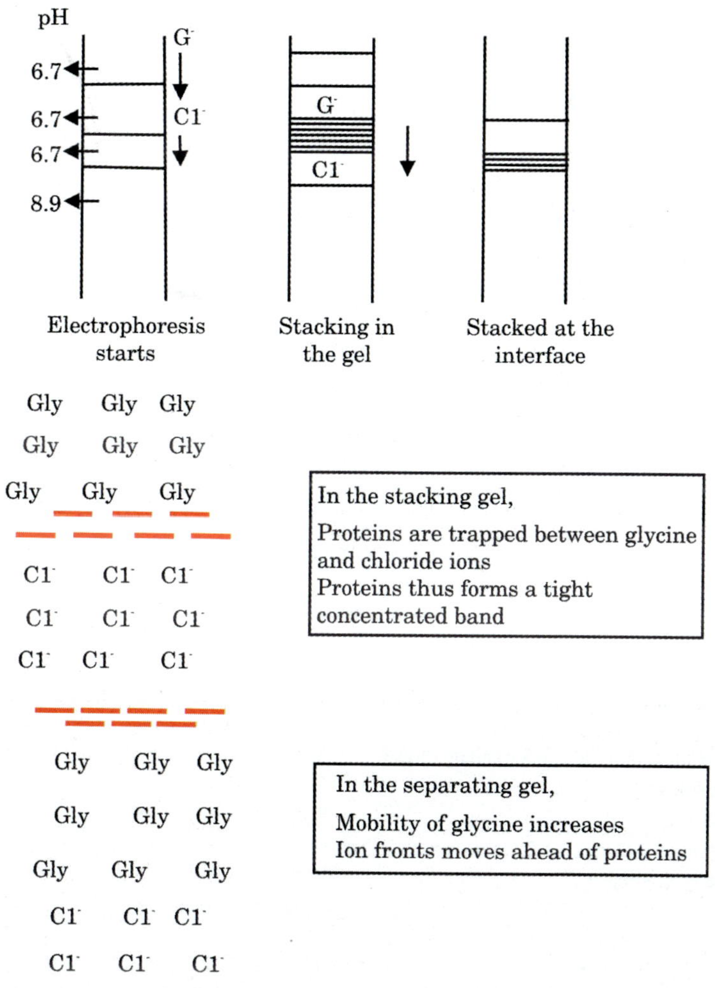

Fig. 4.4: Phenomenon of stacking

Mobility in SDS gel electrophoresis is expressed as relative mobility (Rf)

$$Rf = \text{distance protein migrated} \div \text{gel length}$$

The length of the gel is often defined by the migration of a substance such as a small molecular weight tracking dye (*e.g.* bromophenol blue) which is not impeded by the matrix. This mobility can then be used to calculate the size of proteins. Protein standards of known size are used to generate a standard curve by plotting the log of the molecular weight against the Rf values. The molecular weight of an unknown protein can be extrapolated from its Rf value. Such a calculated molecular weight is designated as Mr to indicate that it is a relative molecular weight based on comparisons to other proteins.

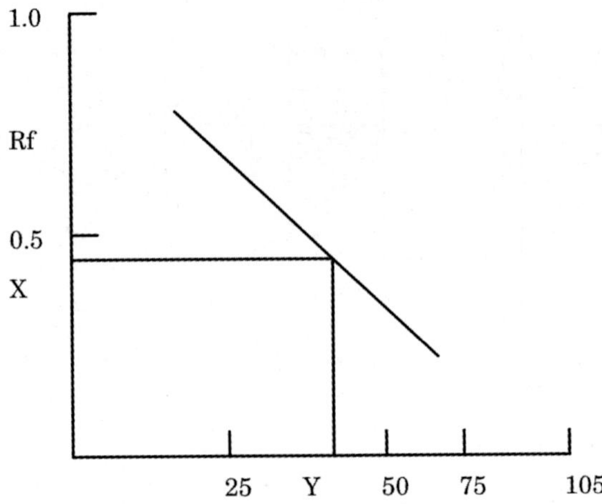

Fig. 4.5: Determination of molecular weights of proteins from polyacrylamide gels.

X = R_f of test sample; y– molecular weight of test sample.

Table 4.3: Commonly used Protein Standard Markers

Protein	*Source*	*Molecular weight (daltons)*
Myosin	Rabbit muscle	212000
Maltose binding protein and beta galactosidase	*E. coli*	158194
Beta galactosidase	*E. coli*	116351
Phosphorylase b	Rabbit muscle	97400
Serum albumin	Bovine	67000
Glutamic dehydrogenase	Bovine	55561
Ovalbumin	Hens egg white	45000
Maltose binding protein	*E. coli*	42710
Lactate dehydrogenase–M	Porcine	36487
Carbonic anhydrase	Bovine	29000
Triose phosphate isomerase	Rabbit	26600
Trypsin inhibitor	Soybean	20040
Alpha lactalbumin	Bovine	14500
Lysozyme	Hens egg white	14313
Aprotinin	Bovine	6517
Trypsin inhibitor	Bovine lumg	6500
Insulin beta chain	Bovine	3400
Bacitracin	*Baccilus licheniformis*	1400

SDS PA gel apparatus consists of a mould to form the gels, an apparatus to hold the gel with buffer reservoirs and a power supply capable of delivering the required voltage or current. Polyacrylamide gels are run in a vertical fashion and agarose gels tend to be run in a horizontal position. Gels can either be formed as cylinders by using glass tubes as a mould (often called tube gels) or formed as rectangular slabs (slab gels). These slab gels are formed by polymerizing the acryamide–bis mixture between glass plates separated by spacers. Typically the gel is 0.75–1.5 mm thick. At the top a 'comb' is used to form sample wells. Slab gels allow multiple samples to be compared on the same gel, thus eliminating gel-to-gel variations.

The first step in electrophoresis is to pour the separating gel after fixing glass plates separated by spacers, whose thickness would determine the thickness of the gel and ensuring that there are no leaks. After pouring the separating gel, the butanol is layered over the poured gel to prevent release of oxygen which inhibits polymerization. Once polymerization is achieved, a distinct demarcation is seen at which time the butanol is discarded and the stacking gel is poured over it after placing the combs. The stacking gel is poured immediately prior to electrophoresis to minimize diffusion between the two gels.

The cast gel is placed into the apparatus so that the top and bottom of the gel are in contact with chambers containing buffer. These chambers contain electrodes which are connected to a power supply. Thus an electric field is generated across the gel when a voltage is applied. Pre cast gels are also commercially available.

Gradient gels can be used in situations where it is necessary to examine both high and low molecular weight proteins on the same gel (Fig. 4.6).

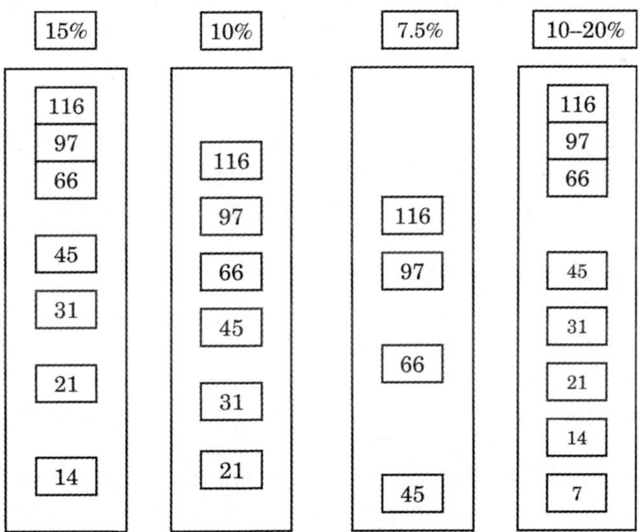

Fig. 4.6: Gradient gels-note separation achieved for a wide range of molecular weights in gradient gels.

Samples are loaded into the wells after arranging the gel in the tank and buffer is poured. If the samples are loaded and buffer is added, the sample may tend to float out or mix with samples in adjacent wells. Hence it is safer to mark the wells before setting up the apparatus. After loading the samples into the wells of the gel an electric field is applied across the gel.

The mobility of proteins in an electric field is proportional to field strength (E/d), or simply the voltage (E) since the distance (d) is determined by the electrophoresis apparatus. Electrophoresis will proceed faster at higher voltages but would generate heat in proportional to the amount of power, which is the product of voltage and current (P = EI). Excessive heating may result in proteins precipitating within the gel or a "smile effect" in which the movement is affected and gives an appearance of a "smiling face". Electrophoresis is usually carried out under constant voltage or constant power to minimize the resulting increase in heating that occurs during electrophoresis. These electrical parameters change during electrophoresis because the ions migrate to the anode and cathode buffers, and therefore lead to an increase in resistance (R). Resistance affects the voltage and current (E = IR). A tracking dye (bromophenol blue) is included in the sample. When this dye reaches the bottom of the gel or some predetermined time afterwards the power is turned off and the proteins detected. Gels are usually 'fixed' before staining with an acetic acid and methanol solution which precipitates proteins into the acrylamide matrix. A common way to detect proteins after electrophoresis is to stain the gel with Coomassie blue, a dye that binds proteins. Coomassie blue G-250 (0.1% dye in 3.5% perchloric acid) can be used as a fast stain (for 20 minutes) followed by de-staining (10% methanol and 7% acetic acid) for 30–60 minutes.

Coomassie blue R-250 (0.1% Coomassie-blue R-250 in 50% methanol + 10% acetic acid) is used as a fast stain (for at least 3 hours) followed by de staining (10% methanol and 7% acetic acid) for 30–60 minutes.

Silver staining is generally 10–100X more sensitive than Coomassie-blue staining. Three basic types of silver staining methods are used diamine (ammonical), non diamine and photo development. All three methods are based upon binding silver ions to proteins and reducing the Ag2+ to metallic silver. The silver interacts with primary amines or sulfhydryls.

In the diamine method, silver diamine complexes are stabilized with ammonium ions and the free amine groups of proteins. The silver bound to protein is then reduced to metallic silver with formaldehyde. In the non-diamine method, AgNO3 reacts with protein under acidic conditions, followed by reduction to metallic silver with formaldehyde under alkaline conditions.

Photo development relies on light (photons) to reduce silver ions to metallic silver.

The results obtained from gel electrophoresis tend to be qualitative.

One possible way to quantify the amount of a specific protein is to electrophorese known amounts of a protein and to compare the staining intensities with that of the unknown protein using scanning densitometry. Gels, autoradiographs, or even photographs are scanned and the peak height and areas of bands are determined. The values are then used to calculate the amount of protein based on standard curves.

The stained protein bands could also be excised, the dye extracted with a solvent and the amount of dye determined with a spectrophotometer. The absorbance values could then be used to generate a standard curve. However, individual proteins bind different amounts of Coomassie blue and there will be gel-to-gel variations.

Similarly radioactive proteins can be excised from the gel, the gel slice solubilized and the amount of radioactivity determined by liquid scintillation counting. This method is laborious.

4.2 Isoelectric Focusing

Isoelectric focusing (IEF) separates proteins based on their isoelectric points. The isoelectric point is defined as the pH at which a protein has zero net charge (*i.e.*, the number of negative and positive charges are equal) and is a measure of the protein's net charge. Separating proteins according to their net charge is accomplished by generating a pH gradient in an electric field. The effect of protein size on mobility is minimized by carrying out the electrophoresis in gels with large pore sizes such as low acrylamide concentrations (*e.g.*, 3.5%) or agarose in which there is no sieving effect.

A pH gradient is generated with carrier ampholytes. These ampholytes are a mixture of aliphatic amines and either carboxylic or sulfonic acid. They have a high buffering capacity, low molecular weight (300–600 Da) and a range of pK_a values. Initially the pH of an ampholyte solution will be the average of the pK_a values of the mixture. Application of an electric current will cause the ampholytes to migrate toward the electrodes according to their charges. The ampholytes will continue to migrate until they reach a position in which the local pH equals their pK_a (*i.e.*, no net charge). The end result is a pH gradient in which the most basic ampholytes are found at the cathode, a dilute alkali solution (*e.g.*, NaOH), and the most acidic ampholytes are at the anode, a dilute acid solution (*e.g.*, H_3PO_4). Carrier ampholytes with defined pH ranges are available commercially and are mixed with the gel while pouring and they form a pH gradient in response to electric field. Proteins are also ampholytes and will migrate within the pH gradient until they reach a pH equal to their isoelectric point.

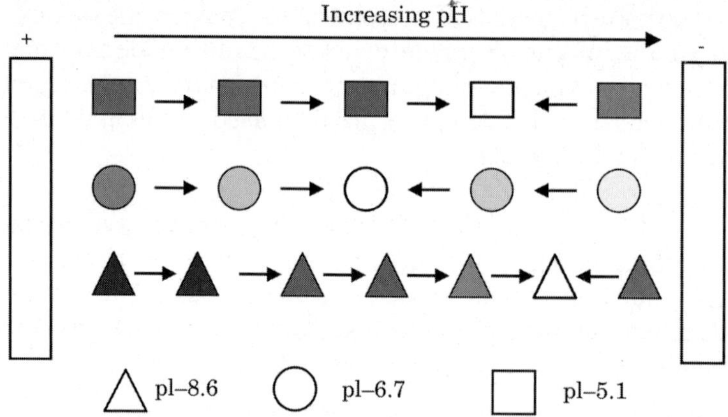

Fig. 4.7: Isoelectric focusing and two dimensional electrophoresis.

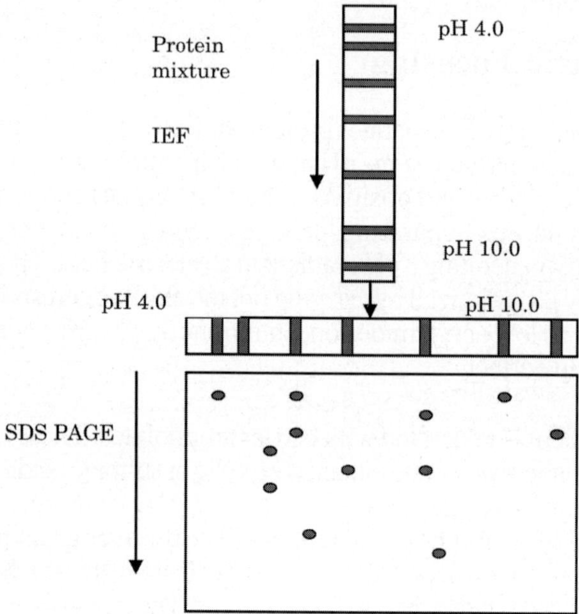

Fig. 4.8: Two dimensional electrophoresis–IEF in the first direction and SDS PAGE in the other direction.

4.3 Autoradiography and Fluorography

Radioactive proteins can be detected by exposing X-ray film to the gel. Radioactivity emitted from the proteins will activate silver grains in the film emulsion which will be converted into metallic silver during development. The reduction to metallic Ag will result in a dark spot or 'band' appearing on the film in positions which correspond to proteins. Table 4.4 gives commonly used radio active elements.

Table 4.4: Properties of Commonly used Radio Active Elements

Radio isotope	*Half life*	*Radiation*	*Energy (MeV)*
C^{14}	5570 years	â	0.155
H^{3}	12.3 years	â	0.0176
Ca^{45}	165 days	â	0.254
S^{35}	87 days	â	0.167
P^{32}	14.5 days	â	1.701
I^{131}	8 days	â	Â–0.608, B–0.354

Fluorography refers to the exposure of film to secondary light emitted by either intensifying screens or fluors upon their exposure to radiation.

Gels are dried before carrying out autoradiography or fluorography. A gel dryer removes all of the water and solvent from the acrylamide matrix by heating the gel while under vacuum. This results in the matrix collapsing into a thin layer. The dried gel is placed next to a sheet of X-ray film in a light tight cassette and exposed for an appropriate amount of time depending on the isotope and the amount of radioactivity. The exposed film is developed.

Some emissions of high energy isotopes (*e.g.*, ^{32}P and ^{125}I) will pass through film without exposing it. An intensifying screen is placed on the opposite side of the X-ray film from the dried gel. Emissions passing through the film will then interact with the intensifying screen which will fluoresce. The light from this fluorescence will expose the X-ray film. Using an intensifying screen will usually decrease the exposure time by a factor of 7–10 ×. The efficiency of the intensifying screen is highest at –70ºC.

Emissions from low energy isotopes (*e.g.*, ^{3}H) and some medium energy emissions (eg. ^{14}C and ^{35}S) are not energetic enough to escape the dried gel matrix. In this case a scintillation fluor is impregnated into the gel before drying. The radioactive emissions interact with the fluors resulting in fluorescence. The fluorescence will then expose the X-ray film.

Phosphor-imager machines use screens containing storage-phosphors as a replacement for the use of film. These phosphor-imager screens trap the energy of radioactive emissions and are sensitive to both beta particles and gamma rays, but insensitive to visible light.

The storage phosphor captures energy with efficiency around 100% for any particle that strikes the screen. Subsequent scanning the screen with a laser beam releases the stored energy as blue light. This blue light is converted into an image file for display and quantitation by the phosophor-imager's computer. Such high efficiency makes it possible to detect low levels of radioactivity after short exposure times. The phosphor screens can be used repeatedly by 'erasing' the screen following scanning.

4.4 Western Blotting

Western blotting is the process of transfer of the separated proteins from gels onto membranes. Southern blotting refers to transfer of separated DNA from gels to membranes since it was developed by Ed Southern in 1975 it is known after him. Following this, the transfer of RNA was called as Northern blotting and proteins as Western blotting (Towbin *et al*., 1979). It has nothing to do with directions.

Following separation of nucleic acids or proteins in gels, the identity of the separated molecules needs to be confirmed by using a known antibody or probe.

If this needs to be done on the gel itself it suffers from some disadvantages, the primary one being accessibility. In order for the primary antibody to bind to the separated proteins it needs to enter in to the pores of the PA gel. The IgG antibody is 180 kDa. It is very difficult to remove the unbound antibodies from the small pores. Then the anti-species antibody coupled to enzyme needs to be added. This binding seems unlikely to occur through the pores of the gels. The other problems would be diffusion of the separated proteins, excessive amounts of reagents, lengthy washings and high backgrounds.

However if the biological activity should be studies, a technique called as zymography is done on the gels directly, using a simple technique of creating a replica copy of the separated proteins that was found on the PA gel on a membrane, the problems of accessibility would be solved. In addition other advantages of blotting include lowered volumes of reagents, easier handling of membranes compared to gels, increased local concentration of proteins as it is localized on to a narrow zone on the membrane and removal of SDS so that biological activity would be regained.

Membranes used for Western blotting include nitrocellulose (NC) or polyvinyl difluoride (PVDF). Nitrocellulose is a linear polymer of nitrate esters of cellulose. The level of nitration varies. High level of nitration is explosive but the membranes have a lower level of nitration and are still flammable. Several characteristitics of the membranes are detailed in Table 4.5.

Table 4.5: Membranes used for Western Blotting

Characteristics	***NC***	***PVDF***
Protein binding	100 ug/cm^2	300 ug/cm^2
Strength	Fragile	Sturdy
Solvent resistance	No	Yes
Binding in presence of SDS	Poor	Good
Rapid Immuno detection	No	Yes
Edman sequencing	No	Yes

Steps in the blotting include:

- The separated proteins are immobilized on the membrane by transfer (Transfer process)
- Vacant sites on the membrane are blocked
- Addition of primary and enzyme labeled secondary antibody
- Substrate addition, colour development and visualization of bands.

Transfer is normally carried out by solvent flow/capillary transfer or application of electric field. Capillary transfer by drawing the molecules out of the gel onto a membrane is achieved by drawing the solvent through the gel thereby dislodging the molecules that in turn is trapped by the membrane placed just above the gel. This is possible with agarose gel with its larger pore size but not so applicable for smaller pored PA gels and proteins.

Electro blotting is applicable for proteins wherein, the gels and the membranes re-sandwiched between supports that have electrodes on each side to provide an electric field across the gel. The electric field drives the molecules out of the gel and they get trapped by the membrane. In electro blotting systems, the distance between the electrodes are small but the surface area is large, hence the current is high and the transfer times are longer. Under electro blotting both 'wet' and 'semidry' methods are used. The wet systems uses large volumes of buffer and is vertical in arrangement. The semidry systems have only buffer in the thick filter papers and are horizontal. The wet systems have better temperature control and transfer of low, medium and high molecular weight proteins are possible. Semidry systems can provide higher voltage gradients than wet systems and hence rapid transfers are possible. In semi-dry blotting the electrodes are placed directly in contact with the gel/nitrocellulose membrane sandwich ensuring a fast, efficient transfer and a only minimum requirement of transfer buffer for equilibration of the gel and membranes (hence the term 'semi-dry').

Assembly of the Western blotting cassette is as follows:

(a) Positive side gel cassette, (b) Scrotch brite pad, (c) Sponge, (c) 2 pieces of blotting paper, (d) Membrane, (e) Gel, (f) 2 pieces of blotting paper, (g) Sponge, (h) Scotch brite pad, and (i) Negative side of the gel cassette.

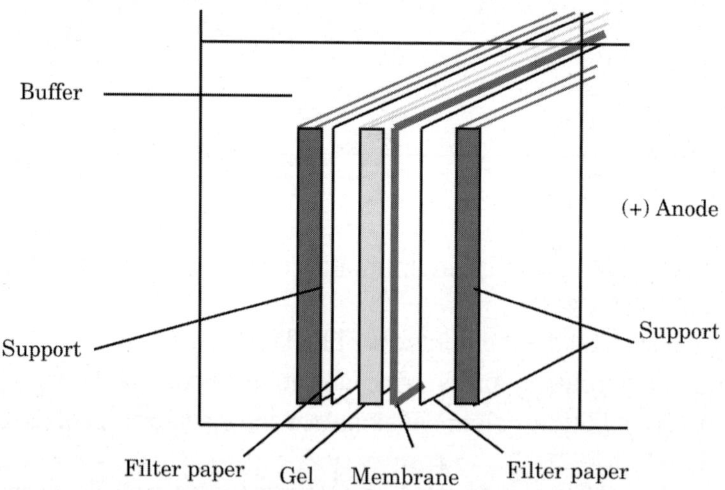

Fig. 4.9: Arrangement for 'wet' western blotting.

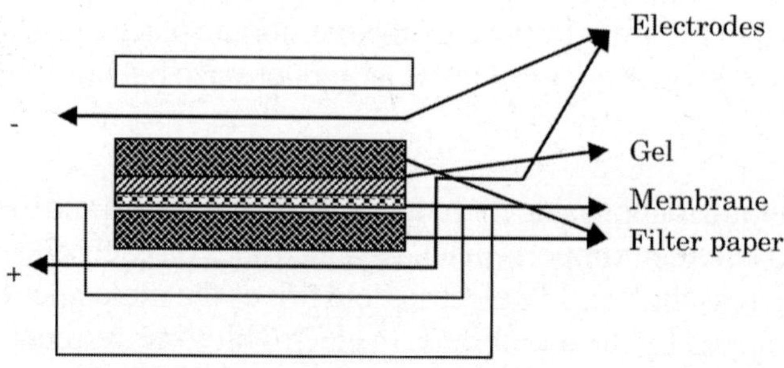

Fig. 4.10: Arrangement for 'semi dry' western blotting.

Extreme care should be taken to avoid air bubbles between any layers since the bubbles would prevent transfer of proteins in that area.

The transfer buffer used should have

- Good buffering capacity (hence concentrations ate often about 20 mM)
- Low conductivity and heating (low dissociation species such as Tris or HEPES and not phosphate useful)
- Low reactivity (Glycine inclusion not recommended if used for amino acid analysis)

- Neutral pH to minimize sample changes
- Addition of methanol to enhance binding of proteins to NC membranes

The common transfer buffer is 25 mM Tris, 192 mM glycine with 0.1% SDS and 20% methanol.

During Western blotting two opposing systems are in operation–one force needs to pull out the proteins from the pores of the PA gels, the other requirement is to bind the dislodged proteins onto membranes. If we give high current expecting to pull out all the proteins, it is possible that the dislodged proteins pass through the membranes also into the buffer. If we favour conditions that bind proteins to the membrane it is possible that a lot of proteins get retained in the gel itself. Thus, inclusion of SDS in buffers would favour movement of proteins out of the gel by making the proteins more negative charged but the binding to NC is decreased since the binding is hydrophobic. Similarly addition of methanol would aid binding of proteins to NC membrane by displacement of SDS and reduction in charge but would retard movement out of the gel since the gel shrinks thereby reducing the pore size further. What is the remedy under such situation. Optimization of transfer conditions for each proteins being handled. It needs to be optimized for the proteins you intend to transfer and is largely dependent on the size and nature of the proteins.

Efficiency of transfer can be assessed by many ways before probing the membrane

1. Following transfer the membrane can be stained with dyes such as Ponceau S but it has limited sensitivity
2. Staining of the transferred gel with Coomassie blue to ensure there is no protein bands left on the gel
3. Use of pre stained single colored or rainbow markers that can be directly visualized on the membranes.

Once the proteins are efficiently transferred onto the membrane, the unbound sites need to be blocked so that the primary or secondary antibody does not bind directly onto the membrane but only through the protein fraction. This is normally achieved by the addition of unrelated inert proteins or non-ionic detergents that would not interfere with the immunological reaction. The blocking agent should have a greater affinity for the membrane than the antibodies. It should not displace the target protein from the membrane. The most common blocking agents used are bovine serum albumin (BSA, 0.2–5.0%), non-fat milk, casein, gelatin, and dilute solutions of Tween-20 detergent (0.05–0.1%). Other detergents, such as Triton X-100, SDS and Nonidet P 40, are sometimes used but can disrupt interaction between proteins. The blocker should result in a high signal to noise ratio, which is measured as the signal obtained with a sample containing the target analyte as compared to a sample with out the target analyte.

It is also recommended to use the serum from the species in which the secondary antibody is prepared. After blocking the primary antibody (mAb to be tested) is added, if using a tissue culture fluid at high concentrations, neat fluids (low dilutions) or appropriately diluted if using ascitic fluids.

Secondary antibodies depend on the species of animal in which the primary antibodies are made. If testing mouse mAbs, secondary antibody must be anti-mouse antibody obtained from a host other than mouse is used. The optimal dilution of the secondary antibody needs to be determined experimentally by titration; however $^1/_{100}$ to $^1/_{500000}$ dilutions can be used beginning from a 1mg/ml stock. The principle of western blotting is illustrated in (Figs. 4.11 and 4.12).

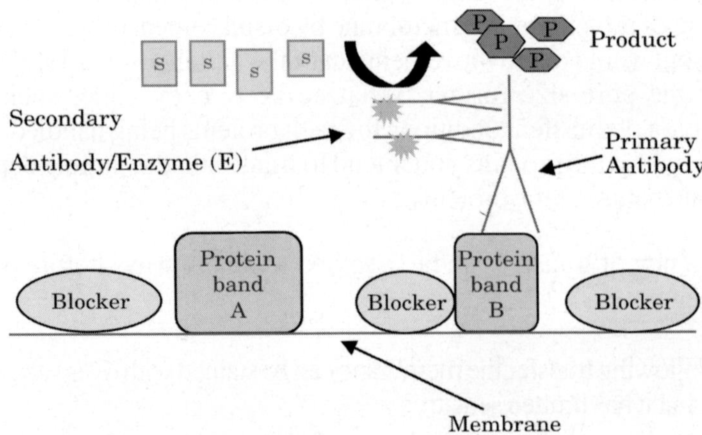

Fig. 4.11: Principle of western blotting.

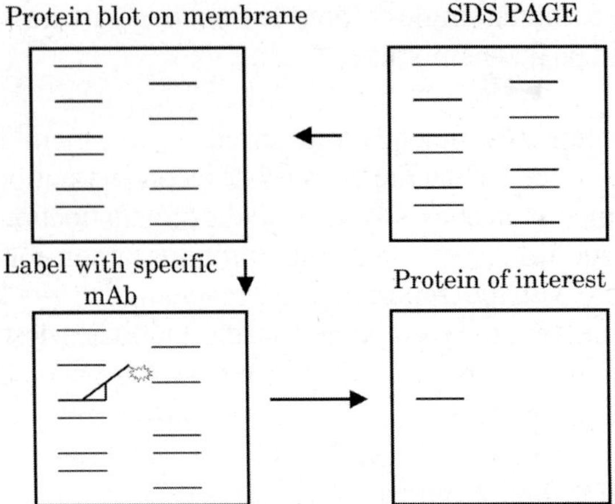

Fig. 4.12: Western blotting-method.

4.4.1 Antibody labels

Many types of labels can be coupled to antibodies radioisotopes require special handling, have short half-life and are expensive Other labels include biotin, fluorophores and enzymes The two most commonly used enzymes include alkaline phosphatase (AP) and horse radish peroxidase (HRPO). AP is 140 kDa and has a pH optimum at 8–10 HRPO is 40 kDa and has a pH optimum at 5–7. AP catalyzes the hydrolysis of phosphate groups from a substrate molecule resulting in a coloured or fluorescent product or release of light. HRPO catalyses the oxidation of substrates by hydrogen peroxide resulting in a coloured or fluorescent product or release of light. Chromogenic substrates get converted in to insoluble coloured product that precipitates on the membrane where the enzyme has been bound.

Substrates used with HRPO include 3, 3' diaminobenzidine tetra hydrochloride (DAB) brown bands, 3, 3', 5, 5' tetra methyl benzidine (TMB) Blue bands, 4-chloro – 1- napthol (CN) blue-purple bands.

Substrates used with AP include nitro-blue tetrazolium chloride (NBT), 5-bromo 4-chloro 3'indolyl phosphate p-toluidine salt (BCIP) and Fast Red.

Chemiluminescence is the process of release of energy from a substance in the form of light because of a chemical reaction. Oxidation of luminol by peroxide results in an excited state product called 3-aminophthalate. This product decays in to a lower energy state by releasing photons of light.

The chemiluminescent reactions differ from the chromogenic substrate reactions in that light detected is a transient product of the reaction that is only present when the enzyme-substrate reaction is occurring, while coloured precipitates remain on the membrane after the enzyme substrate reactions have terminated.

This label has recently become the method of choice for the following reasons

- High signal to noise ratio
- Rapid substrate processing of blots
- No health hazards
- Results are captured on X-ray films
- The X-ray film can be scanned using a CCD camera for quantitative analysis
- The probe can be stripped off and the membrane re probed.

4.4.2 Far western blotting

A far-Western is a blotting method designed to detect protein interactions. Like conventional Western blotting, the proteins are first transferred from gel to membrane. However, the probe in far-Western analysis is not an antibody, as in classical Western blot detection. Hence the term "*far*" was added. This is also known as ligand blotting or West-Western. The separated proteins are probed with a pure protein known to interact or putatively interact with one or more proteins transferred to the membrane. The protein probe or "bait" protein is isotopically labeled and the interaction with the "prey" protein is detected on the membrane.

4.5 Specificity of the Monoclonal Antibodies

The part of the antigen to which the developed mAbs bind is one of the important aspects of characterization of the mAbs. It can be done at different levels based on the requirement. For example, first it must be confirmed that the mAbs bind to our antigen of interest against which the mAbs was prepared and not to other related antigens. Then it is possible to determine the protein specificity of the mAb–find out to which protein on the target organism the mAb binds. At a slightly finer level, we can determine to which part of the protein mAb binds through a process of generation of deletion mutants. Finally it can be determined to which amino acids the mAb exactly binds (epitope). Although the ultimate binding site of a mAb would be a set of continuous or discontinuous amino acids of about 8–12 residues on the target antigen it may not be required to know the exact epitope that the mAb binds all the time.

For example, if mAbs were prepared against peste des petitis rumaints virus (PPRV), a virus affecting sheep and goats and belonging to the *Paramyxoviridae* family and Morbilli virus genus. The other members of the Morbilli virus include the rinderpest virus (RPV), measles virus, canine distemper virus (CDV) and some other dolphin and seal viruses also. If mAbs were prepared against PPRV for diagnosis, it needs to be ensured that it binds to some epitope on the PPRV which is not shared by other related viruses. Hence initial screening of clones can be done with the purified form of the whole virus. The positive clones need to be checked for cross-reactivity with the other viruses to ensure specificity of the mAbs to the antigen of interest.

As a further characterization requirement, it may be needed to know to what protein of the virus the mAbs are binding to. PPRV has six structural proteins, the nucleoprotein, haemagglutinin, polymerase, matrix proteins etc. This protein specificity of the mAbs can be identified using PAGE followed by western blotting.

The purified virus may be fractionated into individual proteins and western blotted on to a membrane. Then it would be probed with the mAbs followed by anti-mouse enzyme conjugate and an insoluble substrate (contrast it with a soluble substrate for ELISA). If a band of about 65 kDa is seen after Western blotting, it is likely that the mAbs binds to some epitope on this protein.

When this extra characterization of mAbs is needed?

Suppose you intend to develop an antigen capture ELISA for the detection of PPRV antigen. Then there is the requirement of a coating or capture antibody and a detection antibody. The coating antibody is first coupled to an ELISA plate followed by the addition of the sample suspected to contain the PPRV antigen. If the antigen is there in the suspected sample, it would get trapped by the coating antibody. Then the detection antibody is added which may be coupled to the enzyme. In such a case the coating and detection antibodies should bind to different epitopes.

If they are shown to bind to different proteins it obviously means that it is binding to different epitopes present in the respective proteins. For example, the coating antibody can be against the matrix protein and the detection antibody against nucleoprotein. In such instances, western blotting is sufficient evidence about protein specificity. But one point that should be rept in mind is that in SDS-PAGE the proteins are denatured and hence if the mAbs are directed against conformational epitopes then it would not bind to the relevant denatured protein. For instance, find that a clone is positive in ELISA while screening but negative in Western blotting then such a possibility exists.

This is after ensuring that there are no technical errors in the experiments performed which could be more likely the case.

Then how to find that?

Non denaturing polyacrylamide gels can also be tried. There are other techniques such as radio immuno precipitation wherein the antigen is labeled and allowed to bind to the antibody before any electrophoresis is done. For example, the PPRV is allowed to replicate in Vero (African green monkey cell line a permissive cell line for replication of PPRV) and labeled with ^{35}S methionine. Prior to labeling it is better to deplete the cell culture medium of methionine by using a methionine deficient medium that can be either prepared or is commercially available.

Now when the virus is replicating which means that the viral proteins are getting synthesized, the ^{35}S isotope would be incorporated. This would also happen with the cellular proteins that are being synthesized. Hence primarily we need to differentiate between viral and cellular proteins. Now allow the mAbs that you have prepared and are characterizing to react with this mixture of labeled proteins. This would bind to whatever proteins in which its epitope is present.

Now since the viral proteins are in its original conformation even mAbs against conformational epitopes would still bind to it. The labeled antigen/mAbs complex that is formed needs to be separated from the rest of the unbound antigen.

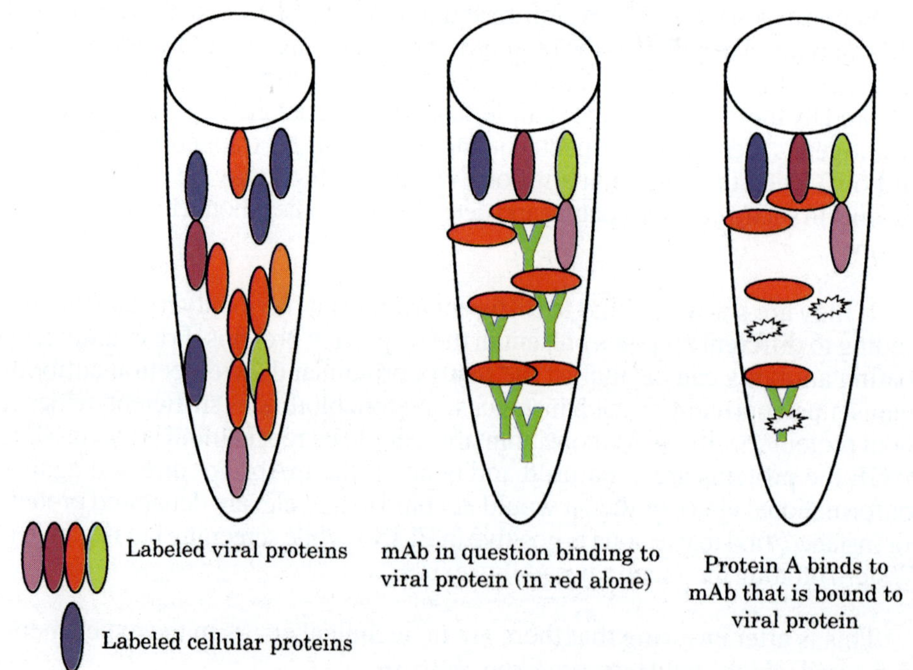

Fig. 4.13: Radio immuno precipitation assay

Since this complex is too small for separation by centrifugation (we need to centrifuge at 100000 g for separation of such complexes), with the aim of increasing the size of the complex, another molecule, mostly protein A is added that would bind to the mAbs or mouse antibodies through their Fc portion.

Now the labeled antigen-mAbs-protein A complex can be separated by centrifugation at around 15000 g in a normal refrigerated centrifuge. After adequate washing, to totally remove the unbound labeled antigen, it is run on a SDS-PAGE. Now from this complex what do you expect to see in SDS-PAGE?

Since this complex is denatured, you should see 4 bands, one band of the labeled antigen, two bands of the denatured mAb and one band of the protein A, provided you stain the gel.

The labeled viral protein + mAb + protein A sepharose is separated by pelleting and disrupted and run on PAGE to identify the protein specificity of mAb

However, it is unlikely that the antigen band is visible by staining because of its low concentrations. But if we use autoradiography, exposure to an X-ray, how many bands would be expected? Only one band that of the labeled antigen that got precipitated by the mAbs. The other mAbs and protein A bands are not visible since they are not labeled. Since a radio isotope was used to pull down a particular protein fraction to which the mAbs bind it is called radio immuno precipitation (RIPA) assay. Since the mAbs are allowed to bind before they are denatured for PAGE, it is possible to detect conformational epitopes.

This test is also sensitive as compared to Western blotting due to the use of radio label. In case we use a polyclonal serum against PPRV in the RIPA assay, how many bands would we expect?

If antibodies are available to all viral proteins, six bands should be seen. While using protein A also make sure whether it binds to the immunoglobulins of the species which you are using or not. Mouse antibodies bind protein A very well while chicken antibodies do not react with protein A. There are other proteins such as protein G or L that can be substituted. The other possibility is what if we do not have access to radio isotope and we need to use immunoprecipitation.

The viral proteins can be labeled using biotin instead of ^{35}S isotope and following western blotting it can be visualized with streptavidin peroxidase conjugate. There is also a technique that can combine immunoprecipitation and western blotting. Following viral infection in permissive cells, the cellular lysates are prepared and precipitated with the mAb to be tested and protein A/G. The unbound proteins are washed out. This complex of viral protein– mAb–protein A is denatured and loaded on to PAGE followed by western blotting. On PAGE, the viral protein band, denatured mAb and protein A bands would be seen, if the gel is stained.

After western blotting, the membrane is probed with hyper immune serum against the same antigen of interest and the anti-species enzyme conjugate in which the hyper immune serum has been prepared. This would light up only the antigen faction that has been pulled down by the mAb that was being tested and thus the protein specificity of the mAb can be established.

Table 4.6: Synposis of the Methods for Analysis of the Protein Specificity of the mAb

Western blotting	*Radio immunoprecipitation*	*Combined immunoprecipitation and western blotting*
Antigen isolation and purification	Radioactive labeling of antigen	No labeling of antigen–antigen captured by mAb followed by protein A

Table 4.6: *(Contd...)*

Table 4.6: (*Contd...*)

Western blotting	*Radio immunoprecipitation*	*Combined immunoprecipitation and western blotting*
SDS-PAGE	Antigen captured by use of mAb and protein A	Complex denatured and SDS-PAGE
Transfer on to membrane	Complex denatured and SDS-PAGE	Western blotting
Staining with mAb	Visualization by autoradiography/ fluorography	Probed with hyper immune serum against the antigen of interest and anti-species conjugate
Visualization of bands–enzyme substrate reactions		Visualization of bands–enzyme substrate reactions

4.5.1 Finding out to which part of the protein the mAb binds–use of deletion mutants

Once the protein specificity of the mAb is identified, the gene coding for the protein can be truncated into different portions by the use of appropriate restriction enzymes sites present in the particular gene and then used for cloning and expression in a suitable vector. The expressed proteins can be then western blotted and the reactivity of the mAb assessed.

Lack of immunoreactivity is taken as an indication that the site of deletion mutation was part of the epitope. For example the nucleoprotein gene of PPRV codes for 525 amino acids. Deleted mutants were prepared say be deleting the last 170 amino acids (mutant A–coding for the initial 355 amino acids of the N protein) and the first 130 amino acids (mutant B coding for the last 395 amino acids of the N protein). These deleted genes were cloned and expressed in a prokaryotic expression vector to produce appropriate sized protein products. When the mAb reactivity was assessed it was found that the mAb reacted with the original nucleoprotein (N) of 525 amino acids and also reacted with the mutant B but not with mutant A. This would mean that the epitope for the mAb lies in the stretch of 225 amino acids which is common to both the original protein and mutant B but not with mutant A. This technique can also be made more fine by mutating only a specific amino acid and looking for immuno reactivity to more precisely identify the epitopic region.

This information is one step ahead of the whole antigen (virus), whole protein (PPRV–Nucleoprotein) and the stretch of amino acids on the PPRV N protein to which the mAb was found to bind (225 amino acids), closer to the ultimate goal of finding the exact stretch of amino acids to which the CDRS of the heavy and light chain of the mAb binds. Overlapping peptides covering the entire sequence of the protein identified by the mAb can be prepared and the immuno reactivity of each peptide fraction can be determined in ELISA. This would help us to identify the exact sequence of the amino acids involved in mAb binding.

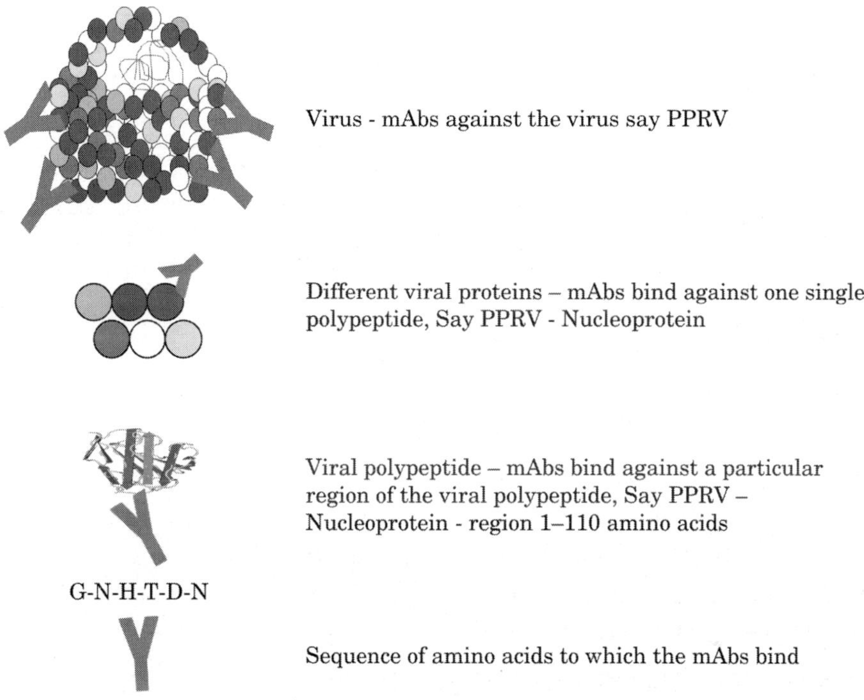

Fig. 4.14: Different stages of analyzing the protein specificity of the mAbs.

This is an expensive method since to look mAb binding to the now reduced 225 amino acid portion of the PPRV-N protein about 19 peptides need to be synthesized with an overlap of 8 amino acids as follows:

First 1–20 amino acids as one peptide, then 12–32 amino acids, 24–44 amino acids, 36–56 amino acids, 48–68 amino acids, 60–80 amino acids and so on till 204–224 amino acids and lastly 216–236 amino acids. With say immuno reactivity to say the third peptide (24–44 amino acids) and to the fourth peptide (36–56 amino acids) is only seen, then it would mean that the stretch of amino acids between 36–44 amino acids would be the most likely epitope for this mAb. This could for example be a stretch of amino acids 'WNPADYGG'. Thus at last we have determined the epitope specificity of the mAb being tested.

Most of the times this information is not required for direct application of the mAb in any diagnostic, therapeutic or research platforms.

It should also be borne in mind that the epitopes that are going to be presented and elicit an immune response would vary with the major histocompatability complex (MHC) of the animal being tested and obviously with the species being tested also.

4.6 Isotyping of Monoclonal Antibodies

The class and subclass of mAbs is important because several immunochemical and functional properties of antibodies depend on the isotype. Determination of the heavy chain isotypes is more important because the light chain isotype κ is the more abundant species comprising 95% with ë isotype being present only in 5% of mouse antibodies.

4.6.1 Why isotyping of mAbs is needed?

Isotyping of mAbs determines the following

- Applicability in particular immunoassays
- Protein A/protein G binding
- Methods for mAb purification and conjugation
- Complement binding
- Valency and avidity
- Kinetics of digestion with papain or pepsin
- Clearance from serum and half-life *in vivo*
- Detect contamination with any other antibody
- Control for lot-to-lot consistency
- Identify hybridoma switch variants

The protein A and G binding ability of mouse isotypes are:

Table 4.7: Protein A and Protein G reactivity of IgG of Human, Mouse and Rat

Species/sub-class	*Protein A*	*Protein G*
Human		
IgG1	++++	++++
IgG2	++++	++++
IgG3	–	++++
IgG4	++++	++++
Mouse		
IgG1	+	++++
IgG2a	++++	++++

Table 4.7: (*Contd...*)

Table 4.7: (*Contd...*)

Species/sub-class	*Protein A*	*Protein G*
IgG2b	+++	+++
IgG3	++	+++
Rat		
IgG1	–	+
IgG2a	–	++++
IgG2b	–	++
IgG2c	+	++

For purification of mAbs belonging to IgA and IgM gel exclusion or immunoaffinity separation columns is the method of choice. Mouse IgG2a and IgG2b are purified with immobilized protein A at pH 7–8, while mouse IgG1 binds best to protein A at pH 8-9. Immunoglobulin that contains kappa light chains can be purified using immobilized protein L.

Isotyping methods include double immuno diffusion, ELISA and lateral flow based methods and several commercial kits are available for this purpose. The main reagent needed for isotyping is class-specific antibodies capable of binding to a particular class and sub class of mouse heavy chains and class of light chains. This is mainly developed as a polyclonal serum using the individual heavy chain isotypes as immunizing antigen and adsorbing out any cross reacting antibodies that would be present using immuno globulins belonging to other isotypes.

This means the polyclonal serum raised against mouse IgG2a subclass should bind to only to epitopes present specifically in the IgG2a subclass of immuno globulins and should not cross react with epitopes present in any other isotype.

The conventional method of testing is the Ouchterlony (double diffusion) assay. This method uses a thin layer of agarose in which several wells are punched in a circular pattern around a centered well. The mAb to be isotyped is added in the central well and antiserum to the different isotypes is added in the peripheral wells. A precipitation line will form between the mAb well and one particular antiserum well indicates the isotype. This assay is inexpensive and simple to use. However, the sensitivity can be low and at least 24–48 hr may be required to obtain results. If a negative result is obtained, the proportion of the antigen–antibody (mAb–anti-isotype antibody) needs to be adjusted before a clear negative result is given, since disproportionate antigen antibody could also result in lack of precipitation line formation.

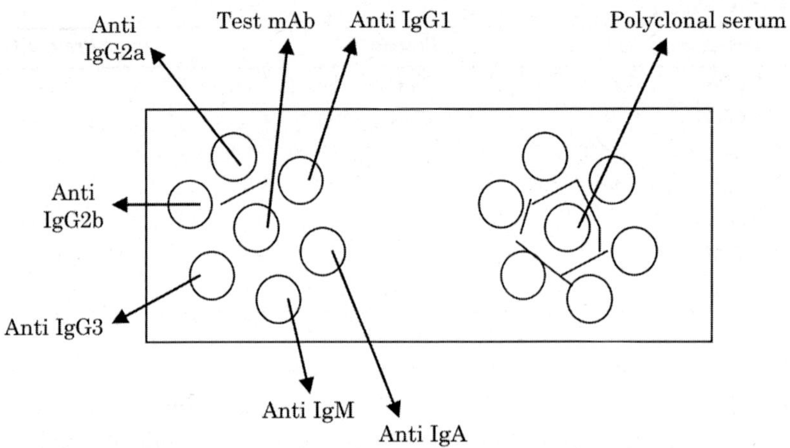

Fig. 4.15: Isotyping of mAbs in Ouchterlony immunodiffusion assay.

Lateral flow based assay based strips are available with strips containing immobilized antibody to mouse IgG1, IgG2a, IgG2b and IgG3 and also IgM and IgA and kappa and lambda light chain isotypes. If these pre coated strips are dipped in the mAb to be tested, a coloured line would be seen only in the particular isotype to which the mAb belongs.

The lateral flow assay, more commonly called as 'strip tests' or 'immuno chromatography assay' essentially consists of an absorbent pad, a capture zone and a control zone. The absorbent pad has the detector reagent impregnated onto it, which is the antibody against the target analyte (epitope 1) coated onto either coloured latex micro spheres or to colloidal gold. When the strip is dipped in the solution containing the potential analyte, the detector reagent binds to the antigen and moves laterally. It is then immobilized by the capture regent *i.e.* antibody against the target analyte (epitope 2) immobilised at the capture zone. Since the micro spheres are dyed, a line appears at the capture zone (if the antigen is present) simply due to the localization of the coloured antibody in a narrow zone (contrast it to the enzyme substrate system of the conventional ELISA). The control zone contains the species-specific anti-immunoglobulin against detector reagent. Some of the micro spheres cross the capture line and moves to the control line where they bind and produce a coloured line. This is needed to ascertain that the detector reagent has moved till the control line. Thus it acts as an internal control to ensure that the test is performing well. Hence the appearance of two lines, one on the capture zone and the other on the control zone indicates a positive result while only one line in the control zone indicates a negative result. If no line is seen in the control zone also, the test is invalid.

In the context of isotyping, the immobilized antibodies are the isotype specific ones and the anti-mouse immunoglobulin whole molecule is coupled to gold/latex beads. The mAb binds to this coloured immunoglobulin (irrespective of the subclass) and moves along till it meet the specific anti-subclass antibody (*e.g.* say anti-IgG2b) then it is captured there forming a coloured line.

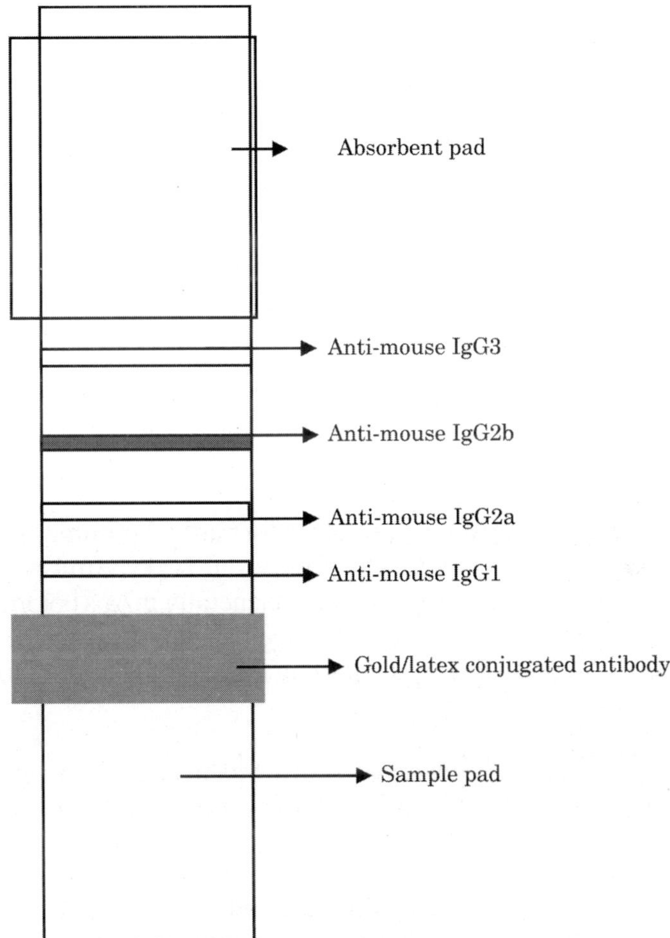

Fig. 4.16: Isotyping of mAbs using lateral flow assay.

ELISA based methods use coated anti-isotype antibodies to capture the mAb sample that is being tested and is detected using a anti-mouse Ig whole molecule enzyme conjugate which would bind to all the classes or subclasses of mouse immunoglobulin. If the well containing the anti-mouse IgG1 and the mAb sample added shows, colour development the mAb belongs to the IgG1 isotype.

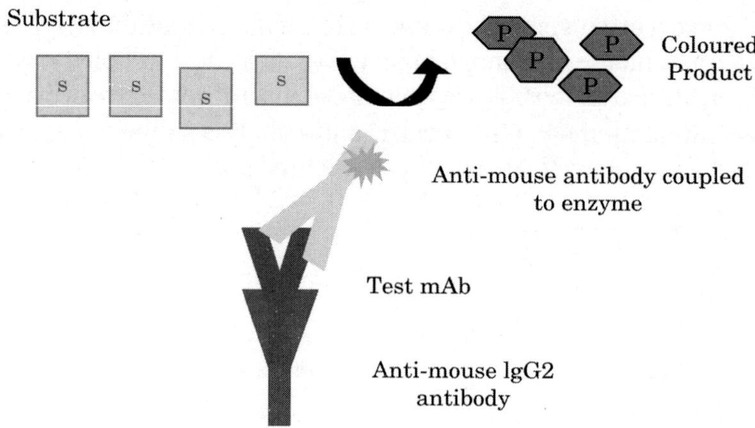

Fig. 4.17: Isotyping of mAbs in ELISA.

If mouse serum is added, which wells would show colour development?

All the wells since mouse serum would contain immunoglobulins belonging to IgG1, IgG2a, IgG2b, IgG3, IgM and IgA with either kappa or lambda light chain isotypes.

Particular isotype of mAbs are preferred for particular immuno assays. For example, if an agglutination test is to be performed, IgM isotype mAbs are preferred since IgM is a better agglutinating antibody. Generally mAbs belonging to IgG isotypes may not be useful in precipitation or agglutination assays since it is against a single epitope and have a lower valency that may not favour immune complex (lattice) formation.

If there is a particular requirement of mAb to a particular isotype, immunization protocols may be modified to favour such isotype availability after fusion and screening procedures.

Although one lymphocyte can produce antibody belonging to one particular class only, it is possible that two clones are present in the same well that is secreting mAbs belonging to the same isotype. Hence showing cell culture supernatants as belonging to a single isotype is not confirmatory evidence that the antibody is monoclonal.

The proof that the antibody is monoclonal can be achieved only by isoelectric focusing. The hybridoma clones can be labeled with ^{35}S methionine and used in the isoelectric focusing gel followed by autoradiography. A single family of bands is confirmatory evidence that the antibody is monoclonal.

4.7 Affinity of the mAbs

Affinity of mAbs is an important criterion for use in some applications which involves quick binding to the corresponding antigen such as lateral flow assays.

The only way to measure the affinity is to experimentally determine a binding curve. This involves measuring the amount of antibody-antigen complex as a function of the concentration of the free antigen. There are two common methods of performing this measurement:

i. *Equilbrium dialysis (haptens and small antigens)*: Antibody is placed inside a dialysis bag and hapten is added to the outside of the bag. When equilibrium is reached the excess hapten inside the bag is due to the formation of antibody-antigen complexes.

ii. *Surface Plasmon Resonance (Biacore)*: Antibodies are bound to a conductive surface, binding of antigen affects the electrical properties of conductive surface.

For a given concentration of antibody molecules, the greater the fraction of ligand bound by them, the greater the affinity for the ligand.

This value can be expressed as an association constant, *K*. At equilibrium

$$K = \frac{[Ab - Lg]}{[Ab][Lg]}$$

where the terms in brackets represent the concentration of:

- Antibody-ligand complexes [Ab–Lg],
- Unbound antibody [Ab], and
- Unbound ("free") ligand [Lg].

A more convenient form of this equation is the Scatchard equation

$$K = \frac{r}{(n - r)(c)}$$

where

- r = the ratio of the concentration of bound ligand to the concentration of antibody molecules placed in the system,
- n = the number of ligand binding sites on the antibody molecule (*i.e.*, its valence), and
- c = the concentration of unbound ("free") ligand.

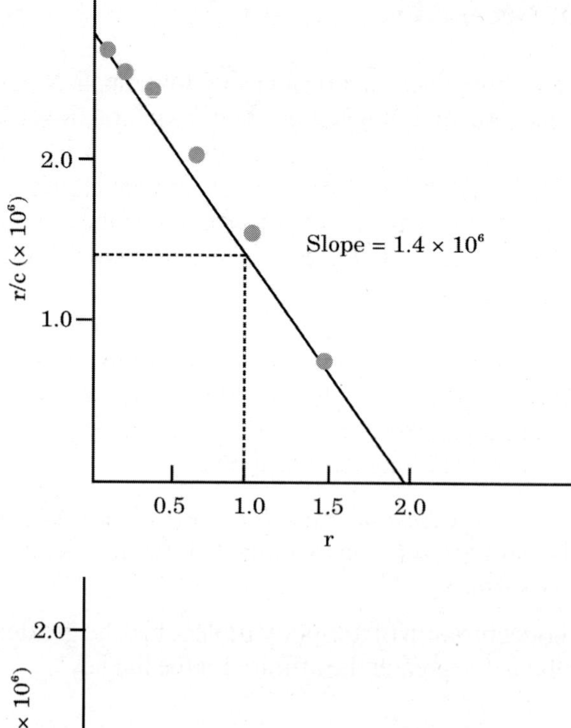

Fig. 4.18: Scatchard plot

A useful way of presenting the resulting data is to plot the ratio *r*/*c* as function of *r*. Such a graph is called a Scatchard plot and if K is constant, such a plot would produce a straight line, the slope of which is –*K*.

This Scatchard plot above with a hapten and mAb shows that the antibodies had an affinity for the ligand of 1.4×10^6 liters/mole (M^{-1}). In addition, it is seen from the graph that the maximum value for *r* (the *x* intercept) is 2. At infinitely high concentrations of ligand, each antibody molecule can bind a maximum of 2 ligand molecules; that is, the valence of these antibodies is 2.

They were IgG antibodies

If a polyclonal serum was used in such equilibrium dialysis, the heterogeneity of binding is also revealed by this Scatchard plot which reveals that the slope of the line is continuously changing as the concentration of ligand in the chambers increases.

Due to the heterogeneity of affinities in most antisera, average affinity (K_0) is used to characterize such reagents. K_0 is the value of K when the ligand concentration is such that one-half the antigen-binding sites are filled. For antibodies such as IgG whose valency is 2, this would occur when $r = 1$.

Thus,

$$K_0 \frac{1}{(2-1)c}$$

or $1/c$.

Thus, the average affinity is the reciprocal of the concentration of free ligand (c) when $r = 1$. This value can be read directly from a Scatchard plot because when $r = 1$, $r/c = 1/c = K_0$. For the antiserum tested above, $K_0 = 6.0 \times 10^5 M^{-1}$.

Often an antibody with a very high affinity for one epitope will have a substantial affinity for a related epitope as well. Such an antibody while highly efficient would actually have a low specificity.

4.7.1 Avidity measurement of serum

The differential assay for high avidity and low avidity antibodies can be used as an alternative or as complementary to the IgM antibody detection. In protein denaturing avidity ELISAs, the sample IgG is allowed to bind to its antigen, followed by elution with or without a protein denaturant such as diethyl amine. Diethyl amine dissociates weakly bound antibodies to their specific antigens but strongly bound antibodies remains intact. Thus the proportion of IgG remaining antigen-bound indicates the time of primary infection or occurrence of reinfection. But the most critical issue is the calculation of cut-off point between low and high avidity IgG responses.

An avidity index is calculated as

$$\text{Avidity index (\%)} \frac{\text{OD of wells with 35 mM diethyla min e}}{\text{OD of wells wash buffer (no DEA)}}$$

4.8 Characterization of the mAbs for intended use

This is the most critical requirement that is going to govern its applicability for the purpose for which it was prepared. The proof of the pudding is in the eating. Hence the mAb has to be tested ultimately in the assay format that is to be used with this highly specific reagent.

For example, if mAbs were to be prepared with an aim of differentiating PPRV from other closely related viruses in say an antigen detection method and an antibody detection method. Let us assume the antigen detection method would be a sandwich (antigen capture ELISA) and the antibody detection method would be a competitive or blocking ELISA.

The following steps are to be followed for development of cELISA for detection and quantitation of antibodies to PPRV in sheep or goat serum

1. Selection of mAbs suitable to the test system
2. Fixing of optimal dilutions of mAbs and test serum
3. Establishing a baseline cut-off value
4. Comparison of the performance characteristics with the gold standard (serum neutralization test)

4.9 Selection of mAbs

The mAbs can be titrated by the addition of different dilutions to antigen-coated plates an running an indirect ELISA. Choose the mAb giving higher OD values even at lower dilutions. Choose three dilutions of the mAb corresponding to 100%, 75% and 50% of the plateau (saturation) OD on the titration curve.

4.9.1 Fixing of optimal dilutions of mAbs and test serum

The criterion to be used for the selection of the optimal dilution of serum and mAbs would be the positive negative differential (P-N differential). The PN differential is calculated by the difference in the percent inhibition (PI) values in blocking ELISA of known PPR positive (SN positive) and known PPR negative (SN negative) serum samples.

The chosen dilutions of mAbs are to be tested against different dilutions of the serum. For each positive and negative serum dilutions (say 1:10; 1:20 and 1:50 dilutions) test 1:10, 1:50 and 1:100 dilutions of mAb. Then calculate the PN differential and plot with PN differential on the Y-axis and serum dilutions on the X-axis for each dilution of mAb. Identify the dilution of serum and mAb giving the maximum PN differential.

Once the dilutions are arrived at, try to do a preliminary testing with sera collected from sheep vaccinated with a known vaccine. This should result in increasing titres over time.

4.9.2 Establishing a baseline cut-off value

Calculate the mean PI values of thousands of known PPRV negative samples. Sera samples negative by the gold standard test (SN test) can also be used. Calculate the mean and standard deviation (SD) of these samples. Choose a cut off based on either mean and 2 times SD or mean and three times SD or twice the mean. This means that after determining the likely mean PI of many known negative samples, a buffer is given to rule out any possible higher mean PI values. Then a cut off is fixed to say that above this value a serum sample is positive for PPRV antibodies. Never forget that this cut-off value is a mathematical derivation and is likely to change as more samples are being tested. If the cut off fixed is 50% samples showing a PI of above 50% are positive. What if a sample is showing a PI of 49%? Would you consider that as a positive or negative sample?

In case of doubts, test another sample after a week or 10 days and if it shows an increase in PI value, the sample is surely a positive sample. If the cut-off values are fixed at a higher level, the specificity of the test increases but the sensitivity would come down. This means that the false positives are rare while false negative could occur. If the cut off is fixed at a lower value, the sensitivity would be higher but specificity would become lower. This means that the false positives can occur while false negative would be rare.

Comparison with the gold standard (serum neutralization test)

Test1 Test 2	*Positive*	*Negative*
Positive	a	b
Positive	c	d

The sensitivity, specificity and accuracy of the cELISA in detecting PPRV antibodies in the samples compared with the SN test can be calculated using a 2 × 2 contingency table using the following formula:

Sensitivity = a/(a+c),
Specificity = d/(b+d),

Accuracy = a+d/(a+b+c+d), where 'a' positive infected, 'b' positive uninfected, 'c' negative infected, and 'd' negative uninfected.

Example,

SN test cELISA	*Positive*	*Negative*
Positive	345	7
Positive	11	428

Sensitivity	=	345/356 = 96.9%
Specificity	=	428/435 = 98.4%
Accuracy	=	(345+428)/(345+7+11+428) = 97.7%

At a quantitative mode, correlation can also be made with PI values and SN attires and a correlation coefficient of close to 1.0 indicates better correlation between the two tests being compared. For use in immuno capture ELISA, one of the prerequisites of coating and detecting mAbs are that they should bind to different epitopes.

To determine whether mAbs recognize the same or different epitopes, alternate rows of an ELISA plate is coated with the purified antigen. Then it is incubated with different dilutions of unlabeled mAb followed by the addition of each biotinylated mAbs at 70 to 80% saturating concentration. After washing, the binding of biotinylated mAbs was detected using peroxidase-labeled streptavidin and substrate reduction as in any ELISA method.

The optical densities (OD) were converted to percent inhibition (PI) values for each mAb pair by using the following formula:

PI=[(100–OD with mAb pretreatment) × 100]/(OD without mAb pretreatment).

Two mAbs (*i.e.*, unlabeled and labeled) were considered to share (overlap) an epitope when 50% or higher reduction occurred.

The relative immunogenicity of each of the epitopes identified by the mAbs can also be measured using a blocking ELISA. First, ELISA plates are coated with the recombinant antigen (PPRV nucleoprotein) followed by the addition of anti-PPRV field caprine sera diluted low or high. Then the plates are incubated with each unlabeled mAb at 70 to 80% saturating concentration followed by peroxidase-conjugated anti-mouse immunoglobulins.

PI value for each serum was calculated by using the following formula:

PI = [(100–OD in the presence of test serum) × 100]/(Mean OD in the presence of negative sera).

When 50% or higher inhibition was observed, the epitope recognized by the mAb of interest was considered to be blocked.

The degree of immunogenicity of each mAb-reactive epitope is determined by comparing PI values of mAbs with 1:20 and 1:400 dilutions of PPR sera. When the binding of a mAb was blocked by 1:400 dilutions of the sera then it is likely that the epitope is highly immunogenic.

CHAPTER 5

MASS PRODUCTION OF MONOCLONAL ANTIBODIES

5.1 Expansion of the Hybridomas Secreting Monoclonal Antibodies

Once the hybrid cells are screened and cloned thrice, they are in 24–well or 96–well plates. They have to be expanded step-wise to higher surface area and larger volumes slowly ensuring all the time that they continue to secrete the mAbs of desired specificity (checked by screening assay) and also freezing a stock of cells, in case the cultures are contaminated or lost during the scaling-up process. Cells can be transferred from wells in 96-well plates (about 0.3 ml/well) to wells in 24 well plates (2–3 ml/well) and subsequently to 12 well and 6 well plates. Culture vessels with surface areas of 25 cm^2 (10 ml), 150 cm^2 and 225 cm^2 are available and can be used to grow the hybridoma cells.

Fill in the required quantity of the complete growth medium (with FCS, antibiotics and HT, if needed) in the 24-well plate. Then gently pipette out the cells from the 96-well plates and suspend it in the medium in the 24-well plate. But make sure that there are enough cells that can sustain growth in the larger surface area without the need for feeder cells. If the cell counts become low in relation to the surface area, the cultures would take a long time to establish and sometimes would be lost. The cells should be regularly fed with fresh medium based on the pH change and their growth.

The hybrid cells can grow vigorously that may quickly change pH, deplete nutrients and increase the waste products that could become toxic. Hence continuous monitoring of the growth with appropriate decisions to moving the cells to larger volumes would allow for continued vigorous cell growth and reduce the frequency of medium changes. Similar procedure may be followed for transfer from the 24-well plates in to $25cm^2$ flasks. Other specialized bulk culturing techniques (*e.g.*, roller bottles, hollow fiber, fermenters, etc.) can be employed if large quantities of antibodies are desired.

5.2 *In vivo* Production of mAbs

Although the original discovery of mAb production was an *in vitro* work; they did conjecture that hybridoma cells produced can be grown *in vitro* in massive cultures. Due to mouse myeloma cells being used as a fusion partner, it was possible to grow the hybrid cells producing desired mAbs in the abdominal cavity of histo compatible mouse, which was called the ascites production.

Since the mAbs could be produced in large quantities in the ascites fluids of mice without contaminating heterologous proteins such as FCS proteins and was viewed as a simple and inexpensive method, it became popular. But unfortunately the animal ethics was overlooked and with the greater availability of alternative methods that could also generate such high amounts of mAbs being produced and the availability of serum free medium, the ascites production has been almost totally replaced with alternative *in vitro* methods.

However, mice are still needed for immunization for production of mAbs and alternatives in the form of *in vitro* immunization procedures have not gained momentum except in case of human hybridoma where there is no other alternative.

For acsites production, the hybridoma cells are inoculated into the peritoneal cavity of the mice following pristine or incomplete Freund's adjuvant (IFA) priming. They grow so vigorously that the abdomen of the mouse becomes very swollen. The peritoneal fluid, containing hybridoma cells and a high concentration of antibodies are aseptically removed from the animal. The antibodies can be isolated from the fluid/cell mixture. The hybridoma cells can be cultured *in vitro*, if desired.

In addition to being a method for producing high concentrations of antibodies, inoculating the hybrid cells into the peritoneal cavity of mouse is useful for removal of contaminated cultures especially mycoplasma-contaminated hybridomas. The macrophages in the peritoneal cavity probably phagocytose the mycoplasma and cleanse the cultures. Continuous *in vitro* culturing of cells can be avoided and cells get invigorated facilitating better secretion of mAbs.

Pristane $C_{19}H_{40,}$ 2,6,10,14-tetramethylpentadecane is obtained primarily from shark liver oil from the Basking Shark (*Cetorhinus maximus*), from which its name is derived (Latin *pristis*, "shark").

Pristane facilitates tumour growth by suppressing the immunological function of the host. It also induces an inflammatory response recruiting immune cells which secrete growth promoting cytokines that may favour hybridoma cell growth. It also induces autoimmune diseases in rodents. Synthetic pristane is also available. BALB/c mice are preferred for ascites production since the myeloma cells have also been derived from it so there would be no rejection as they are histocompatible. Sometimes, F_1 crosses between BALB/c and SW or MF1 mice also are used.

7–11 weeks old male mice are preferred. It is thought that testosterone favours tumour production. Retired breeders whose abdominal musculatures have been stretched can be more useful for ascites production. 0.5 ml of pristine is injected intra peritoneally. 10^6 to 10^7 cells have to be injected. The time interval between pristine injection and cell inoculation can be 7–20 days.

Sometimes solid tumour formation is seen. It may also be related to the type of clone inoculated. However increasing the time period between pristane inoculation and cell injection may be tried (up to 24 weeks) with inoculation of higher number of cells (10 millions).

An alternative to pristane is IFA. Some of the advantages of IFA over pristine include:

- Injecting hybridoma cells as early as one day after IFA priming
- Less stress to the animal
- Fewer animals may be required.

Another agent used for priming for ascites production is the trypan blue.

Trypan blue must be dialyzed against distilled water for 48 hr before use for priming to reduce low molecular weight impurities. Priming with trypan blue is carried out 24 hr and again one hour prior to injection of the hybridoma cells.

About 3–5 weeks after injecting the cells into a pristane-primed mouse, the animal's abdominal area will be greatly distended. The cells and fluid in the peritoneal cavity will be ready for collection (Fig. 5.1).

The fluid can be tapped by inserting a sterile 18-gauge needle into the peritoneal cavity and allowing the peritoneal fluid (containing cells, including some red blood cells) to flow into a sterile 15 ml centrifuge tube that already contains a few mls of sterile balanced salt solution.

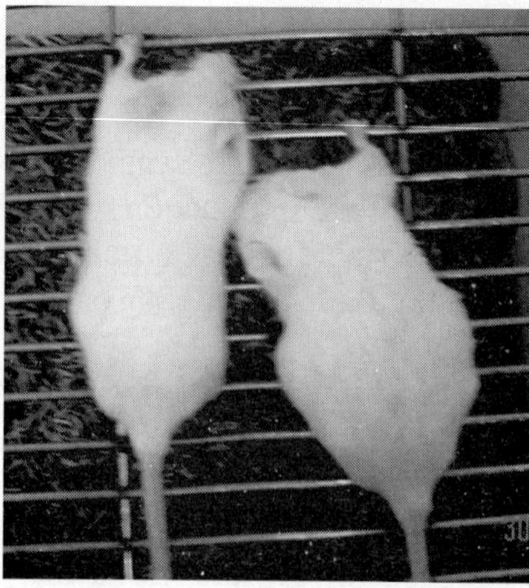

Fig. 5.1: BALB/c mice with ascites (see bulging of the abdomen).

The supernatant can be collected following centrifugation at 200 × g for 5 minutes for antibody testing. The cell pellet can be washed and transferred into culture flasks for further propagation. On an average, a mouse produces approximately 0.5–10 mg/ml of mAb in ascites fluid, and it is possible to harvest about 2 ml ascites fluid per tap. Based on these estimates, the number of animals that need to be used can be arrived at.

To rule out the presence of adventitious agents in the mAb-producing hybridoma cell lines, the mouse antibody production (MAP) test needs to be done.

This involves injecting a sample of cells/tissue into mice, and after 3–4 weeks, testing its serum for antibodies to a panel of known adventitious agents such as lymphocytic choriomeningitis virus, mouse hepatitis virus etc.

5.2.1 Advantages of ascites method

- High concentrations of mAbs are achieved so that further concentration procedures that could denature antibody are avoided.
- Heterologous serum contaminants possible in *in vitro* culture fluids are avoided
- Need for cell culture facilities for bulk production and technical expertise are not required

5.2.2 Disadvantages of ascites method

- Requires continuous supply of mice and daily observation
- Cause significant pain or distress in mice

- Requirement of laboratory animal facility
- mAb produced by *in vivo* methods can contain various mouse proteins
- Possibility of solid tumour formation with little or no ascites fluids

The chances of solid tumour formation can be avoided by collecting the non-attached tumour cells from the peritoneal lavage of the mice with solid tumours. Then such non-attached cells can be passaged and injected into another primed mouse for ascites production.

Despite these disadvantages, under some conditions *in vivo* method of ascites production is still favoured because hybridomas are 'idiosyncratic' and *in vitro* methods are not always suitable. Some of the occasions when ascites production is necessitated are listed below.

- *In vitro* methods produce mAb from over 90% of hybridomas but the rest 10% may require *in vivo* growth
- When concentrated mAbs are needed for *in vivo* protection or therapeutic assays or blocking a receptor ligand interaction
- When purification techniques need to be avoided since purification may result in loss of biological activities such as complement binding
- Some rat hybridoma cell lines do not generate ascites efficiently in rats, but does so in immunocompromised mice
- The amount of production of mAbs by some hybridoma cell lines is reduced under serum-free or low serum concentration conditions
- The positions of glycosylation of mAbs vary between culture and ascites that could alter the epitope binding characteristics
- Contamination of yeast or mycoplasma can be removed by passage of hybrid cells through mice peritoneal cavity

The bulk production of mAbs using ascites method should be avoided unless shown to be absolutely necessary.

5.3 *In vitro* Production of mAbs

As an alternative, *in vitro* methods of mAb production are available; such alternative *in vitro* methods should possess the following characteristics.

- Should be equally or less expensive,
- Does not require special culture conditions,
- Produce high concentrations of mAbs,
- Be free from contamination,

- Require a short period of time to produce,
- Produce relatively pure mAbs in adequate quantities.

The *in vitro* method of mAb production is largely driven by the application of the mAb that in turn determines the quantity and purity of the mAb required

In vitro systems for mAb production include:

- Single compartment systems that permits low-density cell culture
- Double compartment systems that allows high-density cell culture, which results in increased mAb concentration.

Based on production requirements a range of *in vitro* culture options are available, that can be classified as

- For very small-scale production (< 10 g) the simple low density cell culture systems are used. Examples include culture flasks, roller bottles, spinner flasks, gas permeable bags and hollow-fiber bioreactors.
- For small-scale and medium-scale production (10–100 g), double-compartment, high-density cell-culture systems are used. Examples include hollow-fiber systems.
- For high-scale production (> 100 g) homogenous suspension culture systems are used. Examples include large deep-tank stirred fermenters, perfusion-tank systems, airlift reactors.

If limited quantities of mAbs are needed, hybridoma cells can be grown in stationary cell cultures in a variety of flasks ranging from 25 cm^2 to 175 cm^2 and bottles in different batches. Typical cell yields from a 175cm^2 flask range from 1×10^7 cells for an attached line to 1×10^8 for a suspension line. However exact yields depend on the particular cell line. Cells are grown in conventional tissue-culture flasks under standard growth conditions for about 10 days and mAbs are then harvested from the medium.

The following table presents the surface area of conventional cell culture flasks.

Table 5.1: Various Cell culture Dishes Available for Culture of mAbs at Various Stages

Dishes	*Surface area (mm^2)*	*Seeding density ($\times10^6$ cells)*	*Cells at confluency ($\times10^6$ cells)*	*Growth media (ml)*
6 well plate	962	0.3	1.2	3–5
12 well plate	401	0.1	0.4	1–2
24 well plate	200	0.05	0.2	0.5–1.0
T 25 flasks	2500	0.7	2.8	3–5
T 75 flasks	7500	2.1	8.4	8–15
T 160 flasks	16000	4.6	18.4	15–30

Such cultures produce mAbs generally below 20 mg/ml. Most research applications require mAb concentration of 0.1–10 mg/ml, much higher than mAb concentrations in batch tissue-culture methods.

5.3.1 Advantages of batch culture method of producing mAbs

- Technically easy to perform
- Low startup costs
- Have a start-to-finish time of 3 weeks
- mAb concentrations similar to that produced in ascites fluids but albeit in large volumes of fluids.

5.3.2 Disadvantages of batch culture method of producing mAbs

- mAb present in large volumes of tissue-culture media
- Contaminating bovine immunoglobulins (from FCS) present unless serum-free media are used
- Concentration of mAb is low
- Possibility of denaturation of mAbs during downstream purification methods.

Modifications of mAb production methods involve:

- Improved nutrient supply and waste removal,
- Improved stirring,
- Continuous mAb harvesting, and
- Increased hybridoma cell densities.

Using methods to increase the concentration of dissolved oxygen in the medium, increased cell viability and hybridoma cell density can be achieved thereby increasing the mAb concentrations.

Some techniques are used in roller bottles and spinner flasks that keep the culture medium in constant circulation and thus permit nutrients and gases to distribute more evenly in large volumes of cell-culture medium.

Roller bottles are cylindrical vessels that revolve slowly (between 5 and 60 revolutions per hr) which bathes the cells that are attached to the inner surface with medium. Roller bottles are available typically with surface areas of 1050 cm^2.

Spinner flasks are either plastic or glass bottles with a central magnetic stirrer shaft and side arms for the addition and removal of cells and medium, and gassing with CO_2 enriched air. Inoculated spinner flasks are placed on a stirrer (100–250 revolutions per minute) and incubated under the culture conditions appropriate for the cell line.

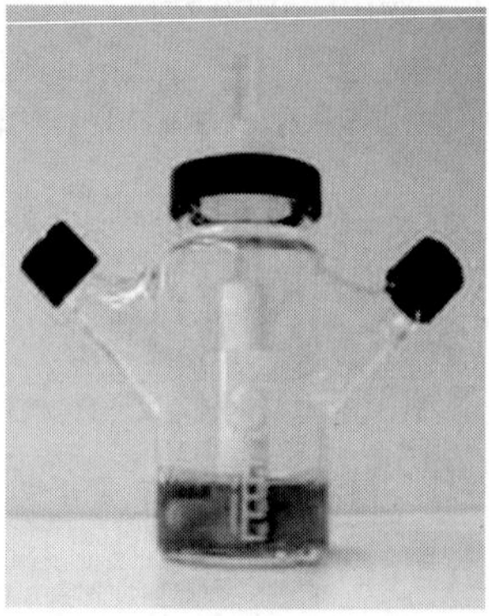

Fig. 5.2: Spinner flask.

In semi-permeable membrane based systems, the hybridoma cells and mAb are produced in a small chamber that is separated by a semi-permeable membrane barrier from a larger compartment that contains the culture media.

Hollow fibers are generally made of cellulose and have a molecular weight cutoff of 45–50 KDa, well below that of immunoglobulin.

This compartmentalization makes it possible to achieve mAb concentrations comparable with those in mouse ascites by the growth of hybridoma cells to high densities (> 10^8 cells/ml). Additional advantages include supplementation of medium with numerous growth factors for optimal growth of the hybridoma, replacement of the medium without affecting the cells, harvesting of the cells and mAbs independently of the growth medium, less or no contamination with FCS. A disadvantage is that the mAb may be contaminated with dead cell products and the technical requirement is larger than batch culture methods.

The hollow-fiber cartridge is composed of semi permeable multiple fibers that run through a chamber that contains hybridoma cells. The hollow-fiber bioreactor consists of a hollow-fiber cartridge, gas-permeable tubing that oxygenates the media, and a medium reservoir from which the medium is continuously pumped through the circuit. The cell can be grown at very high densities, start up costs are high and involved higher degree of technical expertise but yields are as high as 500 mg mAbs.

The essential requirements of a fermenter include automated sterilizing the vessel and process control of temperature, pH, stirring speed and dissolved oxygen. Only if cultures are maintained homogenously, high transfer rates of nutrients and metabolites can be maintained. Hence, mixing needs to be achieved without affecting the sensitive hybridoma cells. This is done either by a stirrer or by a directed flow of gas. Fermenters using continuous gas flow such as air lift reactors are more acceptable since they do not require motors and agitators.

Normally, a bioreactor is inoculated once with cells and during further culturing no other substances are added. This is called batch culture. The cell densities achieved are lower, about $1–2 \times 10^6$ cells/ml. In the fed-batch method, nutrients are added continuously or at intervals which lead to higher cell densities. In split batch fermenters, the initial cell density is maintained during the exponential growth phase.

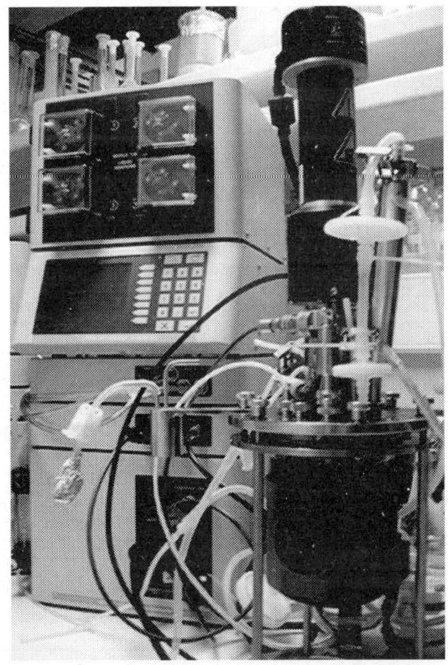

Fig. 5.3: A fermentor used for bulk production of mAb.

Compact autoclavable or disposable fermenters are available now. For example, BIOSTAT® A plus and BIOSTAT® CultiBag STR 200 stirred tank disposable system from Sartorius, CELL-tainer® disposable bioreactor.

Table 5.2: Characteristics of Hollow fibre and fermenter systems for Bulk production of mAbs

Characteristics	*Hollow fibre*	*Fermenter*
mAb production	Medium amounts	Large amounts
Medium requirement	High	Low
Inoculation density required	High	Low
On line measuring techniques	Not present	Available
Usage	Continuous	Continuous and discontinuous
Running costs	High	Low

5.3.3 Advantages of *in vitro* methods

- Animal welfare considerations applied
- Better reproducibility and ease of production
- mAb concentrations as high as those found in ascitic fluid can be produced
- mAbs are free of mouse ascitic fluid contaminants

5.3.4 Disadvantages of *in vitro* method

- Some hybridomas do not grow well in culture
- Supplementation with FCS required mostly that can limit its applications
- Batch culture methods have lower concentrations of mAbs that require down stream purification that may alter affinity or denature mAbs
- Membrane based methods achieve high concentrations of mAbs but could be contaminated with dead cells and their products
- mAb glycosylation can vary during *in vitro* growth as compared to *in vivo* production
- *In vitro* culture methods are generally more expensive than the ascites method for small-scale or medium-scale production of mAb
- Validation of mAbs produced by *in vitro* methods can be cost prohibitive
- Mechanical failure and microbial contamination possible.

Table 5.3: Characteristics of Various Production Systems for Bulk Production of Cells

Production system	*Culture type*	*Maximum density (× 10^6 cells/ml)*	*Concentration (mg/ml)*	*Production time required (weeks)*
Ascites	*In vivo*		< 20	2–3
Cell culture flasks	Static	0.5–1.0	0.01–0.03	2–6
Roller bottle	Stirred	1–2	0.01–0.05	2–6
Spinner flasks	Stirred	1–2	0.01–0.1	2–3
Membrane (dialysis)	Stirred	10–20	0.1–0.3	2–4
Hollow fibre		100–1000	0.5–1.0	3–12
Batch fermenter	Stirred	1–2	0.01–0.03	2–6
Split batch	Stirred	0.5–1.0	0.01–0.03	2–6
Fed batch	Stirred	2–3	0.03–0.1	2–6
Air lift ferementer	Gas agitated	1–5	0.1–0.4	2–6

Some of the commercial devices available for *in vitro* production of mAbs include:

***Stationary suspension culture system*:** CELLine 1000 from Integra Biosciences, Switzerland. This membrane-based disposable cell culture system is composed of two compartments, a cultivation chamber (20 ml) and a nutrient supply compartment (1000 ml) separated by a semi permeable dialysis membrane (10 kDa molecular weight cut-off), which allows small nutrients and growth factors to diffuse to the production chamber. Oxygen supply of the cells and CO_2 diffusion occur through a gas-permeable silicone membrane. Antibodies concentrate in the production medium. This culture system requires to be used in a CO_2 incubator.

***Rotation suspension culture systems*:** Mini PERM from Vivascience, Germany –This is a modified roller bottle two-compartment bioreactor in which the production module (35 mL) is separated from the nutrient module (450 mL) by a semi permeable dialysis membrane. Nutrients and metabolites diffuse through the membrane, and secreted antibodies concentrate in the production module. Oxygenation and CO_2 supply occur through a gas-permeable silicone membrane at the outer side of the production module and through a second silicone membrane extended into the nutrition module. The miniPERM must be placed on a roller base inside a CO_2 incubator.

***Hollow fiber bioreactor systems*:** Cell-Pharm® system 100 (CP100) from Bio-Vest, USA is a fully integrated 0.14 m^2 hollow fiber cell culture system. It does not require a CO_2 incubator because air and CO_2 bottles are connected directly to the system while temperature and pH (air/CO_2 flow) are set on the control unit. The cell culture unit consists of two cartridges: one that serves as a cell compartment and the other, as an oxygenation unit.

Fiber cell from Fibercell Systems Inc., USA is a hollow-fiber cell culture system is composed of a culture medium reservoir (250 ml) and a 60-ml fiber cartridge (1.2 m^2), both connected to a single microprocessor-controlled pump. It is possible to prolong the media supply cycles by replacing the original medium reservoir with a 5 litre flask. In contrast to the Cell-Pharm® systems, the Fiber Cell bioreactor is used inside a CO_2 incubator. Oxygenation occurs by gas permeable tubing.

Tecnomouse from Integra Biosciences, Switzerland is a cell production unit that provides separation of cultivation (12 ml) and nutrient (10 litre) chambers via hollow fibers in combination with two thin gas-permeable silicone membranes to enable oxygenation. Tecnomouse is the only compartmentalized system in which five different hybridoma cell lines can be cultured in parallel in separate cell culture cassettes. A single cassette should be inoculated with 400×10^6 cells. The system can be used as basic equipment running in a CO_2 incubator. With the thermohood accessory, no extra incubator is required for the cell unit. One Tecnomouse bioreactor fits into a standard 180 litre CO_2 incubator. The system requires skilled personnel and a large starting investment, is well suited to for applications requiring 200–1000 mg of mAb.

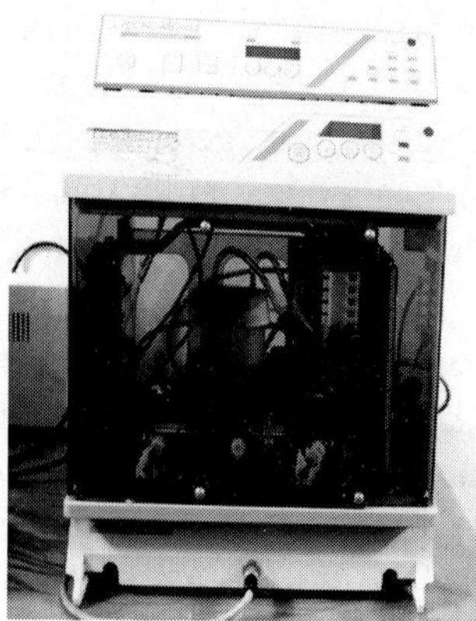

Fig. 5.4: Tecnomouse system for bulk production of mAbs.

5.4 Serum-free Media

Serum-free media (SFM) are media designed to grow a specific cell type or perform a specific application in the absence of serum. The use of SFM allows cell culture to be performed with a defined set of conditions without the variable components present in the FCS. Use of SFM does not require supplementation with serum, but may contain certain other discrete proteins or growth factors.

The use of serum containing medium is not preferable in mAb production because

- FCS has undefined composition that varies with batches
- Contamination with bovine immunoglobulins of about 50μg/ml
- Interferes with down stream purification strategies
- Prone to virus and mycoplasma contamination
- FCS is expensive

5.4.1 Advantages of SFM

- Defined media
- High reproducibility
- Easier purification and downstream processing
- Increased growth of cells and mAb production

SFM is prepared containing additives such as selenium, insulin, transferring and ethanolamine, purified serum fractions such as human or bovine albumins, lipid sources, growth factors, brain pituitary extract, colostrums fractions, cytokines and trace elements.

The application of SFM needs to be optimized for every hybridoma clone using criteria of cell growth, clone stability and above all mAb productivity.

A rich basal medium is used such as DMEM/F 12 at 1:1 ratio and the additives added should be tried empirically. A thumb rule would be

Insulin	=	0.1 to 10 µ/ml
Transferrin	=	0.5–100 µ/ml
Selenium dioxide	=	10–10 0 µM
Ethanolamine	=	5–20 µM
2-mercaptoethanol	=	1–10 µM
Albumin extract	=	0.2–5 mg/ml
Linoleic acid	=	0.05–5 µ
LDL	=	0.1–2 µ

Although in most cases, hybridomas growing in 10% FCS can be adapted within four passages to grow in less than 1% FCS or in FCS-free media some cells may never adapt to the low FCS media or may produce lesser quantities of mAbs under the serum-limited conditions. Adaptation is done by reducing the serum content slowly over a number of passages.

CHAPTER 6

PURIFICATION OF MONOCLONAL ANTIBODIES

6.1 Introduction

The principles and methods of purification of any protein are by and large suitable for the purification of mAbs also. The key questions that need to be answered before making a choice of the appropriate protein purification strategy are:

What is the protein required for? For example in the case of mAbs whether it is to be used for diagnosis or therapy. The presence of other contaminating proteins in the purified mAb preparation is permissible as long as it does not interfere with the diagnostic method. However for therapy the aim is to totally get rid of the mAbs of any other contaminating proteins since their presence may lead to antibody production and may lead to anaphylactic shock next time the antibodies may be administrated.

What is the source of proteins? In case of mAbs whether purification has to be attempted from culture supernatants or from ascitic fluids?

What is known about the protein and its assay criterion? Purification strategies could depend upon the isotype of the mAbs and how is the purification efficiency (specific activity) going to be measured. The other determinants to be considered before embarking on a purification strategy include the time taken and the cost of the procedure.

Purification would also involve a series of steps and the more the steps the lower the yields but the purity would be higher. Specific activity of the protein and the total activity may or may not be the same in all instances.

For example while purifying a virus grown in cell culture that was maintained in FCS, then cell lysates would contain viral proteins, cellular proteins and those in the FCS. Total protein concentration measurement would indicate the value for the mixture of all the above proteins. But if you are interested only in the viral proteins, this measurement is not ideal. You should go for a measurement assay that is based on only the viral property such as haemagglutination titre.

Similarly, while purifying mAb from culture supernatants the measurement of activity of mAbs alone using ELISA would be a better measure than total protein concentrations. Specific activity

$$\text{Specific activity} = \frac{\text{Protein of interest (mg)}}{\text{Total protein (mg)}}$$

$$\text{Degree of purification} = \frac{\text{Spefific activity at step 2}}{\text{Specific activity at step 1}}$$

The choice of purification steps required is determined based on the following criteria:

- Purification factor should be greater than 5
- Yields should be more than 30%
- A single step should be not more than 24 hr
- The enriched fractions may must be loaded directly into the next step without laborious intermediate treatments.

This chapter deals with the purification methods of proteins in general followed by methods for purification of antibodies. The purification methods for proteins are also applicable for mAbs and also for purifying antigens against which mAbs are prepared.

6.2 Total Protein Estimation Methods

This is dealt with earlier in Chapter 1, Section 1.5.1. However concise information is presented here for continuity for analysis of the purification strategies employed.

Spectrophotometry

Most proteins have an absorption maximum at 280 nm due to the phenolic group of tyrosine and the indolic group of tryptophan. Although this is relatively an insensitive method, it is rapid and gives a clear idea of the concentrations. The absorbance of the sample at 260 nm is also measured to rule out interference with purine and pyrimidine rings of nucleic acids and a correction factor is employed.

$$\text{Protein (mg/ml)} = 1.55\ A_{280} - 0.76\ A_{260}$$

While amino acids absorb at 280 nm, the peptide bonds absorb at 205 nm. Using a correction factor for tryptophan and tyrosine content by measurement at 280 nm, the concentration can be estimated using the formula

$$E\frac{1\,mg/ml}{205} = 27.0 + 120 \times \frac{A280}{A205}$$

Biuret method

Under alkaline conditions, copper ion binds to peptide nitrogen and produces a purple colour with an absorption maximum at 540–560 nm. The Biuret reagent contains copper sulphate, sodium potassium tartrate and sodium hydroxide. Tris buffers and ammonia interferes with the Biuret reaction hence may not be applicable for fractions after ammonium sulphate precipitation.

Lowry method

The basis of this reaction is the Biuret reaction of proteins with copper under alkaline conditions and the Folin–Ciocalteau phosphomolybdicpho- sphotungstic acid reduction to heteropolymolybdenum blue by the copper catalyzed oxidation of aromatic acids. The reaction results in a strong blue colour and is more sensitive than Biuret method. This reaction is interfered with by different types of detergents that are normally used to solubilize proteins.

Bicinchoninic acid procedure

The BCA assay for total protein is a spectophotometric assay based on the alkaline reduction of the cupric ion to the cuprous ion by the protein, followed by chelation and color development by the BCA reagent.

(A=562 nm)

Cu^{2+} ions reduced to Cu^{1+} ions by aromatic amino acids in protein. Cu^{1+} ions + Bicinchoninic Acid ® Complex is formed with intense absorption maximum at 562 nm. BCA assay has a good combination of sensitivity and simplicity.

Dye binding procedure

The acidic and basic groups of proteins interact with the dissociated groups of organic dyes under appropriate conditions to form coloured precipitates. The Bradford assay is based on the measurement of bound Coomassie dye (Brilliant blue G250). (A = 595 nm). This assay is the most sensitive and easy to use of Biuret, Lowry, and BCA. Another protein estimation assay is based on the ability of the proteins to bind silver. This assay has high sensitivity but should be considered when alternate procedures are not practicable.

6.3 Proteolysis and its Prevention

Extra cellular proteins such as antibodies are generally less sensitive to proteolytic degradation since they can maintain activity in less-controlled environment outside the cell. In contrast, intra cellular proteins when released from the confines of the cell compartments are subject to many inactivating conditions. Inside the cell, the pH is 6.5–7.5, protein concentration is high around 100 mg/ml and reducing potential is high. When released the protein gets diluted, and faces an oxidizing environment. Further the disruption of lysosomes releases proteases and acidifies the solution in which the protein is present.

Thus to keep proteolysis in check, the choice of buffers, addition of reducing agents and increasing the concentrations of protein in solution are some of the remedial measures.

Reducing agents include 2-mercaptoethanol or dithiothreitol 2-mercaptoethanol is normally used at 5–20 mM in the buffer and should be added immediately prior to use since it oxidizes rapidly and is lost with in 24 hr 1–5 mM of dithiothreitol is normally used and it is suitable for addition in storage buffers since its protective agent lasts longer than 2-mercaptoethanol. However, the stock solution should not be frozen thawed more than thrice. This also should be added to the buffer just prior to use only. The presence of metal ions will also inactivate –SH groups. Hence addition of EDTA at 0.1 to 1.0 mM may be added to buffers.

Dilute protein solutions are generally unstable and get adsorbed on to surfaces. Polystyrene matrix should not be used for storing proteins as it can bind to proteins strongly as in the case of ELISA plates. To avoid this, the proteins should be stored concentrated and its contact with surfaces reduced. One way of doing this is by addition of bovine serum albumin (BSA) or non-ionic detergents such as Triton x –100 or Tween 20 to the buffers. A preferred method of storage of proteins in a concentrated form is as its ammonium sulphate pellet.

Glycerol is also added @ 10–20% in buffers and even up to 50% in storage buffers. It reduces the water activity of the solution. During freezing, pure water would separate and freeze first thereby increasing the salt and protein concentrations. Glycerol solutions of above 20% do not freeze at –20°C and hence they can be stored at low temperature with minimal damage.

Protease is an enzyme that cleaves the peptide bonds between proteins using a process called proteolysis. Protease activity is essential to many biological functions, including immune defense, cell death and growth, and blood clotting.

Proteases are currently classified into six broad groups:

- Serine proteases
- Threonine proteases
- Cysteine proteases
- Aspartate proteases
- Metalloproteases
- Glutamic acid proteases.

Speed and maintenance of the protein at low temperature are needed to minimize proteolysis. The other more common method is the use of protease inhibitors. Protease inhibitors are biological or chemical compounds that function by reversibly or irreversibly binding to the protease. However, no single chemical is effective for all types of proteases. Hence a mixture or "cocktail" of several different inhibitor substances are used. Commonly used protease inhibitors are given Table 6.1.

Table 6.1: Commonly used Protease Inhibitors

Inhibitor	***Target class***	***Typical working concentration***
4-(2-Aminoethyl) benzene sulfonyl fluoride (AEBSF) HCl	Serine proteases	0.2–1 mM
Anti thrombin III	Serine proteases	1 U/ml
Trypsin inhibitors	Serine proteases	10–100 ug/ml
Benzamidine	Serine proteases	1 mM
Phenyl methyl sulphonyl fluoride (PMSF)	Serine proteases	0.1–1 mM
Aprotinin	Serine proteases	100–200 nM
Leupeptin	Serine and cysteine proteases	10–100 μM
Bestatin	Amino-peptidases	1–10 μM
E-64	Cysteine proteases	1–20 μM
Pepstatin A	Aspartic acid proteases	1–20 μM
EDTA	Metalloproteases	2–10 mM
Antipain	Thiol proteases	1 μ/ml
Cystatin	Thiol proteases	250 μ/ml

These protease inhibitors can be unstable and toxic under certain circumstances. Typically, proteases require pre-solubilization in organic solvents such as iso-propanol, ethanol or dimethyl sulfoxide (DMSO). Once in aqueous solutions, the protease inhibitors tend to hydrolyze rapidly. Therefore, it is necessary to add additional inhibitors throughout the purification sequence.

The proteolysis may be prevented by preventing the action of proteases and also by stabilization of the proteins concerned. Ectoines (1,4,5,6-Tetrahydro-2-methyl-4-pyrimidinecarboxylic acid) is a natural compound found in several species of bacteria used to protect them against extreme osmotic conditions, They also stabilize proteins against proteases and denaturing. Ectoines have been identified in *Ectothiorhodospira halochloris*, *Marinococcus halophilus, Pseudomonas stutzeri, Halomonas elongata* etc.

6.4. Purification Strategy

Any purification technique should be evaluated on the basis of capacity resolution and protein yield.

Capacity of a technique is defined as the amount of samples volume and protein concentration that can be handled. The early requirement of purification of mAbs from tissue culture is to reduce the volume. So precipitation techniques that have a high capacity are preferred at this stage.

The resolution of a technique determines how efficiently it separates the desired protein from other proteins (contaminants). The precipitation methods have a low resolution as against affinity chromatography that has a higher resolution.

The yields of desired proteins would also vary with the techniques. While ammonium sulphate precipitation methods give 80% yields affinity chromatography methods would give only 60% yields. In addition the cost of the method is also a prime concern. These factors must be balanced to arrive at the right method at a particular stage of purification. While in early stages of purification capacity is a priority, resolution is important at later stages.

The commonly used purification methods with their properties are highlighted in Table 6.2 below.

The first step in purification of an extra cellular protein such as secreted mAbs from hybridoma clones is to separate from cells and any other particles such as precipitated macro molecules. This can be done by centrifugation or micro filtration.

Table 6.2: Summary of the Purification Methods

Technique	*Property*	*Capacity*	*Resolution*	*Yields*	*Cost*
pH precipitation	Charge	High	Low	Medium	Low
Ammonium sulphate precipitation	Hydrophobicity	High	Low	High	Low
Aqueous two phase extraction	Bioaffinity	High	High	High	High
Gel permeation chromatography	Size	Very low	High	High	Medium
Ion exchange chromatography	Charge	Medium	Medium	Medium	Medium
Hydrophobic interaction chromatography	Hydrophobicity	Medium	Medium	Medium	Medium
Affinity chromatography interaction	Protein-protein	Medium	High	Medium	Medium
Lectin affinity chromatography	Bioactivity	Medium	Medium	Medium	Medium

Nucleic acids can be removed from culture supernatants by the addition of protamine sulphate, streptomycin, magnesium chloride, spermine, polyethylenaimine (PEI) or the appropriate nucleases. The use of positively charged anion-exchange resins can also remove nucleic acids but are less efficient for large-scale work.

Surfactants often coat proteins and therefore can limit their accessibility to purification by chromatography. The removal of lipids and surfactants from the protein mixture can be accomplished by the use of trichloroacetic acid (TCA) to precipitate detergents; 2 SM-2 macroporous or hydroxyapatite coated beads, batch or column chromatography or by the addition of polyethylene glycol (PEG) to precipitate the proteins, leaving lipids and surfactants in the supernatant.

The clarification step is usually followed by a concentration step in which the volume of the protein solution is reduced resulting in an increase in protein concentration. Smaller volumes are easier to handle in subsequent steps such as chromatography. Higher protein concentrations would reduce protein losses by non-specific adsorption to column matrices of container walls.

Sample preparation or clean-up refers to a set of techniques aimed at making extracted or purified protein samples suitable for long-term storage or compatible with downstream applications. Dialysis, diafiltration and gel filtration (desalting) are the most broadly applicable methods for sample preparation.

6.4.1 Dialysis

Dialysis is a separation technique that facilitates the removal of small, undesired compounds from the protein of interest in solution by selective diffusion through a semi-permeable membrane. A sample and a buffer solution (called the dialysate, usually 200–500 times the volume of the sample) are placed on opposite sides of the membrane. Sample molecules that are larger than the membrane pores are retained on the sample side of the membrane. The small molecules diffuse freely through the membrane and approach an equilibrium concentration with the entire dialysate volume. In this way, the concentration of small contaminants in the sample can be decreased to acceptable or negligible levels. Normally 12 kDa cutoff value of the dialysis membrane is used. This can be used only for proteins above this size. If you intend to concentrate a protein of 5 kDa the protein of your interest would go through the membrane into the buffer. Dialysis is conventionally used to remove the ammonium sulphate salts followed ammonium sulphate precipitation. It is commonly used to remove low molecular weight compounds and change the buffer composition.

Dialysis can also be used to concentrate proteins. The protein to be concentrated is placed in a dialysis bag which is placed in a solution or powder that draws the water through the dialysis membrane. Solutions of polyethylene glycol (MW > 20000) at a concentration of 20% are normally used. Dry powder can also be used by placing the dialysis bag in a Petri dish covered by the powder. Care must be taken since, if left unattended, the whole solution can be drawn out leaving protein traces adsorbed on to the walls of the dialysis membrane.

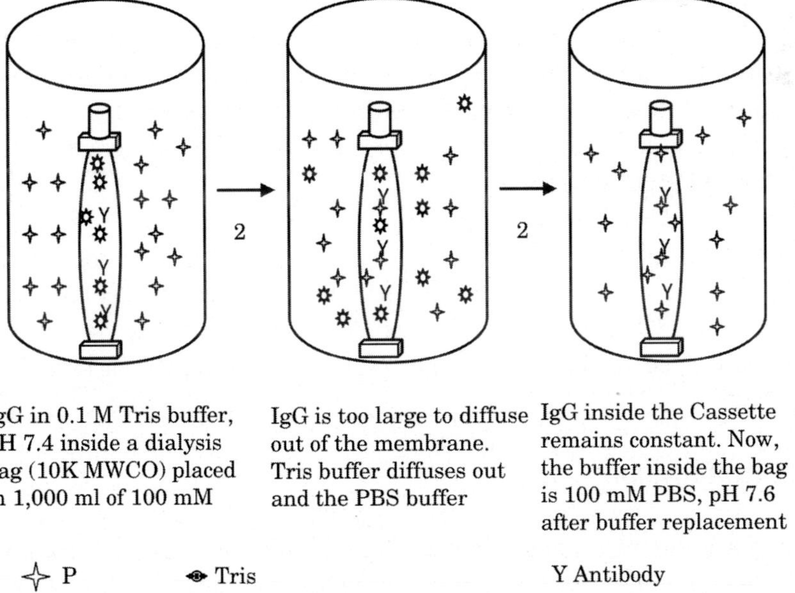

Fig. 6.1: Dialysis.

6.4.2 Diafiltration

In diafiltration, similar to dialysis, a semi-permeable membrane is used to separate macromolecules from low molecular-weight compounds. While dialysis relies on passive diffusion, diafiltration involves forcing solutions through the membrane by pressure (*i.e.*, reverse osmosis, syringe tip sterilization cartridges) or centrifugation (Amicon, Centricon, Vivaspin).

During diafiltration, both water and low molecular-weight solutes are forced through the membrane-filter where they are collected on the other side. Macromolecules remain on the sample side of the membrane, where they become concentrated to a smaller volume. Typical diafiltration devices that involve centrifugation are called concentrators, and this technique is used primarily for concentrating samples.

6.4.3 Desalting and buffer exchange

Desalting refers to the removal of salts from a sample. This is done by equilibration of the column with water. Buffer exchange refers to the replacement of one set of buffer salts with another set. This is performed by first equilibrating with the column resin with a buffer the sample should finally end up in.

In both cases, the buffer constituents in which the protein is dissolved in and is loaded into the column will be replaced by the solution with which the column is pre-equilibrated. Both desalting and buffer exchange are a separation process based on gel filtration, also known as molecular sieve chromatography and results in dilution of the protein sample.

One of the quickest methods of concentration involves addition of a dry inert matrix polymer such as Sephadex G-25 facilitating adsorption of the water and small molecules. The protein of interest has to be of higher molecular weight than the pore size of the matrix. After the matrix is swollen, the remaining protein solution is removed.

6.4.4 Ultrafiltration

In ultrafiltration, water and other small molecules, are driven through a semi permeable membrane by a trans membrane force such as centrifugation of high pressure. The difference between Microfiltration and Ultrafiltration is given in Table 6.3.

Table 6.3: Microfiltration *vs* Ultrafiltration

Parameter	*Microfiltration*	*Ultrafiltration*
Pore size	0.1 to um	1–20 nm; nominal molecular weight cutoff (NMCO)
Pore size distribution	Pore sizes are uniform	Pore sizes are not uniform and vary around the mean
Sieving effect	Allows proteins and other molecules to pass through; retains large cells and particles	Retains proteins above NMCO and
What we need	Is the filtrate	Retentate
Force	Positive or negative pressure	Tangential or centrifugal force

Ultrafiltration differs from dialysis on the following counts (Table 6.4).

Table 6.4: Dialysis *vs* Ultrafiltration

Parameter	*Dialysis*	*Ultrafiltration*
Purpose	Buffer exchange	Protein concentration and buffer exchange
Mode of operation	Diffusion mass transfer driven by concentration differences across the semi permeable membrane	Conventional mass transfer driven by pressure differences applied across the membrane
Membranes	Mechanically not very strong	Mechanically stronger

The cellulose type polymer membranes have low protein binding capacity but may degrade upon exposure to sodium hypochlorite based cleaning solutions. However, polysulfone and polyethersulfone based membranes are more alkali resistant. Most small-scale ultra filtration membrane devices operate in a dead-end mode whereas larger scale systems employ the cross flow mode.

The dead-end applications most commonly include syringe-end filters or centrifugal filters. A membrane disk is placed inside a 15 ml or 50 ml conical centrifuge tube and the permeate is collected at the bottom of the tube under the membrane. The feed sample is driven across the ultrafiltration membrane by centrifugal force leaving concentrated sample above the membrane. Some of the centrifugal ultrafiltration devices available for processing samples from less than 1 ml to 60 ml include Nanosep, Microsep, Macrosep and Jumbosep or Centriplus containing membranes with MWCO ranging from 10 to 100 K. These devices can be used in most centrifuges that can accommodate 50 ml centrifuge tubes, with swinging-bucket or fixed angle rotors.

Ultrafiltration membranes are also incorporated into 96 or 384-multiwell filter plates for high-throughput concentration or buffer exchange of several small samples (80–300 ml).

A stirred-cell based ultra filtration device consists of membrane housing on a support plate sealed at the bottom of a cylindrical housing. The fluid in the stirred device is agitated using a magnetic bar and the air provides the pressure driving force.

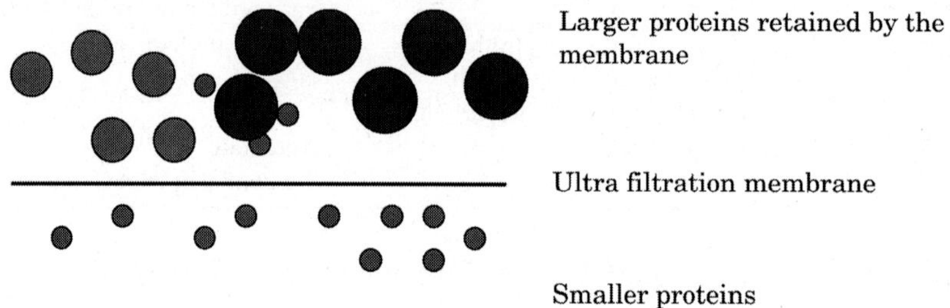

Fig. 6.2: Principle of Ultra filtration

6.4.5 Lyophilization

The boiling point of a solution is the temperature at which the vapour pressure of the solution equals the atmospheric pressure. Solvents can be brought to boil either by increasing solution temperature or by lowering the headspace air pressure by application of vacuum. This latter technique is called vacuum concentration.

Lyophilization involves lowering the temperature of the solution to the point where the solution freezes and solvents are removed by sublimation. The freezing and vacuum step can be performed simultaneously when both heat and headspace gases are removed to concentrate the product of interest.

Lyophilization consists of three steps:

- Freezing
- Primary drying
- Secondary drying.

Slow freezing can cause ice crystals to form which enhances freeze-drying, but may denature labile proteins. Conversely, when sample freezing is performed rapidly small ice crystals form which can impede freeze-drying but protect protein stability.

Primary drying causes conversion of more than 80% of the solvent to vapour phase through sublimation. The residual solvent remains adsorbed on the product as moisture.

This is desorbed during secondary drying to attain a moisture level low enough to inhibit microbial growth or chemical reactions, while still preserving the activity and integrity of the freeze-dried product.

6.5 Concentration By Precipitation

The solubility of a protein molecule in aqueous solvent is determined by the distribution of charged hydrophilic and hydrophobic groups on its surface. These charged groups will interact with ionic groups in the solvent. Proteins aggregate form due to changes in pH, ionic strength or by addition of organic solvents or other polymers or solutes. The precipitates can be separated by filtration or centrifugation. To remove the precipitating agent the precipitate has to be dialyzed, desalted or diafiltered.

If the pH of the solution is equal to the pI of the protein, it precipitates out of solution. At pI, the surface positive and negative charges can each other and hence electrostatic repulsion does not occur resulting in precipitate formation. This method is preferred to remove unwanted proteins in a preparation rather than purifying the protein of interest.

Few proteins can be precipitated by lowering the ionic strength. Precipitation by addition of neutral salts is the most common method for fractionating proteins by precipitation (salting out by increasing the ionic strength). In a protein the hydrophobic areas in normally in the interior of the proteins but some are also exposed on the surface. The water molecules become ordered around these patches. When a salt is added, the water solvates the salt ions and water is removed from around the protein hydrophobic areas thereby exposing these areas which interact with one another and aggregate and precipitate out. Proteins with more hydrophobic patches precipitate first before those with fewer patches.

The salts than can be used for salting out are phosphate > sulphate > acetate > chloride. Multi charged anions are the most effective. Since phosphates are not present in the form of PO_4^{3-} but more as HPO_4^{2-} and $H_2PO_4^-$ at neutral pH, sulphate is a better choice.

Monovalent cations are most effective in the order $NH_4^+ > K^+ > Na^+$.

Thus the most common salt used for this purpose is ammonium sulphate. A saturated ammonium sulphate solution in water is about 4 M. The density of a saturated solution of ammonium sulphate is 1.235 g/ml as compared to the density of a protein aggregate (1.29 g/ml). Higher the difference between the density of aggregate and solution makes separation of the aggregate easier by centrifugation.

Note: Hydrophobic proteins aggregating in the presence of ammonium sulphate

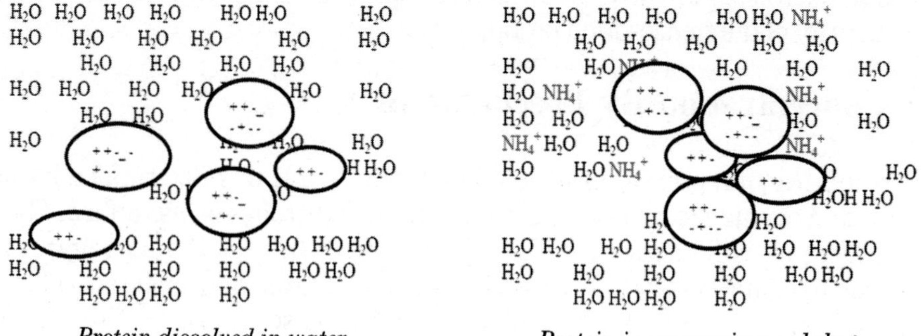

Fig. 6.3: Principle of 'Salting out' Ammonium sulphate precipitation

To find out the amount of ammonium sulphate (g) to add to 1 l at 200°C to

$$G = \frac{532\,(S2 - S1)}{100 - 0.3S2}$$

Where S1 is the starting concentration and S2 is the final concentration. This equation takes in to consideration the increase in the volume of the solution that occurs on addition of the salt.

To determine the optimum ammonium sulphate precipitation conditions the following tables are helpful.

Sample (ml)	10	10	10	10	10
Amm. SO_4 (g)	1.06	1.64	2.26	2.91	3.61
Percent saturation	20	30	40	50	60

Following centrifugation, the ammonium sulphate saturation is increased by another 10% respectively as follows:

Sample (ml)	10	10	10	10	10
Amm. SO_4 (g)	0.55	0.56	0.58	0.60	0.62
Percent saturation	30	40	50	60	70

Now the pellet would be indicative of precipitation at 20–30%, 30–40%, 40–50%, 50–60% and 60–70% saturation. Each of these are measured for its activity and purity and the optimal saturation of ammonium sulphate required can be determined.

Proteins can also be precipitated by the addition of water-miscible organic solvents like acetone and ethanol. These solvents lower the dielectric constant of the solution and thus its solvating power. This decreased solubility favours aggregation through electrostatic attraction.

Precipitation is also achieved by the addition of organic polymers such as polyethylene glycol (PEG). The mechanism is similar to those induced by organic solvents. Conventionally PEG 6000 is used. Strong acids such as trichloroacetic acid (TCA) or perchloric acid can also be used to precipitate proteins especially when the proteins are not required to maintain their activity.

6.5.1 Different precipitation methods

Precipitation agent	*Sample*
Ammonium Sulphate	1 mg/ml proteins especially immunoglobulins
Dextran Sulphate	Samples with high levels of lipoproteins like ascites
Polyvinyl pyrollindone	Samples with high levels of lipoproteins like ascites
Polyethylene glycol	Plasma proteins
Acetone	Peptide precipitation
Polyethyleneimine	Precipitates aggregated nucleoproteins
Protamine Sulphate	Precipitates aggregated nucleoproteins
Caprylic acid	Precipitates bulk of proteins leaving Ig in solution

6.6 Chromatography

Chromatography is the separation of sample components between a mobile and a stationary phase. When a sample containing a mixture of proteins is allowed to pass through a column, the proteins having a greater attraction for the solid phase migrate slower then proteins attracted to the mobile phase.

Capacity is the measure of the amount of protein that is absorbed onto a unit volume or weight of the stationary phase from the solution. High capacity techniques separate proteins from large volumes of solution and are preferred early in the purification strategy.

Selectivity measures the ability of a technique to adsorb a specific protein from a mixture by avoiding contaminants. A highly selective technique such as affinity purification is used during the later stages of purification.

Resolution is a measure of the degree of separation of the desired protein from contaminants. It is a measure of relative separation between two peaks. A single, well resolved peak does not indicate a pure substance. It is possible that the peak may contain a number of closely related components that are not resolved at all by the particular chromatographic technique. Thus methods with high selectivity can separate proteins with a high degree of resolution.

Throughput is the measure of the purification of maximum amount of protein in the minimum amount of time. Throughput can be increased by the use of high capacity matrices and by column matrices useful with high flow rates.

Table 6.5: Different Chromatography Methods

Technique	*Based on*	*Suitable for*
Gel filtration (GF)	Differences in size	Proteins, peptides, polynucleotides
Ion exchange (IEX)	Differences in charge	Proteins, peptides, polynucleotides
Affinity chromatography (AC)	Recognition of specific ligands	Proteins
Hydrophobic interaction chromatography (HIC)	Differences in hydrophobic residues	Lipoproteins

6.6.1 Gel filtration

This technique is also called

- Size exclusion chromatography
- Molecular sieve chromatography
- Gel permeation chromatography.

Separation based on the exclusion of molecules from the pore size of the matrix. Proteins of different molecular sizes are eluted through a column of gel granules, equilibrated with appropriate buffer. Large molecules will be excluded from the pores of these granules and will pass thorough the interstitial space and elute first followed by smaller molecules.

The features of gel filtration include:

- Versatile method of separation with high resolution and can be done under mild conditions
- Different buffer systems can be used as the buffer ions are generally excluded
- Separation is independent of ionic strength
- Can be used for desalting and buffer exchange.

Some of the matrices used as stationary phase are:

***Cellulose*:** This is linear polysaccharide of beta 1–4 linked glucose monomers. Each glucose residue has three hydroxyl groups which make the matrix very hydrophilic. The pores in the polymer of cellulose occur at places where the hydrogen bonds are fewer. Alkali treatment of the cellulose powder with 0.5 M alkali is required to swell the matrix and open the pores.

***Agarose*:** Agarose is a polysaccharide composed of the polymeric chains of the disaccharide agarobiose (D-galactose and 3,6, anhydro–1-galactose).

***Dextran*:** consists of glucose residues linked by alpha 1-6 bonds. Each residue has 6 hydroxyl groups providing a very hrdrophilic matrix. The exclusion limit for dextran is 300 kDa lower than that of agarose. Unlike cellulose the pore sizes are uniform and gel does not need any pre-treatment.

Matrices based on agarose are more porous than dextran. Thus the speed of separation may be increased but there is less selectivity.

A second polymer was grafted onto a preformed matrix thereby preparing composite gels. Sephacryl is formed by cross linking allyl dextran with N N' methylene bisacrylamide. Superdex consists of dextran chains covalently bound to a highly cross linked agarose matrix.

Table 6.6: Gel Filtration Media

Name	*Type*	*Fractionation range (kDa)*
Sephadex G 25	Dextran	1–5
Sephadex G 100	Dextran	4–150
Sephadex G 200	Dextran	5–600
BioGel P 30	Polyacrylamide	2.4–40
BioGel P 300	Polyacrylamide	60–400
Sepharose 6 B	Agarose	10–4000
Sepharose 4 B	Agarose	60–20000

6.6.1.1 *Application of gel filtration technique*

- Desalting removing small molecular weight compounds from protein samples
- Preparative separation of protein
- *Analytical use*: Estimation of molecular size of proteins.

Gel filtration step can be applied

- After ammonium sulphate precipitation stage
- Before ion-exchange chromatography step
- At the end of purification to clean up the preparation (*e.g.* after ion-exchange).

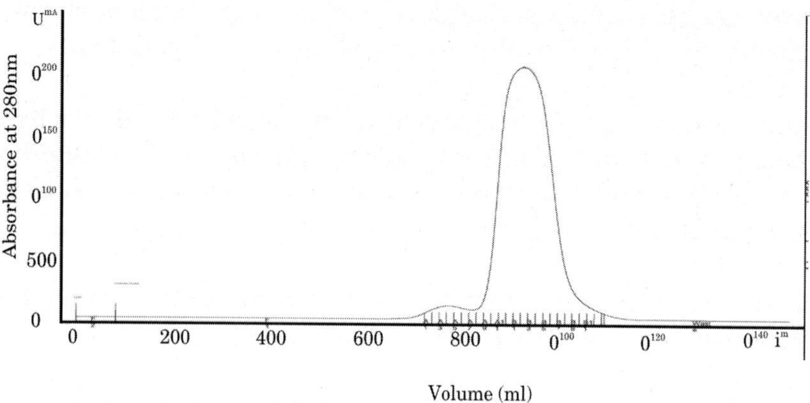

Laboratory scale chromatogram recorded using Superdex 200 size exclusion column of 5 cm diameter , 85 cm bed height. Note sharp increase in absorbance whole fractions can be pooled and used for checking in PAGE

Fig. 6.4: Chromatogram of gel filtration.

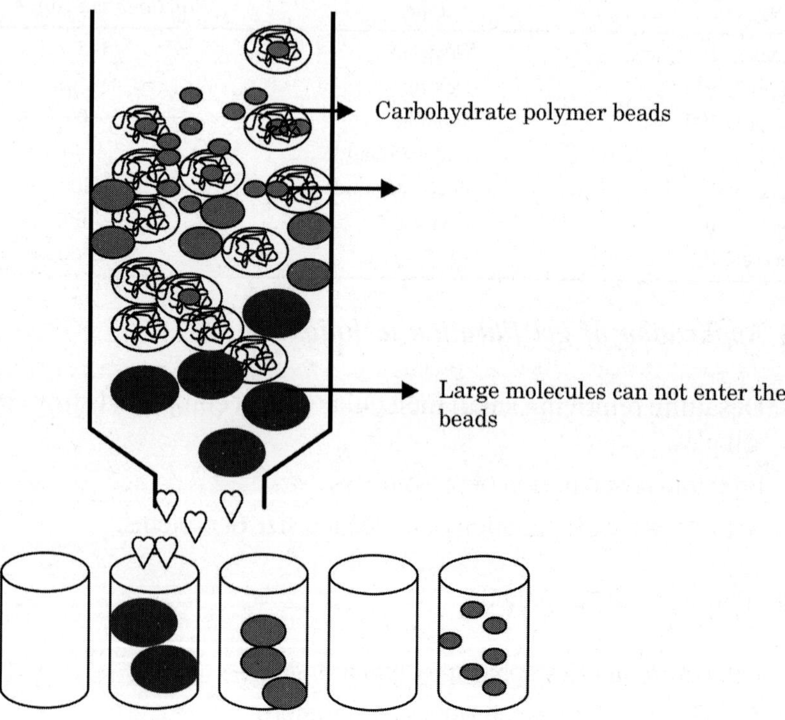

Fig. 6.5: Principle of gel filtration or size exclusion chromatography.

6.6.2 Ion-exchange chromatography

Separation of molecules by ion-exchange chromatography depends on differences between the net surface charges on the solute molecules. Amino acids contain side chains which can ionize to varying extents depending on the pH of the solution. Hence the net surface charge of a protein will undergo a change as the pH of their environment varies.

At the isoelectric point (pI) of the protein the protein will have little or no tendency to bind either to a cationic stationary phase (that is, one which has positively charged groups) or to an anionic stationary phase (one that has negatively charged groups).

At pH value below the pI, the protein will have a net positive charge, and will tend to bind reversibly with to the surface of a cation-exchange resin, that is, one that has negatively charged groups at that pH. A cation-exchange resin is anionic, having negatively charged groups, while an anion exchange resin is cationic, since it has positively charged groups.

On applying the sample, conditions are chosen so that unwanted solutes do not bind to the resin, leaving only the molecules of interest bound to the top of the column. When all the unwanted solutes have been eluted, the composition of the buffer is gradually altered, either by increasing the ionic strength, or, less commonly, by changing the pH of the eluting buffer. This is called gradient elution. The bound solutes are eluted at different values of the ionic strength, as buffer ions compete with the bound molecule for cationic or anionic sites on the resin.

If the elution process is carried out using the same buffer that was used in applying the sample, the elution is said to be isocratic.

Alternately, if the elution is carried out with a buffer and then the buffer is changed, it is called step-wise elution.

There are a variety of commercially available matrices that can be classified as follows:

Table 6.7: Anion and Cationic Exchangers

Anion exchangers	*Type*	*Functional group*
Quaternary ammonium (Q)	Strong	$-OCH_2N^+(CH_3)_3$
Diethylaminoethyl (DEAE)	Weak	$-OCH_2CH_2NH^+(CH_2CH_3)_2$
Diethylaminopropyl (ANX)	Weak	$-OCH_2CHOHCH_2NH^+(CH_2CH_3)_2$
Cation exchangers	***Type***	***Functional group***
Sulfopropyl (SP)	Strong	$O-CH_2CHOHCH_2OCH_2CH_2CH_2SO_3^-$
Methyl sulphonate (S)	Strong	$O-CH_2CHOHCH_2OCH_2CHOHCH_2SO_3^-$
Carboxymethyl (CM)	Weak	$O-CH_2COO$

Generally speaking, a protein will bind to a cation exchange resin if the buffer pH is lower than the isoelectric point (pI) of the protein, and will bind to an anion exchange resin if the pH is higher than the pI.

Strong ion-exchangers do not show any marked change in their ionic states with changes in pH. They remain fully charged over a broad range of pH values.

Ion-exchange chromatography can be used after salt precipitation step or after gel-filtration. The sample requires dialysis of sample prior to ion-exchange and can be used directly after gel filtration.

Separation of dextran blue from cytochrome C - Dextran Blue is a large non-ionic polysaccharide (500000 MW) while cytochrome C is positively charged (12400 MW), Cytochrome C is a cation and solid matrix has a negative charge.

Potassium acetate is a positively charged eluant.

- Add sample mixture
- Add 0.01 M KO Ac first
- Remove (elute) dextran blue
- Add 0.5 M KO Ac next
- Remove (elute) cytochrome c

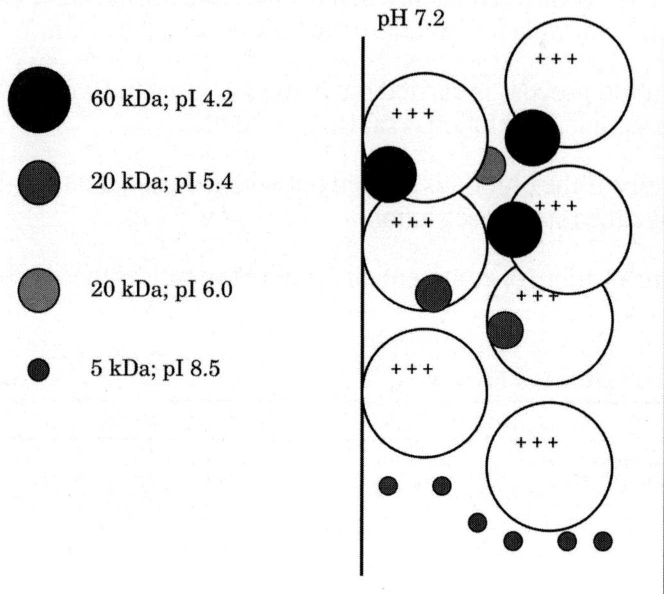

Fig. 6.6: Principle of ion exchange chromatography

6.6.3 Affinity chromatography

Affinity chromatography is based on the highly specific biological interaction between two molecules, such as interactions between enzyme and substrate, receptor and ligand, or antibody and antigen, one of which is bound to an insoluble inert matrix. For example, an enzyme would bind to ligand sites on the matrix if it mimics the substrate of the enzyme. Affinity chromatography is capable of achieving a purification of 100–1000 folds in a single step.

The following Table 6.8 lists the major types of application.

Table 6.8: List of Ligand–target Molecule Interactions used for Affinity Chromatography

Biomolecule	*Ligand*
Enzymes	Substrate, inhibitor, cofactor
Antibodies	Antigen, virus, cell surface antigens
Nucleic acids	Complementary base sequence, histone, nucleic acid polymerase
Hormones	Receptor, carrier protein
Lectins	Polysaccharide, glycoprotein, cell receptor
His Tags	Metal ions

The affinity matrix is the solid support onto which ligand is immobilized. This matrix should have the following characteristics

- Macroporous with uniform pore size
- Should selectively bind the target of interest
- High degree of chemical and physical stability
- Low nonspecific binding
- Good flow properties.

The affinity matrix may be commercially available or can be made by attaching a suitable ligand to a solid support via the appropriate chemistry. Some of the commercially available matrices include Sepharose CL4B (agarose), Sepharose CL6B (agarose), Biogel A (agarose), Biogel P 100 (polyacrylamide) and Perloza MT 100 medium (cellulose).

The ligand used for affinity chromatography should have specific but reversible affinity for the substance to be purified and it should possess chemically modifiable groups that facilitate binding to the affinity matrix. The preferred dissociation constant (Kd) for the ligand-binding molecule complex is in the range of 10^{-4} to 10^{-8} M. If the affinities are higher then elution retaining the activity becomes difficult. When the affinities are lower the binding is weak for efficient binding and elution. Sometimes a spacer arm is needed to be present between matrix and ligand for effective binding by overcoming steric hindrance.

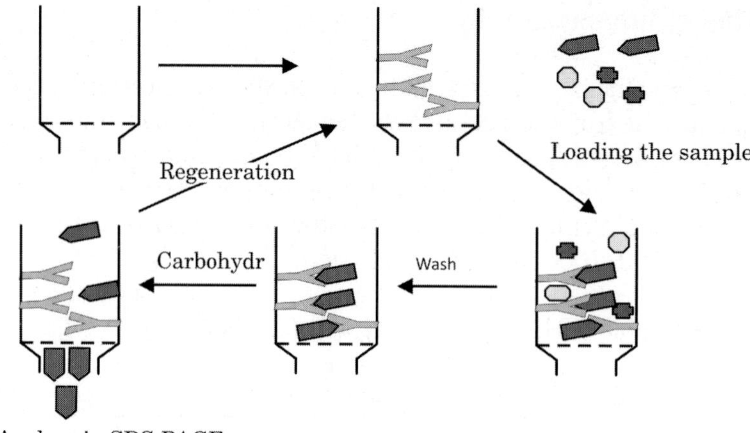

Fig. 6.7: Immunoaffinity chromatography.

Conventionally the ligand is attached to a matrix, through covalent coupling so that it does not leach during purification. But alternate ligand binding based on nonspecific adsorption or bio-specific interactions as in biotin-streptavidin are also used in the absence of reactive groups or to reduce the risk of ligand denaturation. Group specific adsorbents are designed to have affinity for a group of related molecules. Commonly used group specific adsorbents are given in Table 6.9.

Table 6.9: Group Specific Adsorbents

Ligand	*Specificity*
Cibacron Blue	Albumin, kinases, dehydrogenases, enzymes requiring adenylyl-containing cofactors, NAD^+
Blue B	Kinases, dehydrogenases, nucleic acid binding proteins
Orange A	Lactate dehydrogenase
Green A	Dehydrogenases
Biotin	Streptavidin, Avidin
Gelatin	Fibronectin
2'5'ADP	Enzymes with $NADP^+$ as cofactor
Poly A	Nucleic acid with poly U sequences
Lectins	Glycoprotein, polysaccharides
Protein A	Fc region of Ig
Protein G	Fc region of Ig
Protein L	Kappa light chain of Ig

Table 6.10: IgG Binding Proteins from Bacteria

Protein	*Source*	*Binding*
Protein A	*Staphyloccus aureus*	Strong, Fc region
Protein G	Groups C and G *Streptococci*	Strong, Fc region
Protein L	*Peptococcus magnus*	Binds to kappa light chains
Protein P	*Clostridium perfringens*	Binds to kappa light chains
Protein D	*Branhamella catarrhalis*	IgD. Binds small amounts of IgG
Protein P	Group A *Streptococci*	IgA. Binds weakly to IgG

The albumin binding region of protein G is deleted genetically to avoid undesired reactions involving albumin. There are two IgG binding domains per ligand. The high affinity and specificity of protein G for IgG makes this a method of choice for purification of mouse or rat mAbs from cell culture supernatants (Table 6.10). The general procedure is to centrifuge the cell culture supernatant at 10000 g for 10 min to remove cell debris and cells followed by filtration in 0.45 μ membrane filters. Pack the protein G column @ 1 ml of gel per 5 mg IgG. Equiliberate the column with 2-3 bed volumes of 0.02 M sodium phosphate buffer pH 7.0. Apply sample to the column, wash the unbound proteins using the start buffer until no protein is detected in the effluent as checked by lack of absorbance at 280 nm. The bound mAbs is eluted by glycine –HCl buffer pH 2.7. Collect the fractions in tubes containing neutralization buffer (1M Tris HCl pH 9.0). Regenerate the column with elution buffer followed by start buffer. When not in use, store the column in buffer with bacteriostat such as 0.04% sodium azide or 20% ethanol.

Protein L (*Peptostreptococcus magnus*), which has ability to interact with kappa light chains without affecting the antigen-binding site of antibodies makes protein L uniquely suited for purification of antibodies lacking Fc regions. In most cases, good binding to antibodies can be achieved at or near neutral pH, but the optimal pH for sample application can differ depending on the protein used. Protein A binds antibodies strongest at pH 8.2, protein L at pH 7.5 and protein G at pH 5 but protein G can also be used at pH 7–7.5.

6.6.3.1 *Lectin affinity chromatography*

Lectins are proteins that bind specifically and reversibly to sugar residues. This specificity is used in affinity purification or enrichment of carbohydrate moieties of complex glycoconjugates, such as polysaccharides, glycolipids, and glycoproteins. They also allow for a specific isolation of different glycolforms of a specific protein depending on the nature of glycosylation.

Table 6.11: Lectins and their Sources useful in Affinity Chromatography

Lectin	*Source*	*Specificity*	*Features*
Conacanavalin A (ConA)	*Canavalia ensiformis*	a-D-mannose, a-D-glucose, and N-acetylglucosamine	Requires the presence of divalent metal ions, Ca^{2+} and Mn^{2+}
Wheat germ lectin		Sialic acid and N-acetyl-D-glucosamine residue	Stable in 0.07% SDS and 1% deoxycholate
Jacalin		a-D-galactosyl groups	Binds O-glycosylated proteins
Helix pomatia lectin	Snail – *Helix pomatia*	N-acetyl a D-galactos-aminyl residues	Purification of T-cells
Lentil lectin	*Lens culinaris*	a-D glucose and a-D mannose	Binds even in the presence of 1% sodium deoxycholate; preferred for purification of viral envelope proteins or detergent solubilized membrane proteins

Coupling of lectin onto resin is done at neutral pH in the presence of sugar to preserve sugar binding site. Binding to the target molecule is also usually carried out in neutral pH. Elution is achieved by the addition of excess specific sugar molecule to the elution buffer. After elution, the free sugar should be removed by dialysis or size exclusion chromatography.

ConA sepharose is used for the separation and purification of glycoproteins, polysaccharides and glycolipids. It is also used for purification of enzyme antibody conjugates, isolation of cell surface glycoproteins and determine changes in composition of carbohydrate containing substances.

6.7 Biomimetic Ligands

Most of affinity chromatography ligands are naturally occurring. They are highly selective and have a high capacity of binding, but are less stable. This led to the development of synthetic or altered affinity ligands, biomimetics, which mimic the structure and binding of natural biological ligands. The popular biomimetic ligands include the synthetic polycyclic dyes, Cibacron Blue and Procion Red. They are structurally similar to cofactors such as NAD^+ and $NADP^+$ which enable them to bind to a wide range of enzyme proteins such as kinases, dehydrogenases etc. Other proteins such as albumin, interferon, and blood coagulation factors bind less specifically by electrostatic and/or hydrophobic interactions. Elution is achieved by the use of free cofactor.

Heparin is a highly sulphated glycosaminoglycan which binds to mast cell protease, serine protease inhibitors, growth factors, nucleic acid binding proteins etc. It also acts as a cationic exchanger due to its high content of anionic sulphate groups thereby interacting with nucleic acid binding proteins by mimicking the polyanionic structure of nucleic acids.

6.8 Covalent Affinity Chromatography

Affinity chromatography is based on the reversible interaction between the target molecule and the ligand. In contrast, covalent chromatography is also used especially for the isolation of thiol-containing proteins and peptides. A thiol containing target molecule is covalent bound with an activated thiol immobilized onto purification matrix. Bound protein can be eluted by reducing the cysteine disulphide with 2-mercaptoethanol, TCEP, or dithiothreitol.

A similar covalent binding-based purification has been developed based on the specific covalent interaction between a chloroalkane ligand and HaloTag. HaloTag is a 34-kDa monomeric protein fusion tag which can be genetically fused to any protein of interest either at its C- or N-terminus. HaloLink, is the resin carrying the chloroalkane ligand that enables efficient capture of target proteins even at low abundance. The bound protein can be eluted by specific protease (TEV) as the TEV recognition site is present between the HaloTag and fusion target protein. Upon cleavage, HaloTag stays bound to the resin while the fusion partner is released yielding highly pure protein free of tag.

6.9 Magnetic Affinity Beads

Use of magnetic affinity beads has several advantages such as

- Less sample dilution in contrast to column based elution
- Quick retrieval of affinity beads at each step
- Useful even on viscous materials that might clog columns
- Eliminated sample pre treatment
- High throughput.

Paramagnetic particles are available as unmodified, modified with common group-specific affinity ligands like streptavidin, protein A, etc., and conjugated particles with specific recognition groups such as monoclonal and polyclonalantibodies. These magnetic particles can also be used to immobilize a target protein which then acts as a bait to pull down its interaction partner(s) from a complex biological mixture. For example a magnetic particle bound to a antibody to green fluorescent proteins (GFP) would pull down GFP tagged expressed protein and with it any signaling molecules or other novel proteins interacting with the protein of interest.

The amine group on the ligand is bound to the amine reactive group on the ligand that is an imindocarbonate formed as a result of the reaction of cyanogen bromide activated surface. Other alternative attachment chemistries involve the use of N-hydroxysuccinimidyl ester or the use of a coupling agent N-ethyl N' (3-dimethyl aminopropyl) carbodiimide (EDC).

Following binding, nonspecifically bound proteins can be removed by washing. Reduction of ionic interaction can be achieved by increasing salt concentration or pH. Hydrophobic interactions can be reduced by decreasing salt, altering pH or adding surfactants such as triton X-100. Low concentrations of competitive reagents can also be used to remove contaminants.

6.10 Protein Tags

Recombinant proteins are prepared with additional residues or tags engineered on either the N- or C-terminal end of the protein during the cloning step. These tags are used to improve protein production or to confer new additional properties to the protein that can be used for its characterization. The term "fusion protein" is also used instead of the term "tag," and both terms are interchangeably used (Table 6.12 to 6.14). The production of recombinant proteins in prokaryotes cause problems of low expression, and misfolding of the expressed protein into insoluble aggregates called inclusion bodies. Tags used to improve the production of recombinant proteins can be are classified as purification and solubility tags. The purification tags are used along with affinity chromatography to allow rapid and efficient purification of expressed proteins. The solubility tags are added to enhance proper folding and solubility of a protein.

Table 6.12: Enzymes to Remove Protein Tags

Protease	*Cleavage site*
Enterokinase	Asp-Asp-Asp-Asp-Lys ▼
Factor Xa	Ile-Glu/Asp-Gly-Arg ▼
Thrombin	Leu-Val-Pro-Arg ▼ Gly-Ser
Human rhinovirus 3C protease)	Leu-Glu-Val-Leu-Phe-Gln ▼ Gly-Pro
TEV (tobacco etch virus) protease	Glu-Asn-Leu-Tyr-Phe-Gln ▼ Gly
SUMO protease	recognize the tertiary structure of the ubiquitin-like (UBL) protein, SUMO
PreScission	Leu-Glu-Val-Leu-Phe-Gln ▼ Gly-Pro

Table 6.13: Common Solubility Tags

Tag	*Size*
Maltose-binding protein (MBP)	396 amino acids
Thioredoxin (Trx)	109 aa
IgG domain B1 of streptococcus Protein G (GB1)	56 aa
Mutated dehalogenase (HaloTag)	300 aa
Small ubiquitin modifier (SUMO)	100 aa
N-utilization substance (NusA)	495 aa

Table 6.14: Common Affinity Tags

Tag	*Affinity matrix*
His-tag 6–10 Histidine	Immobilized metal ions Ni, Co, Cu, Zn
MBP (maltose binding protein)–396 aa	Cross-linked amylose
GST (glutathione-S-transferase)–211 aa	Glutathione resin
FLAG-tag 8 aa (DYKDDDDK)	Anti-FLAG mAB
Strep-II-tag 8 aa (WSHPQFEK)	Modified streptavidin
Protein A–280 aa	Immobilized IgG
Chitin-binding domain–51 aa	Chitin
Halotag–300 aa	Chloroalkane
Calmodulin binding protein–26 aa	Immobilized calmodulin

Immobilized metal affinity chromatographic (IMAC) is used for purification of His-tagged proteins. Metal ions are immobilized using Ni (II)-nitrilo triacetic acid

(Ni-NTA) or Co^{2+}carboxymethyl-aspartate linkages to resins or beads. IMAC has binding capacities of about 5–40 mg of His-tagged protein/ml and is cheap. The nickel ions can be stripped using buffers with EDTA and recharged for multiple cycles. Cobalt based resins such as Talon from Clontech Inc., use stable proprietary linkages and hence cannot be recharged; but are more specific for polyhistidine tags and does not cause metal leakage during protein elution. Tagged protein bound on IMAC media can be easily eluted using elution buffers with imidazole (100–250 mM) or low pH (4.5–6).

The features of IMAC include:

- IMAC can be used under denaturing conditions, since the His-tag does not need a specific protein conformation for metal binding
- Binding to IMAC resins is stronger under denaturing conditions as the His-tag becomes more exposed
- A low level of imidazole (5–20 mM) may be included in loading and wash buffers to minimize nonspecific binding
- Samples loaded on IMAC columns should not contain any EDTA. To minimize proteolysis, only EDTA-free protease inhibitor cocktails should be used
- Tris salts weakly chelate metal ions as well, and the use of Tris buffers should be minimized to concentrations of 50 mM or less.

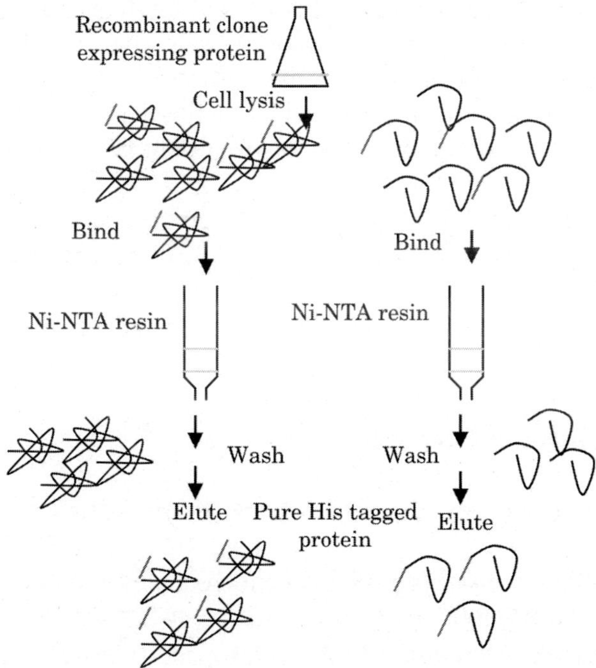

Fig. 6.8: Purification of His-tagged recombinant protein.

6.11 Hydrophobic Interaction Chromatography

Separation of molecules by hydrophobic interaction chromatography (HIC) relies on differences in hydrophobic groups on the surface of solute molecules. In turn, these hydrophobic groups tend to bind to hydrophobic groups on the surface of an insoluble matrix. The legend on the right will identify the salient features of the diagram on the left. The reversible interaction between the solute and the matrix is increased at high ionic strength. Hence, typically, protein solutes are introduced onto the column at high concentrations of ammonium sulphate, and eluted by running a decreasing gradient of this salt. The hydrophobic ligands on the matrix can be chosen with differing binding strength: a strongly hydrophobic matrix will have phenyl or octyl groups, while weakly hydrophobix matrices may bear ether or isopropyl groups. Hydrophobic interaction chromatography is best used as an intermediate purification technique. For example, after precipitation with ammonium sulphate, a mixture of proteins may be brought back in solution by decreasing the concentration of ammonium sulphate to about 1.5M, and applied to the column. Washing with this solution will remove unbound material. Gradually decreasing the concentration of the eluting solution will then elute the different components.

6.12 Thiophilic Interaction Chromatography

SH containing ligands are immobilized on divinyl sulphone activated matrices to form T-gels which are useful for purification of selective proteins by interaction with their thiophilic regions promoted by the presence of salt. T-gels are particularly useful for purifying Igs wither from polyclonal antibodies or mAbs. Desorption of the bound proteins is achieved by omission of salt from the buffer.

The advantages of T-gels are mild elution conditions at neutral pH unlike low pH required for protein A or protein G gels and low cost of the adsorbents.

Disadvantages include less specific adsorption and presence of high salt in binding buffer.

6.13 Purification of mAbs

The likely contaminants in mAb production include the following

- ***Cell culture containing FCS*:** Phenol red, albumin, transferrin, bovine IgG, á2-macroglobulin, other serum proteins, viruses
- ***Cell culture without FCS*:** Albumin, transferrin (serum-free supplements)

- ***Ascites***: Lipids, albumin, transferrin, lipoproteins, endogenous IgG, other host proteins

A combination of methods is preferred for purification of antibodies

- Salting out
- Affinity chromatography
- Ion exchange chromatography.

The need to purify mAbs would depend on the

- Source
- Intended use.

Culture supernatants would contain bovine serum while ascites would have mouse serum proteins from the donor. Since ascites fluids are used at high dilutions, the normal mouse proteins may be too dilute to interfere.

Tissue cultures containing mAbs would also have bovine IgG from the FCS and application of protein A chromatography would lead to purification of not only the mAb of interest but also the bovine IgG from FCS. This problem can be avoided:

- By the use of serum free medium
- Depletion of bovine IgG from the FCS prior to the addition to tissue cultures.

Why we need pure antibodies?

- For diagnosis, substances in the source material may interfere with the detection process
- For conjugation of mAbs with radioisotopes, fluorochromes, enzymes etc
- For therapy
- For purification of antigens
- For proteolytic fragmentation of antibodies
- For calibration of protein content
- Sequence determination
- Finding inhibitors
- Kinetic studies

Every antibody is unique
Antibodies are multifunctional

Purification methods involving affinity chromatography can harness the following features of antibody molecule.

- Specificity of antigen binding
- By targeting the Fc part of the antibody.

The common affinity based methods used for purifying mAbs may include

- Affinity purification using antigen
- Affinity purification with anti-antibodies
- Bacterial Fc receptors
- Protein A mimetic ligands
- Lectin affinity chromatography
- Metal affinity chromatography
- Histidine ligand affinity chromatography
- T-gels
- Using affinity tags.

Use of immobilized antigen as affinity ligand is widely used for purification of mAbs of desired affinity. This can also be used for purification of antigens using immobilized antibodies. Anti-antibodies can also be used as affinity ligand and purification achieved by targeting the constant domains of heavy and light chains of antibodies. It can also be used to remove contaminating antibodies from the mAb source. For example, the presence of bovine antibodies can be removed from the cell culture supernatants by passing it through the anti-bovine antibody coupled affinity columns, leaving the mouse antibodies intact in the flow through.

Protein A mimetic ligands include low molecular weight compounds able to bind Igs, like protein A. For example, the peptide TG19318 binds Igs from human, rat, goat, mouse and horse and rat and mouse mAbs. This ligand also has affinity for mouse monoclonal IgE or IgM.

Some antibodies have an innate affinity for metal due to the presence of histidine rich sequences. Murine IgG1 contains a metal affinity site near the carboxy terminus of the H chain. Murine IgG1 had 60% purity following purification through metal affinity with transferrin as a major contaminant.

The following is the basic protocol for purification of mAbs from hybridomas

1. Use protein G affinity column for mouse IgG1 and protein A for mouse IgG2a, IgG2b, IgG3 (Table 6.15).
2. The volume of protein G sepharose column prepared is based on the fact that the culture supernatants contain 20–50 μg/mL antibody and 1 mL of wet beads bind approximately 10–20 mg antibody.

3. Wash column with 100 mM Tris-HCl pH 8.0
4. Adjust cell culture supernatant pH by adding $^{1}/_{10}$ volume of 1.0M Tris-HCl pH8.0, and pass it through protein A column at speed of 2 ml/min.
5. Wash column with at least 10 column volumes of 100 mM Tris-HCl followed by 10 mM Tris-HCl
6. Elute the column with 50 mM glycine (pH3.0), collect elute fraction into tubes containing 100 ul 1M Tris-HCl for immediate neutralization of antibody solution
7. Estimate the protein content using Bradford or BCA assay
8. Check 5 ul of each fraction on 11% SDS-PAGE gel to assess the purity of antibody
9. Combine the fractions containing antibody, determine the antibody concentration by measuring OD 280nm (1 OD = 0.75 mg/mL)
10. Make series of dilutions of antibody, perform western blot or ELISA to determine the optimal titre of the antibody, based on the antigen used.

Table 6.15: Binding and Elution Conditions for Protein A affinity Chromatography

Species	*Subclass*	*Protein A binding pH*	*Protein A elution pH*
Human	IgG1	6.0–7.0	3.5–4.5
	IgG2	6.0–7.0	3.5–4.5
	IgG3	8.0–9.0	< 7.0
	IgG4	7.0–8.0	3.0–6.0
Mouse	IgG1	8.0–9.0	4.5–6.0
	IgG2a	7.0–8.0	3.5–5.5
	IgG2b	7.0	3.5–4.0
	IgG3	7.0	3.5–5.5
Rat	IgG1	> 9.0	7.0–8.0
	IgG2a	> 9.0	< 8.0
	IgG2b	> 9.0	< 8.0
	IgG3	8.0–9.0	3.0–4.0

6.14 Purification of mAbs used for Various Applications

A suitable purification protocol has to be designed for each mAb based on the following properties ascertained for that mAb

- pI
- stability
- hydrophobicity
- glycosylation
- likely impurities
- aggregate formation tendency.

Large scale mAb purification conventionally consists of a protein A-based capture step followed by one or two additional chromatography steps. The protein

A affinity chromatography yields highly pure mAbs (typically > 99%) with high recovery rates. Other chromatography methods such as cation/anion exchange chromatography, or hydrophobic interaction chromatography are considered for the intermediate and polishing steps. The polishing step is the final step in a purification strategy where low or trace levels of contaminants are removed. While purifying mAbs these contaminanats would include IgG aggregates and/or dimers.

Protein dimers or aggregates tend to form at high protein and salt concentrations. These aggregates can lower the biological activity of the sample. Gel filtration is used at laboratory scale for removing aggregates and is hence used as the final polishing step in many purification strategies.

For therapeutic purposes, the mAbs should meet very high standards of purity. Contaminants such as DNA, host cell proteins, culture media components, viruses and endotoxins have to be completely removed. Antibody-based therapies are increasingly being used and this requires large quantities of mAbs to be purified.

In the past 15 years, protein A affinity chromatography has been the gold standard in antibody manufacturing. Protein A isolated from *S. aureus* and purified over a human IgG column have been replaced with recombinant ones and purification is no longer performed using any human or animal-derived products. However with increases in protein yields in the range of 8–10 g per litre, protein A binding capacities of 30 mg/mL at linear flow velocities of 200 cm/hr still leaves scope for improvement.

Ion exchange is certainly amenable to large-scale purification of mAbs and is used as the primary capture step for the purification of Humira®, a human mAb against tumour necrosis factor indicated in rheumatoid arthritis. This technique has higher capacities and cleaning and sanitization steps are easier. However, yields were best for the protein A affinity chromatography, although capacities were with on-affinity chromatography.

Most antibody manufacturers currently use a three-column platform comprising protein A affinity chromatography for product capture, followed by anion exchange chromatography in flow-through mode to extract negatively charged contaminants such as host cell protein, endotoxins, DNA and leached protein A, and then cation exchange chromatography or hydrophobic interaction chromatography in retention mode to remove positively charged contaminant species such as host cell proteins and product aggregates.

As an alternative to traditional column-based chromatography, membrane adsorbers are gaining popularity particularly because they eliminate cleaning and validation costs, and facilitate scale-ups. Membrane adsorbers are thin, synthetic, microporous or macroporous membranes that are derivatized with functional groups similar to those on the resins (Table 6.16). About 10–15 membranes are stacked in a cartridge which reduces buffer consumption but increases the flow rate. Adsorption is efficient, despite the increased flow rate, because the solutes are transported to their binding sites mainly by convection as against pore diffusion that occurs in resins. Membrane adsorbers have been successfully applied during the purification of Teleukin, fully-human mAb vascular targeting immunocytokine for anionic and cationic exchange chromatography steps (Sartobind Q AEX and Sartorium S CEX adsorbers from Sartorius Stedim Biotech, Göttingen, Germany). The purified mAbs had 90% recovery and 99.9% purity as determined by size exclusion chromatography, cation exchange HPLC, and SDS–PAGE.

Table 6.16: Affinity Membranes for Antibody Purification

Target protein	*Ligand*	*Menbrane*
IgG	Protein A	Surface modified hollow filbres
mAbs and polyclonal	Protein A and G	Cellulose acetate
Antibodies	Protein A and G	Plastic sheets with silica particles
mAbs from cell culture media	Thiophilic	Regenerated cellulose
IgG2	Protein A	Regenerated cellulose
Immunoglobulins	Protein A, TG19318, histidine, metal chelates, thiophilic	BD2, FD and PVA coated membranes, PES, regenerated cellulose

Although membrane adsorbers are presently widely used in antibody purification the bead-based chromatography is still predominant and effective for the capturing step.

An emerging area in pharmaceutical manufacturing is Process Analytical Technology that is also applicable for antibody manufacture. The FDA defines PAT as "a system for designing, analyzing and controlling manufacturing through timely measurements (*i.e.* during processing) of critical quality and performance attributes of raw and in-process materials and processes, with the goal of ensuring final product quality". It encourages manufacturers to innovate and implement the most recent scientific advances into manufacturing processes. The expected benefits include decrease in cycle times, lower wastes, and improved automation with concomitant decrease in human error.

6.15 Purity Testing

Purity is the demonstration that the contaminant in question is below a specified level.

To assess the purity of a sample, the likely impurity that would be encountered has to be identified (*i.e.*, nucleic acid, carbohydrate, lipid, unrelated proteins) and then a characteristic property that can distinguish the putative contaminant(s) in the presence of the protein of interest, need to be applied. The identification of the impurity would largely depend on the sensitivity of the assay method used (Table 6.17). For example, the application of SDS-PAGE followed by Coomassie blue staining may not show up many impurities that would be present in the mAb preparation simply because of the sensitivity of the staining method as against the ore sensitive silver staining.

Impurities may be either process or product-related. Process-related impurities are those that are derived from the manufacturing process, and includes host cell proteins, host cell DNA, cell culture inducers, antibiotics, media components, or the effects of downstream processing and product-related impurities include the "molecular variants arising during manufacture and/or storage, which do not have properties comparable to those of the desired product with respect to activity, efficacy, and safety".

Table 6.17: Methods used to Detect Impurities in a Sample

Method	*Property assessed*	*Quantity*
Electrophoresis (denaturing/native)	Charge/size	ng-ug
Isoelectric focusing	pI	ng-ug
Gel permeation chromatography	Size	ug
Ion exchange chromatography	Net charge	ug
Affinity chromatography	Specific binding	ug
Reverse phase chromatography	Polarity	ug
Sedimentation	Mass/size	ug
Light scattering	Mass/size	ug
Composition	components	variable
Activity	Presence of active site	variable

The purity of the antibody can be tested by several approaches. One such approach is to use SDS PAGE with silver staining. If more sensitive methods are needed isoelectric focusing or two-dimensional gel electrophoresis may be used. The presence of extra bands indicated impurities but may also be due to the proteolytic cleavage of the protein of interest.

The protein of interest may be purified through sucrose gradient centrifugation and the fractions collected can be assessed on SDS-PAGE and also by biological activity. The intensity of the bands following staining of SDS-PAGE can also be measured and related to the biological activity. The intensity distribution across the gradients must correlate with the distribution of biological activity.

Gel filtration would also fractionate the proteins just as sucrose gradient does. The method of choice for detecting impurities depends on the following criteria:

- Quantity of protein purified
- Nature of the impurity

- Accuracy of the estimate needed
- Peculiarities of the protein or its solvent.

If the expected contaminants differ in molecular weight from that of the desired protein, SDS PAGE would resolve the impurity. To resolve impurities that are of the same molecular weight but different amino acid composition, nondenaturing gel electrophoresis can be used. In such cases, isoelectric focusing techniques would also be preferred. It is also difficult to predict the gel concentrations to be used for PAGE in the absence of information of the impurity. Gradient gels can be tried.

6.16 Protein Storage

Proteins are an extremely heterogeneous class of biological macromolecules. The shelf life of proteins depends on the nature of the protein and its storage conditions.

Proteins tend to lose their activity due to proteolysis, aggregation and less optimal storage conditions.

Proteins stored at room temperature leads to degradation mostly due to microbial contamination. Proteins can be aliquoted in clean, autoclaved glassware or polypropylene tubes and stored in solution at 4°C but it may not be stable for more than a few days or weeks. Repeated freeze thawing should be avoided. If the protein is repeatedly needed, store at 4°C. Addition of 50% glycerol or ethylene glycol will prevent solutions from freezing at –20°C, enabling repeated use. In contrast, lyophilization facilitates long-term storage.

Proteins should be stored in a concentrated form since dilute protein solutions containing less than 1 mg per ml proteins get inactivated due to binding to the storage containers.

Common additives added during storage of proteins include

- cryoprotectants such as glycerol or ethylene glycol in the range of 25–50%
- Protease inhibitors
- Anti-microbials - Sodium azide –0.02–0.05% (w/v) or Thimerosal –0.01 % (w/v)
- Metal chelators - EDTA at a final concentration of 1–5 mM
- Reducing agents - Dithiothreitol and 2-mercaptoethanol at final concentrations of 1–5 mM

To sum up, purification of mAbs largely depends on its final application. As mentioned earlier, it is better to use the same screening assay as the intended final application of the mAb so that the idiosyncracy of the mAb is accounted for. Similarly, the purification strategy is largely based on the intended application. For diagnosis, the mAbs can be used as such as tissue culture fluid or ascites, if the extraneous proteins present in each does not interfere in the assay. For coupling of the mAbs affinity purification is largely sufficient to yield a pure form of protein. However, for therapeutic application, more stringent purification procedures amenable for large scale application are needed and more research is being undertaken in this particular application including non-chromatographic modes of purification.

CHAPTER 7

CRYOPRESERVATION OF HYBRIDOMAS

7.1 Introduction

The catalogued and useful hybridomas need to be stored for long periods of time. The most appropriate method available as on date is cryopreservation in liquid nitrogen, although samples may be stored at –70°C (–94°F) for months or even years. However, the chemical reactions responsible for cellular deterioration are not completely stopped at this temperature.

Some of the terms in general use in the field of cryobiology are:

7.1.1 Eutectic

A eutectic is when all the constituents crystallize simultaneously at this temperature from the molten liquid. For example an aqueous solution of sodium chloride will remain a two phase system of ice and a concentrated solution of sodium chloride until the temperature reaches –21.4°C at which temperature the sodium chloride solution will solidify.

7.1.2 Freezing point

The freezing point is the temperature at which the first crystal of ice appears during freezing. Sometimes this can be the same temperature as the melting point. However water and aqueous solutions have a tendency to supercool and ice formation can be delayed to temperatures significantly below the melting point. For example, in carefully controlled conditions water may be cooled to –40°C before ice nucleation becomes inevitable. Because the freezing point depends on the method of freezing, it is more useful to refer to the melting point.

7.1.3 Glass transition temperature (Tg)

The temperature at which a material transforms from a liquid to a glass–this is usually taken as the temperature at which the viscosity of the liquid exceeds 10^{12} poise. The solutions that cells are cryopreserved in have well defined Tg. For example the tertiary system of 300 mOsm NaCl, water and glycerol, Tg is –64°C whilst that of the equivalent tertiary system with dimethylsulphoxide is –123°C. It is the Tg of the solution that the cells are suspended in which determines low temperature stability. The glass transition temperature for water is –132°C.

7.1.4 Melting point

Melting point is the temperature at which the last crystal of ice disappears during warming. For example, the melting point of water is 0°C and for a 10% solution of glycerol it is –2.3°C.

7.1.5 Nucleation

Nucleation is the initiation of ice crystal formation in undercooled water or aqueous solutions.

7.1.6 Seeding

Seeding is the special case of initiation of ice crystal formation in undercooled water or aqueous solutions by the introduction of ice crystals.

7.1.7 Super cooling or under cooling

The tendency of water and aqueous solutions to cool below their melting point before nucleation occurs. The extent of under cooling is the difference between the temperature of unfrozen system and the melting point.

7.2 Cryopreservation

The objective of cryopreservation is to minimize damage to biological materials such as tissues, mammalian cells, bacteria, fungi, plant cells and viruses during low temperature storage.

7.2.1 Principle of cryopreservation

Preservation by cooling is achieved by striking a balance between the beneficial and harmful effects of reducing temperature. The most beneficial effect of cooling is the slowing of chemical reactions and, therefore, the decreased demand for oxygen and other substrates and the conservation of chemical energy. Rapid cooling may be harmful due to thermal shock.

7.2.2 Method of cryopreservation

Water is the major component of all living cells. During freezing, most of the water present inside the cell changes to ice and cellular metabolism ceases. The extent of freezing damage depends on the amount of free water in the system and the ability of that water to crystallize during freezing.

7.2.3 Need for cryopreservation of hybridomas

Each mAb secreting hybridoma has to be cryopreserved as each is unique and hence needs to be stored indefinitely. It may not be possible to reproduce the same hybridomas although it is possible to produce an equivalent one in terms of its class, subclass, epitope specificity and affinity. Cryopreservation is needed for the following reasons:

- Stoppage of mAb secretion following continuous passage
- Contamination by organisms especially mycoplasmas
- Loss of the hybridomas due to incubator failure, lack of CO_2, mislabeling etc
- Transport of hybridomas between laboratories
- Reduction in handling of all the positive hybrids at the same time
- Back up of the clones being handled.

7.2.4 Variety of stresses

During freezing hybridomas cells are exposed to a variety of stresses listed in Table 7.1 below.

Table 7.1: Variety of Stresses

Stress	*Potential effects*
Low temperature	Depolymerisation of the cytoskeleton and changes in membrane lipid phase
Increased solute concentration	Osmotic shrinkage
Increased ionic concentration	Solubilisation of membrane proteins
Dehydration	Destabilization of the lipid bilayers
Changes in pH	Denaturation of proteins
Precipitation of salts	Damage not well defined
Gas bubble formation	Mechanical damage
Solution becomes extremely viscous	Osmosis may become limited
Cells may become closely packed	Membrane damage

7.3 Principle of Cryopreservation

7.3.1 Basics of Cryopreservation

Proper cryopreservation should ensure that the above stresses to the cells are removed or minimized. During exposure of cells to low temperatures, ice formation is initiated in the extra cellular environment. This results in increased salt concentration as water is removed to form ice. This ice formation thus results in an osmotic imbalance. Water then leaves the cells by osmosis, and cellular dehydration results. Cryopreserved cells could be dehydrated sandwiched between extra cellular ice domains. The aim of cryopreservation is two fold:

- Minimizing intracellular ice crystal formation
- Reducing damage due to the high concentration of solutes formed when intracellular water freezes.

This is possible by practicing techniques that perform the following functions. Slow freezing that facilitates water to leave the cell but disfavours ice crystal growth by

- Use of a hydrophilic cryoprotectant to sequester water
- Maintaining appropriate storage temperature to minimize the effects of high salt concentrations causing protein denaturation
- Controlling the thawing rate to minimize ice crystal growth and formation of solute gradients by melting of the residual intracellular ice crystals.

All of these events influence the outcome of cryopreservation.

7.3.2 Cryoprotective agents

The commonly used cryoprotectants include:

- Glycerol
- Dimethyl sulphoxide (DMSO)
- Salts such as magnesium chloride
- Dextrans, glycols, starches, sugars
- Polyvinylpyrrolidone.

Foetal calf serum is also used in cryoprotection solutions but it is not a cryoprotectant. Cryoprotectants exert their action by one of the following mechansisms:

- Minimizing intracellular ice formation
- Reducing high salt concentrations

- Reducing cell shrinkage
- Reducing the volume of the solution frozen at a given temperature.

7.3.3 Cryoprotectants are classified as:

Intracellular cryoprotectants are low molecular weight substances that permeate cells and minimize cell damage. Examples include glycerol and dimethyl sulfoxide at concentrations from 0.5 to 3 M. These are useful for cells cooled at slow freezing rate.

Extracellular cryoprotectants are relatively high molecular weight substances that do not penetrate cells. Examples include polyvinylpyrrolidone and hydroxyethyl starch. These are effective for cells cooled at rapid rates. These agents have direct protective effects on the cell membrane.

Of the two commonly used cryoprotectants, DMSO is more effective, as it penetrates the cell better than glycerol. Concentrations of 7.5% or 10% are commonly used.

The freezing medium used consists of 20% FCS, 10% DMSO and 70% RPMI or DMEM. However, there have been instances of laboratories using 90% FCS and 10% DMSO. However, resuspension of cells in such a medium may lead to trapping of cells due to extensive frothing.

7.3.4 Cell concentration

Cells survive freezing best when frozen at a high cell concentration. This ensures the following effects

- A high seeding concentration despite lowered viability post thawing
- Sufficient dilution of the cryoprotectant after thawing.

Prior to freezing the following factors need to be considered:

- Cells appear healthy and are in the late log phase before the plateau phase
- There is no contamination
- Adequate cell numbers are available.

7.3.5 Vitrification

- Vitrification is this conversion of a liquid into a glass.
- Glass is an 'arrested liquid' or a 'molecular stasis' state wherein the liquid is too cold to flow.

- Vitrification is solidification due to increase in viscosity rather than by crystallization.

Glass transition temperature is the temperature at which a material can be considered as 'glass'. This is usually associated with a sudden change in density that causes cell damage. This can be avoided if the biomaterial is vitrified but stored at, or just below the glass transition temperature.

Vitrification does not have any of the biologically damaging effects associated with freezing and is commonly used to preserve gametes. Ice formation is effectively prevented and cell viability can be retained.

7.3.6 Rate of cooling

The osmotic response of cells is the primary determinant of viability. The extent of the osmotic loss of water during freezing is dependent on the rate of cooling. At 'slow' rates of cooling, cells may remain essentially in equilibrium with the external solution, reaching low temperatures. As the rate of cooling is increased, there is less time for water to diffuse from the cell, which becomes increasingly supercooled until eventually intracellular ice formation occurs this is inevitably lethal.

The optimum rate of cooling is the fastest rate of cooling at which intracellular ice formation is prevented. The response of cells to the hypertonic conditions encountered during freezing is determined by a number of biophysical factors:

- Cell volume and surface area
- Permeability of the cell to water
- Arrhenius activation energy the temperature dependence of the water permeability
- Type and concentration of cryoprotective added
- Cooling rate.

When the rate of cooling is not optimum, the following effects are possible:

- At rates of cooling slower than the optimum, cell death is associated with long periods of exposure to hypertonic conditions essentially the cells become pickled
- At rates of cooling faster than the optimum, cell death is associated with intracellular ice formation.

7.3.7 Nucleation

Nucleation represents the onset of a change of state from liquid to crystalline. This process involves the progressive separation of ice from the remaining unfrozen solution, which increases the concentration of solutes.

7.4 Liquid Nitrogen

7.4.1 Properties of liquid nitrogen

Nitrogen is a colorless, odorless, tasteless and inert diatomic gas at standard conditions, constituting 78.1% by volume of earth's atmosphere. It serves as an inert replacement for air where oxidation is undesirable. Liquid nitrogen is nitrogen in a liquid state at a very low temperature. It is prepared by fractional distillation of liquid air. Liquid nitrogen is a colourless clear liquid with density of 0.807 g/mL at its boiling point and a dielectric constant of 1.4.

7.4.2 Nitrogen blanketing

The inert properties of nitrogen make it a good blanketing gas in many applications. Nitrogen blanketing is used to protect flammable or explosive solids and liquids from contact with air. Certain chemicals, surfaces of solids, and stored food products have properties that must be protected from degradation by the effects of atmospheric oxygen and moisture. Protection is achieved by keeping these items in a nitrogen atmosphere. 'Inerting' or 'padding' are other terms used to describe displacement of air and nitrogen blanketing.

Samples stored at temperatures below the glass transition of water or –130°C (–202°F), can be stored indefinitely.

7.4.3 Advantages of liquid nitrogen in Cryopreservation

The major advantage of a liquid nitrogen storage system is that electrical power is not required to maintain the samples.

The use of liquid nitrogen is favoured because of the following features:

- Chemically inert
- Relatively low cost
- Non-toxic
- Non-flammable
- Readily available.

7.4.4 Liquid nitrogen storage phases

The two liquid nitrogen storage phases are liquid and vapor. Liquid phase storage offers a uniform temperature of –196°C (–320°F). Vapour phase storage offers a temperature gradient, not a uniform temperature. For instance, in a wide-mouth container the temperature range would be normally between –75°C to –100°C gradient from the liquid to the vapor just under the lid.

7.4.5 Storage of cells

Step down freezing is often practiced for storage of cells but is a less automated method. The samples are placed in a refrigerator overnight, transferred to a –70°C (–94°F) freezer for a period of time (3–4 hr), and moved to nitrogen vapor. In some cases, the samples can also be plunged into liquid nitrogen for permanent storage. This freezing process although does not provide the controlled cooling rates and ice nucleation associated with a true controlled rate freezer but is effective in storage of the cells.

7.5 Programmable Freezers

In a programmable freezer, the temperature of the vial is sensed with a probe and liquid nitrogen is added to the freezing chamber at the correct rate to achieve a preprogrammed cooling rate. Programmable freezers (as against step-wise reduction of temperature) ensure that the temperature compensation initiates nucleation and compensate for release of the latent heat of fusion resulting in improved post-thaw cell viability. The major variables involved are rate of chamber temperature decrease, hold temperature and duration, the rate of temperature increase, and the temperature at which chamber cooling is re-initiated.

The methods of controlled rate freezing are as follows:

- Direct temperature feedback
- Timed pulse
- Liquid nitrogen submersion, or plunge freezing.

The advantages of the programmable freezers include:

- Different cooling rates optimized to suit the cells being frozen can be programmed at different phases of the cooling curve
- Seed freezing as the cell suspension reaches the eutectic
- Minimizes the stress of super cooling and
- Can achieve a linear cooling rate.

Programmable coolers are expensive and should be preferred only when the cooling rates need to be varied or the shape of the cooling curve needs to be altered. With the insulated container methods, the cooling rate is proportional to the difference in temperature between the vials and the ambient air.

7.6 Thawing

The rate of rewarming cryopreserved samples can also affect cell viability, but in general this is less critical than the controlled rate of cooling. The cells can survive rapid thawing because they accumulate relatively little solute during rapid cooling, and recrystallization has little opportunity to occur during rapid warming. Cooling rate and warming rate cannot be optimized independently.After thawing, the cells are returned to their normal environment isotonic physiological solutions. This again creates an osmotic gradient across the plasma membrane. Normally after thawing, the cryoprotectant is removed either by centrifugation or by replacing the medium after 24 hr post-thaw.

Cryopreservation of cells can either be done in vials or ampoules clipped on to an aluminum cane, inserted into a cardboard box or placed within cylindrical canisters in the LN_2 container. The advantages of the cane system include:

- Samples can be handled in multiples of six at a time they all could be from the same fusion or from the same master hybridoma clone
- Shifting from the deep freezer to the LN_2 container can be easy and quick
- The canes can be colored and numbered, making location easy
- The samples can be removed for thawing without exposing all the other ampoules to the warm atmosphere.

Storage in rectangular drawers is preferred

- Identification and retrieval can be easy if the drawer number and the coordinate is properly numbered and identified
- More samples can be stored in the containers.

However the total contents of the drawer have to be exposed to higher temperatures during removing even one of the samples required.

Polypropylene cryovials of 2 ml capacity preferably with O-rings are normally used for cryopreservation. They should be labeled with a fine-tipped marker, or labels, which should be alcohol resistant and able to withstand the low temperatures. The labels should be readily interpreted by others and sufficiently comprehensive as the stored cells can easily outlive a researcher's stay in a particular laboratory.

Most cultured cells are cooled at the rate of 1°C/min by compromising between fast freezing minimizing ice crystal formation and slow cooling favouring extra cellular migration of water. Add cells to pre-labeled cryovials, clip the vials on to an aluminum cane and place in an insulated foam tube and transfer to a –70°C freezer overnight. Then transfer the vials to a liquid nitrogen freezer. When removed from the freezing device, they will heat up at a rate of –10°C/min. It is critical that they do not warm up above –50°C as their viability would go down dramatically. Hence transfer to the liquid nitrogen container must be done in less than two minutes.

Improperly closed vials may lead to seepage of liquid nitrogen inside the vials and they may explode when thawed. Such leakages also can lead to cross contamination between vials. Leakage in the vials can be ascertained by placing them in a dish of 1% methylene blue in 70% alcohol at 4°C for 10 min before freezing. If the vials are not properly sealed, the methylene blue will be drawn into the ampoule, and the vial should be discarded.

7.7 Selection of Liquid Nitrogen Containers

Liquid nitrogen containers should be selected on the following criteria

- Cost
- Consumption
- Controls
- Capacity

The competitiveness of the pricing can be determined based on the additional features on offer and the calculation of the cost per storage vial based on the unit price divided by the unit capacity.

To evaluate a unit's vacuum integrity after the manufacturing process, vacuum is pumped down on a unit, and then liquid nitrogen is added. After stabilization overnight the unit is weighed. The unit is weighed again after 24 hr, allowing the evaporation rate to be calculated. This static evaporation rate is used as an indicator of the consumption. However it is not without pitfalls since this is not tested with storage vials that would be using liquid nitrogen as heat is removed from them. Pressure differentiation is the standard method for measuring liquid levels. Most manufacturers offer audible, visible, and remote alarms and recording devices for data validation and documentation. The capacity of liquid nitrogen containers include:

- 16.0", 24.0", 31.0", and 39.5" (40.6 cm, 61.0 cm, 78.7 cm, and 100.3 cm) diameter tanks for long-term storage

- 14.5" to 22.0" (36.8 cm to 55.9 cm) diameter portable containers for short-term storage
- 7.3" to 15.0" (18.5 cm to 38.1 cm) diameter dry shippers.

Liquid nitrogen containers with narrow necks would reduce the rate of evaporation of liquid nitrogen but makes access difficult. Wide-necked freezers are chosen for ease of access and maximum capacity, but tend to have a faster evaporation rate.

7.8 Monitoring and Replenishing Liquid Nitrogen

The levels of liquid nitrogen should be monitored by a strict monitoring regime coupled with electronic liquid level alarms. The levels should be monitored at least once per week with a dipstick and recorded on a chart. Even if refilling is automatic, it should be backed up, with two independent temperature recorders, with alarms if the temperature rises above –170°C and above –150°C.

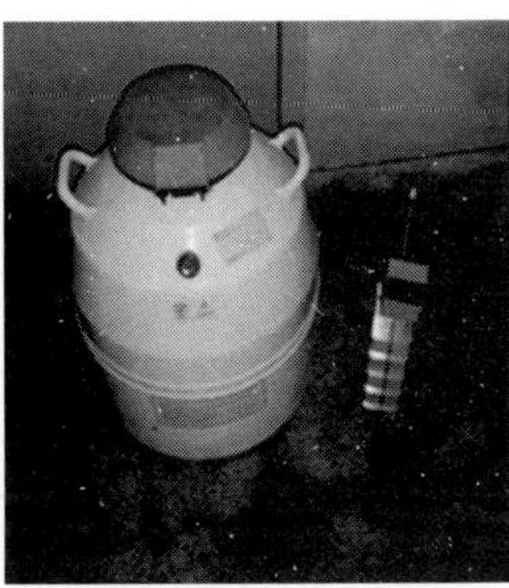

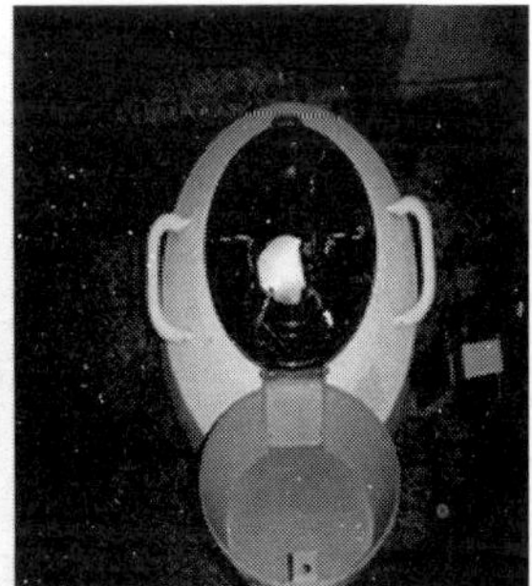

Fig. 7.1: Liquid nitrogen containers (closed and open) with canister with boxes to store cryovials for preservation of hybridomas.

7.9 Transportation of Cells

Cultures are transferred between laboratories in the form of frozen vials or as living cultures. Frozen vials are shipped in solid CO_2, in thick-walled polystyrene foam containers of at least 30 cm × 30 cm × 30 cm dimension that can hold about 5 kg of dry ice. The vial containing hybridoma cells can be transferred from liquid nitrogen containers in to another polypropylene centrifuge tube (15 ml capacity) as quickly as possible covered with absorbent tissues, sealed without leakage and shipped. The cells would remain frozen for 3 days but thawing would be detrimental to cell viability. On receipt the cells may be thawed as usual. The recipient must be well prepared to receive the cultures with information on the media and serum requirement and the subculture regimen for the cells being received.

Alternatively, cells may be shipped as a growing culture. The cells should be at the mid- to late log phase. Confluent monolayers tend to detach during transport. The culture flask should be filled to the top with medium sealed securely with a waterproof adhesive tape and sealed in a polythene bag. The bagged flask can be packed within a rigid container such as a stainless box filled with absorbent packing or in a bubble wrap lined covers.

On receipt, the flask is swabbed thoroughly with 70% alcohol, opened under sterile conditions and the medium is collected in another sterile flask leaving the required volume in the flask containing the cells. The collected medium can be used preferably after 0.22 micron syringe-filtration.

7.10 Protocol for Freezing and Thawing of Hybridomas

Grow the culture to late log phase, prepare a high concentration cell suspension in medium with a cryoprotectant, aliquot into vials and freeze slowly. Cryoprotectant should be free of impurities; DMSO should be stored in a glass or polypropylene vial while glycerol should be fresh and stored in a universal container. Grow the hybridoma culture up to the late log phase, centrifuge, count and resuspend at 2×10^6–2×10^7 cells/ml in freezing medium with 10% DMSO. Dispense the cell suspensions into prelabeled vials, seal them efficiently and place them in a refrigerator for 4 hr and shift to –70°C overnight.

Transfer the samples to the liquid nitrogen containers into the predetermined canister or drawer. This transfer must be done as quickly as possible preferably within 2 min. Protective gloves and a facemask should be worn while placing the samples in liquid nitrogen. Then complete the appropriate entries in the freezer index. Thawing of the cells should be done rapidly and reseed them at a high cell density. Check the location of the vial to be thawed. Prepare the medium and label the culture flask. Then retrieve the vial from the liquid nitrogen container and swab it with 70% alcohol on the outside and place it in sterile water at 37°C in a beaker.

When the vial has thawed completely, again swab thoroughly with 70% alcohol and open it in a laminar-flow hood. Transfer the contents to a culture flask with a 1-mL pipette. Add medium slowly to the cell suspension @ 10 ml over about 2 min added drop wise, then a little faster diluting the cells and cryoprotectant. If centrifugation is used for removal of cryoprotectant, dilute the cells slowly in a centrifuge tube, centrifuge them for 2 min at 100 g, discard the supernatant medium with the cryoprotectants and resuspend the cells in fresh growth medium.

Check after 24 hr for the appearance of the hybridoma in terms of the glistening appearance with lack of granularity and dilute to regular seeding concentration.

CHAPTER 8

CONJUGATION OF MONOCLONAL ANTIBODIES

8.1 Introduction

Two major application of mAbs has been in the areas of (i) diagnosis of diseases and (ii) delivery of drugs which otherwise cannot reach the target directly. This can only be done by chemical modification or coupling of mAbs. It is essential to convert the mAbs into a reporter molecule, which can deliver a 'pay load'.

The application of labeled mAbs include:

- Diagnosis
- Rebuilding the basic structure of antibody
- To introduce effector functions
- Make mAbs into cytotoxic agents.

These applications can be effected only by making conjugates.

A mAb conjugate has three elements

- mAbs
- Molecule to be attached or delivered
- Linkage between the two elements.

It has to be ensured that the coupling agent and the method do not alter the immunoreactivity of the mAbs. It is also important to understand the effects of the increase in size of the conjugated mAbs. For example, conjugation of radio iodine causes insignificant changes in the size of the mAb while conjugation to enzymes increases the size considerably. In case of tumour imaging or therapy, the size is critical in favouring biodistribution and tissue penetration. The size of the conjugate may be reduced by the use of smaller fragments wither by enzyme digestion or genetic engineering. While IgG would be 150000 MW $F(ab')_2$ is about 100000; F(ab') is 50000 and scFv is about 27000 MW.

The molecules that are generally conjugated to mAbs include Radio isotopes, Fluorescent dyes, Enzymes and Low molecular weight compounds.

8.2 Antibody Modification Sites

- Primary amines ($-NH_2$) on lysine residues are abundant, widely distributed and easily modified because of their reactivity and location on the antibody surface.
- Sulphahydryls generated by reducing disulphide bonds in the hinge region of the antibody resulting in sulphahydryl group labeling that will not sterically hinder antigen binding.
- Carboxyls, present on glutamic and aspartic acid residues are abundant and easily accessible, but they do not react as readily as amines and coupling to them requires the crosslinker, *e.g.* EDC.
- Carbohydrates moieties are present on the Fc portion and hence can be labeled without altering antibody activity. Labeling carbohydrates is a two-step process because the carbohydrates must first be oxidized to create reactive aldehydes.

8.3 Radiolabeling of mAbs

The isotopes commonly used for radio labeling include

- ^{125}Iodine or ^{131}Iodine
- ^{111}Indium
- ^{99m}Technetium ('m' stands for metastable nuclear isomer)
- ^{90}Yttrium.

Radioiodination using Pierce Iodination Reagent or Iodogen is a commonly used method for labeling mAbs. Radio iodine is introduced into the tyrosine residues of antibody by oxidation catalysed by 1,3,4,6-tetrachloro-3α, 6α-diphenylglycouril or Iodogen. Antibody and radio iodine are mixed in a tube that has been previously coated with Iodogen. Labeled antibody is separated from free label using gel filtration chromatography.

Bolton Hunter reagent (MW 263.25) increases the amount of ^{125}I on proteins. It introduces tyrosyl moieties through end-terminal α-amino groups or ζ-amino groups of lysine. It is highly useful for the iodination of proteins with no tyrosines, or tyrosines with limited accessibility.

Water soluble Bolton-Hunter reagent (sulphosuccinimidyl-3-(4-hydrophenyl) propionate (MW 365.3) is ideal for labeling cell surface proteins since it is membrane impermeable (Fig. 8.1 and Fig. 8.2).

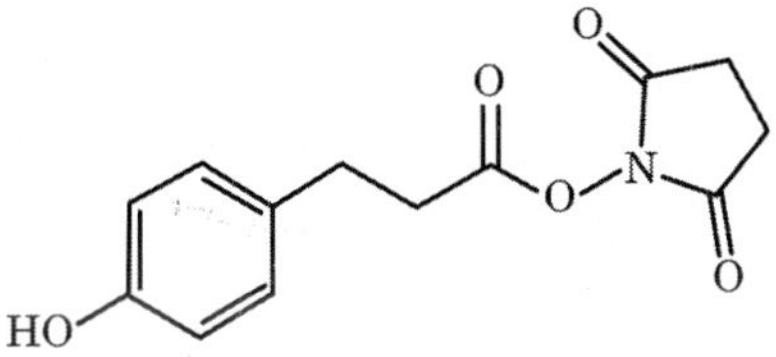

Fig. 8.1: Bolton-hunter reagent.

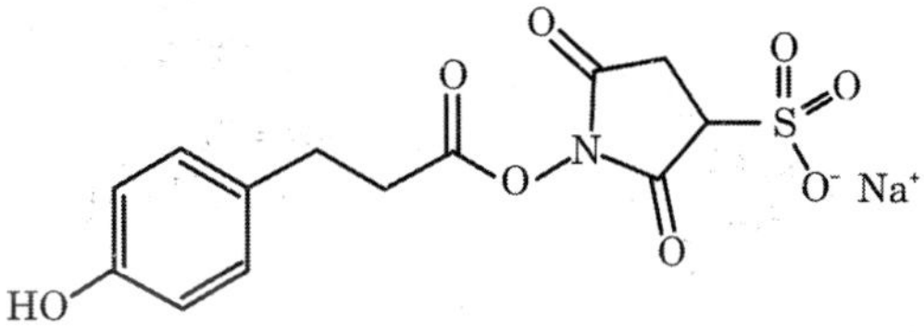

Fig. 8.2: Water soluble bolton-hunter reagent.

For mAbs labeled with radioiodine by conventional methods, the catabolic product is iodotyrosine, which rapidly diffuses from the cell. However, most radiometal conjugates have catabolic products that are trapped within lysosomes and hence are better retained at the tumor site. Such intracellularly retained labels are called residualizing radiolabels. Although the rate of turnover varies depending on the particular cell line, the typical half life is ~2 days.

Antibodies labeled with metals require covalent attachment of the metal binding moiety to the antibody which is able to chelate the radio metal. The chelating agent is diethylene triamine pentaacetic acid (DTPA). Appropriate radiation safety precautions must be taken at all times while using radioisotopes.

8.4 Conjugation of mAbs to Fluorescent Dyes

The fluorochromes commonly used are fluorescein, rhodamine, Texas red, and phycoerythrin. Fluorescein is the fluorochrome of choice in binding assays because of its high quantum yield. Rhodamine has superior sensitivity and less photobleaching than fluorescein. Texas red has a spectrum that minimally overlaps with that of fluorescein; therefore, these two dyes are suitable for multicolor applications. Phycoerythrin is a 240-kDa highly soluble fluorescent protein whose conjugates are among the most sensitive fluorescent probes available. In addition, the newly introduced Alexa fluorochromes are more fluorescent and photostable with excitation/emission spectra similar to those of commonly used dyes.

8.4.1 Fluorescein conjugation of mAbs

Fluorescein is typically excited at 488 nm of an argon laser, and emission is at 530 nm. The reactive isothiocyanate form of fluorescein (FITC) is typically conjugated to proteins via primary amines (*i.e.*, lysines). Usually, between 3 and 6 FITC molecules are conjugated to each antibody; higher conjugations can result in solubility problems as well as internal quenching (and reduced brightness). Optimal concentration of mAbs for FITC conjugation should be at least 2 mg/ml. FITC is highly unstable, hence once it is solubilized, it should be used immediately. It is economical to perform multiple FITC conjugations on the same day since each vial of FITC contains sufficient material for conjugation with ~100 mgs of antibody. When first conjugating an antibody, a range of FITC to antibody concentrations should be titrated. Each conjugate should be evaluated by staining and select the ratio that gives brightest staining with low backgrounds. Normally 40–80 µg of FITC per mg of antibody is used. Before conjugation, sodium acid has to be completely removed from mAb preparations since it will react with the FITC and prevent conjugation.

Commercial kits are available for such conjugation and could be useful for coupling a few mAbs and if not done routinely. Dialyze or exchange over a column (PD-10 or NAP 5 columns of Sephadex G-25M; Amersham), the antibody in the reaction buffer (500 mM carbonate, pH 9.5). Measure the antibody concentration after buffer equilibration. Dissolve 10 mg of FITC in 1 ml anhydrous DMSO immediately before use. Add FITC to give a ratio of 40–80 µg per mg of antibody; mix immediately. Wrap the tube in foil; incubate and rotate at room temperature for 1 hr. Remove the unreacted FITC and exchange the antibody into storage buffer (10 mM Tris, 150 mM NaCl, 0.1% NaN_3, pH 8.2) by gel filtration or dialysis.

Determine F/P and protein concentration by measuring the absorbance at 280 and 495 nm.

- IgG: 1 mg/ml has an A (280) of 1.4; MW = 150000
- IgM: 1 mg/ml has an A (280) of 1.2; MW = 900000
- Fluorescein: 1 mM has an A (495) of 68 and an A (280) of 11.8.
- Protein concentration:
- IgG (mg/ml) = [A(280)–0.31 *A(495)] / 1.4
- IgM (mg/ml) = [A(280)–0.31 *A(495)] / 1.2

F/P ratio:

- IgG: 3.1 *A(495)/[A(280)–0.31 *A(495)]
- IgM: 15.9 *A(495)/[A(280)–0.31 *A(495)]
- F/P values of 3–10 are considered optimal for IgG

Fluorescein isothiocyanate $C_{21}H_{11}NO_5S$; MW 389.382

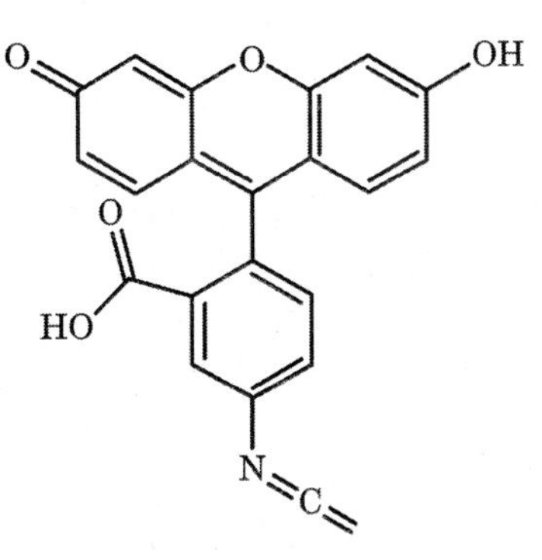

Fig. 8.3: FITC.

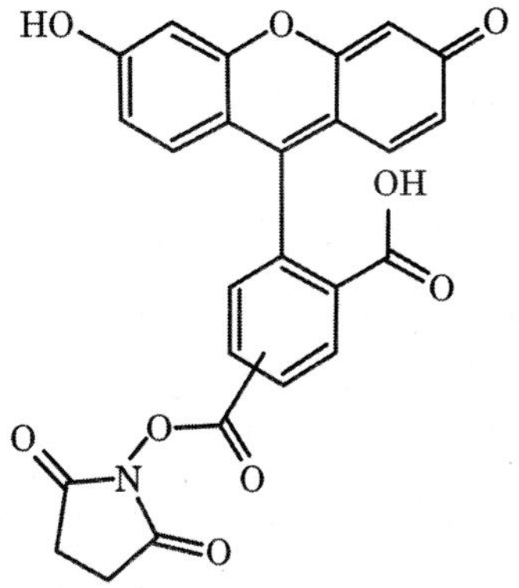

Fig. 8.4: NHS-Fluorescein.

FITC (Fig. 8.3) is the base fluorescein molecule functionalized with an isothiocyanate reactive group (–N=C=S), replacing a hydrogen atom on the bottom ring of the structure. FITC is reactive toward primary amine groups on proteins. A succinimidyl-ester functional group attached to the fluorescein core, creating NHS-fluorescein (Fig. 8.4), is another common derivative that has much greater specificity toward primary amines in the presence of other nucleophiles and a more stable linkage following labeling.

8.4.2 Conjugation of mAbs to phycoerythrin

Phycoerythrin (PE) is one of the most commonly used and brightest fluorescent dyes. It is a large protein 240 kDa MW containing 25 fluors. Typically, only one PE molecule is conjugated to an antibody. It is excited at 488 nm and emits at about 570 nm. Use 3.5 mg of R-PE per mg of IgG to be modified. To check the PE purity and concentration measure the absorbance at 280, 565 and 620 nm (1 mg/ml of PE has an OD at 565nm of 8.2). A 565/620 ratio > 50 indicates adequate removal of contaminating phycocyanin; a 565/280 ratio > 5 indicates adequate removal of all other proteins.

The amino groups on the PE react with the succinamide to yield a maleimide-labeled PE. Prepare a 10 mg/ml stock solution of succinimidyl 4-(N-maleimidomethyl) cyclohexane-1-carboxylate (SMCC, Pierce) in dry DMSO immediately prior to use. Add 11 µl of SMCC per mg of PE while vortexing. Wrap the reaction tube in aluminum foil and rotate at room temperature for 60 minutes. Pass the derivatized PE over a gel filtration column pre-equilibrated with exchange buffer (50 mM MES, 2 mM EDTA, pH. 6.0). The SMCC-derivative is stable and may be stored at 4 °C for several weeks.

The hinge disulphide bonds are reduced to yield free sulphahydryls. Prepare a fresh solution of 1 M DTT (15.4 mg/100 µl) in distilled water. IgG solutions should be at least 4 mg/ml. The reduction can be carried out in buffers such as MES, phosphate and Tris buffers (pH range 6 to 8). Make each IgG solution 20 mM in DTT: add 20 µl of DTT stock per ml of IgG solution while mixing. Incubate at room temp for 30 minutes. Then pass the reduced IgG over a filtration column pre-equilibrated with exchange buffer (50 mM MES, 2 mM EDTA, pH. 6.0). Collect 0.25 ml fractions from the column; determine the protein concentrations and pool the fractions containing IgG as indicated either spectrophotometrically or colorimetrically.

The PE is covalently coupled to the IgG through reaction of the maleimide groups with the free sulphahydryl on the IgG. This has to be done immediately since IgG sulphahydryls will reoxidize. Add 3.2 mg of SMCC-PE per mg of IgG. Wrap the reaction tube in aluminum foil and rotate for 60 minutes at room temp. After 60 minutes, unreacted free sulphahydryls on the IgG must be blocked. Prepare a fresh solution of 10 mg N-ethylmaleimide (NEM; Sigma) in 1.0 ml dry DMSO. Add 34 µg (3.4 µl) per mg of IgG. Wrap and rotate for 20 minutes at room temperature. The product can be either dialyzed or exchanged over a column into a storage buffer (10 mM Tris, 150 mM NaCl, 0.1% NaN_3, pH 8.2). Never freeze the conjugates. It may be useful to spin PE conjugates prior to use in staining, especially if background seems to be a problem (*e.g.*, at 10000 g in a microcentrifuge, at 4ºC).

Other fluorescent dyes used for coupling of mAbs especially for flow cytometry include, Cy7PE, Texas red, Allophycocyanin, Cy5, Alexa fluor etc.

8.5 Cross Linking Agents

Crosslinkers contain at least two reactive groups. Functional groups that can be targeted for crosslinking include:

- Primary amines
- Sulphahydryls
- Carbonyls
- Carbohydrates and
- Carboxylic acids

Coupling also can be nonselective using a photoreactive phenyl azide crosslinker. Many crosslinkers, by virtue of their hydrophobic spacer arms, have limited solubility in aqueous solutions. These crosslinkers are generally dissolved in DMF or DMSO. However, water-soluble and membrane-impermeable crosslinkers are also available. Some crosslinkers contain a spacer arm formed from polyethylene glycol (PEG) subunits to provide water solubility. Other crosslinkers obtain their water-solubility by virtue of charged reactive groups, such as sulfo-NHS esters or imidoesters at either end of the cross linker. Symmetrical cross linking reagent such as glutaraldehyde joins the amines of the mAbs to the amines of the effector molecule.

Bifunctional crosslinking reagents contain two reactive groups for covalently linking two target groups. In homobifunctional crosslinking reagents, the reactive groups are identical. These reagents couple, like functional groups–typically two thiols, two amines, two acids or two alcohols–and are predominantly used to form intramolecular crosslinks. When used to conjugate two different biomolecules, for example an enzyme to an antibody, these relatively nonspecific reagents tend to yield high molecular weight aggregates. In heterobifunctional crosslinking reagents, the reactive groups have dissimilar chemistry, facilitating the formation of crosslinks between unlike functional groups. Although heterobifunctional crosslinking reagents can also form high molecular weight aggregates, but conjugations that use these reagents can be more easily controlled and hence are very useful for preparing conjugates between two different biomolecules.

An additional variation is the "zero-length" crosslinking reagent–a reagent that forms a chemical bond between two groups without itself being incorporated into the product. An example is the water-soluble carbodiimide EDAC, which is used to couple carboxylic acids to amines.

The most common cross linking method involve the coupling of an amine group on one biomolecule to a thiol group on a second biomolecule. The high reactivity of thiols and their relative rarity in most biomolecules make thiol groups ideal targets for crosslinking. If neither molecule contains a thiol group, then one or more can be introduced using one of several thiolation methods. The thiol-containing biomolecule is then reacted with an amine-containing biomolecule using a heterobifunctional crosslinking reagent such as SMCC (see below). Thiol-reactive groups such as maleimides are typically introduced into the second biomolecule by modifying a one or more of its amines with a heterobifunctional crosslinker containing both a succinimidyl ester and a maleimide. The maleimide-modified biomolecule is then reacted with the thiol-containing biomolecule to form a stable thioether crosslink. Chromatographic methods are usually employed to separate the higher molecular weight heteroconjugate from the unconjugated biomolecules.

Succinimidyl-4-(*N*-maleimidomethyl)cyclohexane-1-carboxylate (SMCC) contains an amine-reactive *N*-hydroxysuccinimide (NHS ester) and a sulphahydryl-reactive maleimide group. NHS esters react with primary amines at pH 7-9 to form stable amide bonds. Maleimides react with sulphahydryl groups at pH 6.5-7.5 to form stable thioether bonds. Conjugation using SMCC, the NHS ester is reacted first with the antibody, excess crosslinking reagent removed and then the sulphahydryl-containing enzyme molecule is added. This results in formation of specific antibody-enzyme conjugate.

SMCC; MW 344.32

NH_2

Maleimide activated antibody

HS HS-Enzyme

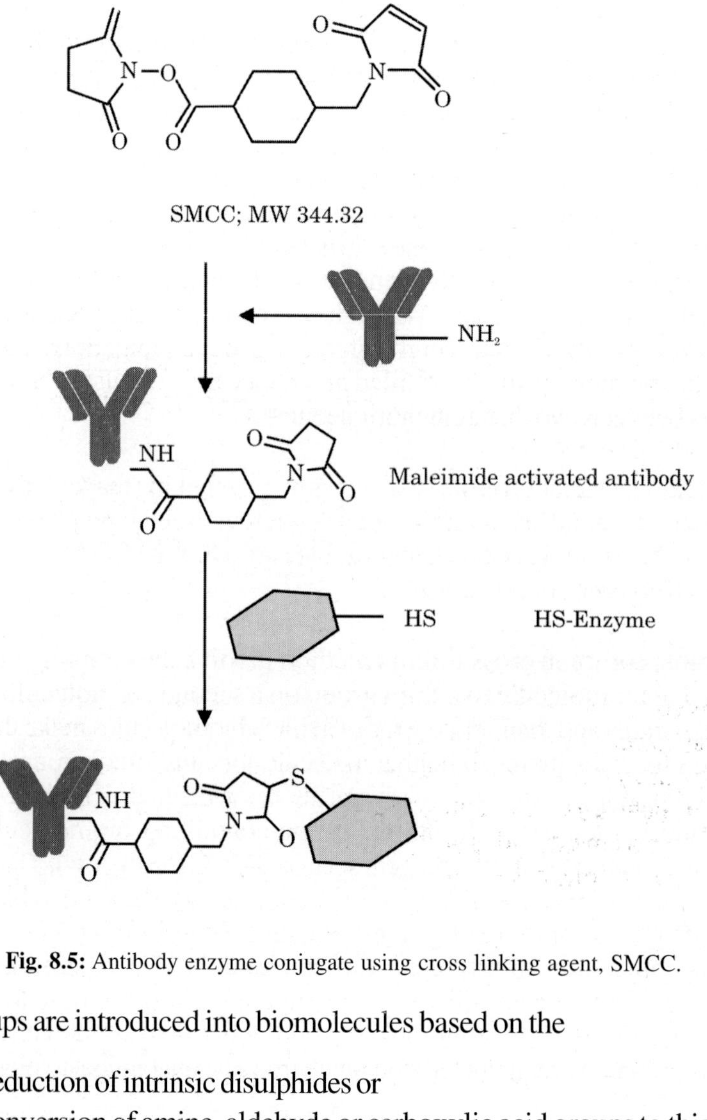

Fig. 8.5: Antibody enzyme conjugate using cross linking agent, SMCC.

Thiol groups are introduced into biomolecules based on the

- Reduction of intrinsic disulphides or
- Conversion of amine, aldehyde or carboxylic acid groups to thiol groups
- Disulphide crosslinks of cystines in proteins can be reduced to cysteine residues by dithiothreitol 1, tris-(2-carboxyethyl) phosphine (TCEP), or

tris-(2-cyanoethyl) phosphine. However, reduction may result in loss of protein activity or specificity.

- Amines can be indirectly thiolated by reaction with succinimidyl 3-(2-pyridyldithio)- propionate 3 (SPDP), followed by reduction of the 3-(2-pyridyldithio) propionyl conjugate with DTT or TCEP.
- Amines can be indirectly thiolated by reaction with succinimidyl acetylthioacetate 4 (SATA), followed by removal of the acetyl group with 50 mM hydroxylamine or hydrazine.
- Thiols can be incorporated at carboxylic acid groups by an EDAC-mediated reaction with cystamine, followed by reduction of the disulfide with DTT or TCEP.
- Tryptophan residues in thiol-free proteins can be oxidized to mercaptotryptophan residues, which can then be modified by iodoacetamides or maleimides.

The use of hetero-bifunctional reagents, such as succinimidyl 6-maleimido-hexanoate (EMCS) or N-succinimidyl-3-(2-pyridyldithio)-propionate (SPDP) are used to introduce the thiol group on to mAbs.

SPDP is a heterobifunctional, water-soluble, thiol-cleavable crosslinker that reacts with an amine-containing biomolecule, yielding a pyridyldithiopropionyl mixed disulphide. The mixed disulphide can then be reacted with a reducing agent such as DTT or TCEP to yield a 3-mercaptopropionyl conjugate or with a thiol-containing biomolecule to form a disulphide-linked tandem conjugate.

DCC is the acronym for N, N'-dicyclohexylcarbodiimide is a carbodiimide that is widely used for amide and ester formation, especially for solid-phase peptide synthesis.

EDC (also **EDAC** or **EDCI**, acronyms for 1-ethyl-3-(3-dimethylaminopropyl) carbodiimide) is a water soluble carbodiimide that reacts with the carboxylic acid groups which can then bond to the amino group in the reaction mixture.

DCC and the water soluble EDCI have been used to crosslink mAbs carboxyl groups with amines and also to activate small molecule carboxyls for conjugation to lysine group in mAbs.

Succinic and glutaric anhydrides convert the amino group to carboxyls and the resultant hemi succinate or hemi glutarate is then activated for conjugation to mAbs.

Only the epsilon amine of lysine and the phenols of tyrosines are sufficiently reactive under conditions that preserve the integrity of mAbs. The phenol groups are mostly used for radiohalogenation.

The reactive groups that have been used to functionalize the mAb lysine are:

- Activated carboxylates
- Aldehydes
- Alpha–haloesters
- Isocyanates
- Isothiocyanates.

8.6 Enzyme Coupling of mAbs

Enzymes are coupled to the amino groups of Igs using reagents such as sodium periodate or glutaraldehyde or by using bifunctional linkers such as SPDP. Sometimes the amino-directed labeling may result in loss of antigen-binding activity. In order to overcome this problem enzyme could be coupled to the carbohydrate moieties of Igs since they are not involved in the antigen binding site. Conjugates are chosen based on the pre-determined OD value expected in ELISA at the lowest initial antibody and enzyme concentrations.

8.6.1 Horse radish peroxidase

Horse radish peroxidase (HRP) is a plant glycohemoprotein found in large amounts in the roots of horse radish. HRP (EC1.11.1.7) is a commonly used enzyme label for immunological detection systems. It is suitable for labeling of mAbs due to its:

- Small molecular weight
- Stability to chemical modification and
- Availability of a range of substrates.

Commonly used coupling methods for HRP include the

- Sodium periodate oxidation method
- Glutaraldehyde methods
- Maleimide-sulphahydryl methods using heterobifunctional coupling reagents.

The coupling methods rely either on the conversion of the terminal sugars in the N-glycan moieties in HRP to aldehyde functions and subsequent linking to amino groups in the mAbs, or are based on exploiting the amino groups of the enzyme molecule and mAbs with succinimide ester functions.

There are six amino groups per molecule of the commonly used HRP preparations. These groups become blocked with allyl isothiocyanate (H_2C=CH–CH_2–NCS) during extraction steps from horse radish roots. Allyl isothiocyanate is the source of the pungent lachrymatory odour associated with horse radish on cutting or shredding which is enzymatically produced from sinigrin. Allyl isothiocyanate reacts with free amino groups at neutral and alkaline pH to produce N-allylthiocarbamoyl amino acids. This is the main reason why the sodium periodate oxidation method remains the principal method of coupling HRP to antibodies and antigens since it was first described.

Cyanuric chloride (2,4,6-tricchloro-1,3,5-triazine) has been used as a coupling reagent as the chlorine atoms in the molecule react with nucleophillic groups (thiol, amino, imino and hydroxyl functions) to form stable linkages. The first chlorine reacts readily at low temperatures and pH, the second at 25–40°C in alkaline pH and the third will react mainly with thiol groups at high temperature and pH. The variations in the reactivity of the 1st and 2nd chlorine atoms and near inactivity of the 3rd atom make cyanuric chloride an efficient heterobifunctional coupling reagent for linking hydroxyl, amino and thiol groups. Cyanuric chloride has been used for labelling IgG with commercial HRP and the producing conjugates with high enzyme and binding activities.

HRP decomposes two molecules of hydrogen peroxide, the natural substrate, into water and oxygen. However, the specificity of HRP for the second molecule of hydrogen peroxide is low and many other electron donors may be substituted. This low specificity has allowed the development of many chromogenic substrates for HRP:

- 4-chloro-1-naphthol (4-CN)
- O-phenylenediamine
- 3-amino-g-ethyl carbazole
- 2,2'-azino-bis(3-ethylbenzthiazolone)
- Hanker-Yates reagent (HYR)
- 3-methyl-2-benzothiazolinone hydrazone hydrochloride (MBTH) + 3dimethylaminobenzoic acid
- 4-aminoantipyrene + a phenol
- 3,3'-diaminobenzidine (DAB) and its derivatives, such as 3,3',5,5'-tetramethylbenzidine (TMB)
- O-dianisidine and
- Dicarboxidine.

8.6.2 Alkaline phosphatase

Alkaline phosphatase (EC 3.1.3.1) from bovine intestinal mucosa is stable, has a moderate size (140 kDa), a high turnover number, and can be assayed using a variety of different substrates which are measured by changes in absorbance, fluorescence, or luminescence. The most common method of labeling IgG mAbs with this enzyme uses the homobifunctional reagent glutaraldehyde. Alkaline phosphatase may also be coupled using heterobifunctional reagents containing the *N*-hydroxysuccinimide and maleimide groups, for example, succinimidyl 4-(*N*-maleidomethyl) cyclohexane-1-carboxylate. However, because the enzyme has no free thiol groups this approach is usually used for the labeling of F(ab')2 fragments of IgG via their thiols.

8.7 Coupling of mAbs with Biotin

The avidin–biotin bond is the strongest known non covalent biological interaction between a protein and a ligand ($Kd = 1.3 \times 10^{-15}\ M$ at pH 5). Hence they are extremely resistant to any type of denaturing agent. Biotin 244 Da vitamin is a small, hydrophobic molecule present in all living cells that functions as a coenzyme of carboxylases. Avidin is a tetrameric glycoprotein of 66000–68000 mol wt, found in egg albumin and in avian tissues.

Avidin has an isoelectric point of 10.5. Because of its positively charged residues and its oligosaccharide component, consisting mostly of mannose and glucosamine, avidin can interact nonspecifically with negative charges on cell surfaces and nucleic acids, or with membrane sugar receptors resulting in high background nosie.

Table 8.1: Biotin Binding Proteins

Parameter	*Avidin*	*Streptavidin*	*Neutravidin*
Molecular weight	67 kDa	53 kDa	60 kDa
Biotin binding sites	4	4	4
Affinity for biotin	10^{-15} M	10^{-15} M	10^{-15} M
Isoelectric point	10	6.8	6.3
Non-specific binding	High	Low	Low

Streptavidin, a near-neutral, biotin binding protein (Table 8.1) isolated from *Streptomyces avidinii,* is a tetrameric nonglycosylated analog of avidin with a mol wt of about 60000. Like avidin, each molecule of streptavidin binds four molecules of biotin, with a similar dissociation constant. The two proteins have about 33% sequence homology, and tryptophan residues are involved in their biotin binding sites. In general, streptavidin gives less background problems than avidin. However it contains a tripeptide sequence Arg-Tyr-Asp (RYD) that mimics the binding sequence of fibronectin Arg-Gly-Asp (RGD), a universal recognition domain of the extracellular matrix that specifically promotes cell adhesion leading to high background in certain applications.

A chemically modified avidin, NeutrAvidin™ (Pierce Chemical Company, Rockford, IL) consists of chemically deglycosylated avidin, which has been modified to reduce the isoelectric point to a neutral value, without loss of its biotin binding properties and without significant change in the lysines available for derivatization.

The valeric acid side chain of the biotin molecule (Fig. 8.6) can be derivatized to incorporate various reactive groups that are used to attach biotin to other molecules including mAbs. The most frequently used biotinylation reagents, *N*-hydroxysuccinimide (NHS) esters and *N*-hydroxysulfosuccinimide (sulfo- NHS) esters, react with primary amines.

Easy-to-use biotinylation kits are commercially available. Some of the kits utilize biotin-*XX* sulfosuccinimidyl ester, which is water-soluble and allows for the efficient labeling of dilute protein samples. Other kits use biotin-*X* 2,4-dinitrophenyl-X lysine succinimidyl ester (DNP-biocytin) as the biotinylating reagent.

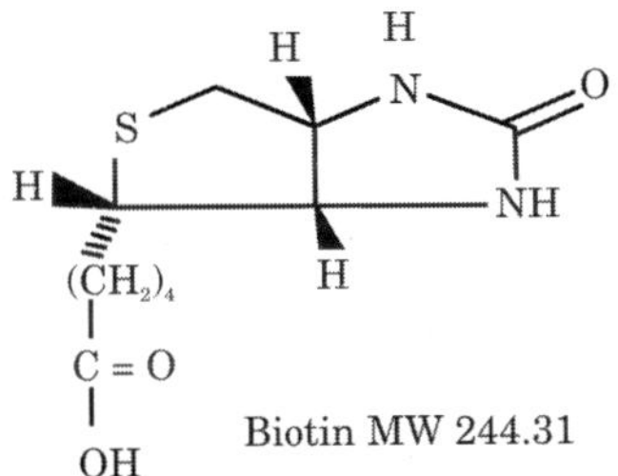

Fig. 8.6: Biotin.

8.8 Coupling to Magnetic Particles

Antibodies labeled with magnetic nanoparticles give magnetic signals (Fig. 8.7) on exposure to a magnetic field. Iron oxide particles ae usually coated with different organic shells including dextran, albumin or polyethylene glycol.

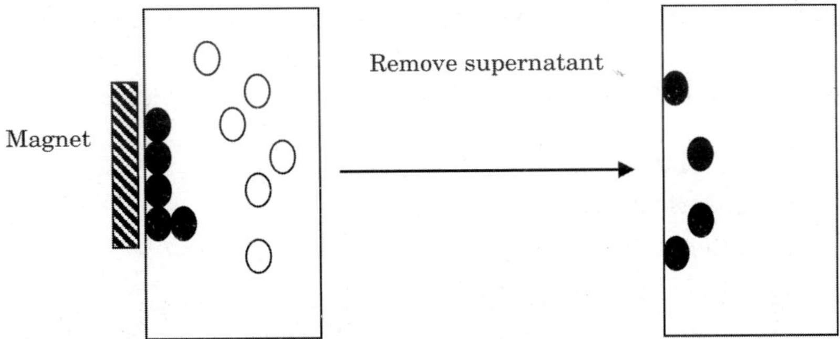

Fig. 8.7: The standard method of magnetic separation–a magnet is attached to the container wall of a solution of magnetically tagged (•) and unwanted (° %) biomaterials. The tagged particles are gathered by the magnet, and the unwanted supernatant solution is removed.

The advantages of magnetic particles are:

- Fast, easy separations
- Easily scalable
- Separation without the need for centrifugation
- Easily automated methodology
- Increased binding kinetics and binding efficiency
- Magnetic particles can be completely resuspended during the washing step of a purification protocol
- Sample sizes can be highly varied.

Magnetic particles are 'paramagnetic' in nature. They are attracted to a magnet when placed in a magnetic field but will not remain magnetized when removed from the magnetic field. This characteristic prevents clumping and allows for easy dispersion of the particles.

Magnetic nanoparticles sizes range from 1–100 nm that can be easily controlled. Compare with the dimensions of these particles with the following entities:

- Cell (10–100μ m),
- Virus (20–450 nm),
- Protein (5–50 nm) or
- DNA (2 nm wide and 10–100 nm long)

This means that they can 'get close' to a biological entity of interest. They can also be coated with biological molecules to make them interact with or bind to a biological entity, thereby providing a controllable means of 'tagging' or addressing it. They can be made to deliver a package, such as an anticancer drug, or a cohort of radionuclide atoms, to a targeted region of the body, such as a tumour.

Magnetic particles coupled to antibodies or other biomolecules are useful in:

- Enzyme immunoassays
- Immunoprecipitation
- IP-western blots
- Nucleic acid hybridization

For example, anti-TSH monoclonal antibody coupled to a magnetic particle was used as a capture antibody. TSH levels can be estimated by reacting with the secondary antibody labeled with ALP and chemiluminescence detection.

Such magnetic particles are useful for the detection of analytes in complex samples using microfluidic or biosensors devices.

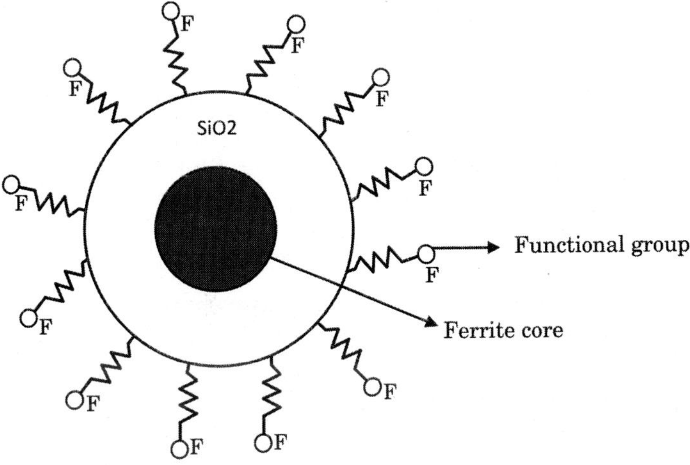

Fig. 8.8: Schematic diagram of a functionalized magnetic nanoparticle showing a core structure with a shell of silica, SiO_2, and functional groups attached to the shell.

8.9 Detection Methods for Coupled mAbs

The most common detection method is using enzyme-labeled antibodies with colorimetric enzyme substrates. To detect increasingly smaller amounts of target molecules more sensitive detection methods such as chemiluminescent and chemifluorescent substrates have been useful. Chemiluminescent and chemifluorescent substrates produce a more intense signal than colorimetric substrates, thereby giving increased sensitivity. Chemiluminescence is the release of energy in the form of light from a substance because of a chemical reaction. Luminol is one of the most widely used chemiluminescent reagents. Its oxidation by peroxide results in creation of an excited state product called 3-aminophthalate. This product decays to a lower energy state by releasing photons of light.

The advantages of chemiluminescent substrates are:

- Higher sensitivity detection limits in the femtogram levels and
- Large linear response for detection and quantitation over a wide range of protein concentrations.

Chemiluminescent substrates are limited by a relatively short duration of light output and lack of stop reagents, such as those available for colorimetric detection.

The signal is a transient product of the reaction that is only present while the enzyme-substrate reaction is occurring. As the substrate gets exhausted, light production decreases and eventually ceases. This is in contrast to substrates that produce a stable, colored product; that persist in the well even after the enzyme-substrate reaction has terminated.

ELISA conditions should be re-optimized when changing the substrate. Higher dilutions of a conjugate are used with a chemiluminescent substrate than with a colorimetric substrate. When the antibody is not diluted sufficiently, too much enzyme is present and the substrate is used up quickly resulting in an unstable output of light.

Chemifluorescence is the enzymatic conversion of a fluorogenic substrate to a fluorescent product. Fluorogenic compounds (non-fluorescent or weakly fluorescent substances that can be converted into fluorescent products) are available for use with a wide variety of enzymes. Chemifluorescent substrates offer the best characteristics of both detection methods. Chemifluorescent substrates are more sensitive than colorimetric substrates and produce a stable signal when stopped, so that the fluorescent signal can even be evaluated at a later time. Fluorogenic substrates, such as 10-acetyl-3,7-dihydroxyphenoxazine (ADHP), are useful for quantitative analysis in ELISAs than their colorimetric counterparts.

ADHP is non-fluorescent but it produces a fluorescent product, resorufin, upon reacting with HRP, with excitation/emission maxima of 570/585 nm. The long-wavelength emission spectrum of resorufin reduces interference from lower wavelength autofluorescence (*e.g.*, blue and green), making it an ideal substrate for quantifying target molecules in biological samples. The fluorescent signal remains stable for several hours which is advantageous in high-throughput ELISA applications.

Chemiluminescence is linear over a ten-fold range while chemifluorescence is linear over about a 50-fold range. This method also eliminates the need for dark room, film and chemiluminescent screens.

Table 8.2: Comparison of Colorimetric, Chemiluminescence and Chemifluorescent Detection Chemistries

Colorimetric	*Chemiluminiscent*	*Chemifluorescent*
Spectrophotometer	Luminometer	Fluorometer
Medium/low sensitivity	High sensitivity	High sensitivity
Enzyme catalyzed quickly	Enzyme catalyzed quickly	Enzyme activity maintained
Slow signal generation	Rapid signal generation	Rapid signal generation
Small linear range	Large linear range	Large linear range
Many substrates	Few substrates	Few substrates

Comparison of detection chemistries of colorimetric, chemiluminescence and chemifluorescent is given in Table 8.2.

8.10 Anti-tumour Therapy using mAbs

The two classes of anti-tumour drugs that have been conjugated with mAbs include Anthracyclines–such as doxorubicin and daunorubicin and Dihydrofolate reductase inhibitor methotrexate.

Antibody drug conjugates (ADCs) are mAbs attached to biologically active cytotoxic drugs by chemical linkers. By combining the unique targeting of mAbs with the cancer killing ability of cytotoxic drugs, ADCs will permit specific discrimination between healthy and diseased tissue. The ADC should retain the binding activity of the mAb as well as the biological activity of the drug.

The drugs used for conjugation include:

- Alkylating agents
- Antimetabolites
- Anti-tumour antibiotics
- Topoisomerase inhibitors
- Corticosteroids and
- Mitotic inhibitors.

The characteristics of ADC include:

- Targeted delivery of potent drugs
- High therapeutic activity
- Efficacy at low dosages
- Reduced undesirable side effects of chemotherapy.

An ADC, approved by the FDA in 2000 for the treatment of relapsed acute myelocytic leukemia in adults was Gemtuzumab Ozogamicin (Mylotarg; Wyeth). The drug payload in this ADC is N-acetyl-g-calicheamicin which binds in the minor groove of DNA and causes double strand DNA cleavage resulting in target cell death.

The cytotoxicity of maytansine analogues DM1, DM4 and monomethyl auristatin E (MMAE) is related to their ability to inhibit cell division by binding tubulin which arrest the target cell in G2/M stage of the cell cycle resulting in apoptosis (cell death). These very potent drugs will indiscriminately destroy both healthy and diseased tissue by stopping mitosis so accurate targeting is required to realize the full potential of these exciting new cancer drugs. Another ADC consists of the anti-microtubule agent (MMAE) conjugated to chimeric anti-CD30 mAbs.

The conjugation of mAbs is driven through availability of commercial kits or contract services. However, the conjugation method should ensure that the biological activity of the mAbs is retained and the size does not spatially hinder the penetration ability for therapeutic or binding efficiencies in case of diagnostic applications. The rise of antibody-based therapeutics further illustrates substantial changes in the paradigms of pharmaceutical development.

CHAPTER 9

APPLICATION OF MONOCLONAL ANTIBODIES

9.1 Introduction

The application of mAbs is wide and varied depending on the requirements and context it may be hard to give a total and exhaustive list of its applications. Generally, the mAbs could be applicable where ever polyclonal sera or antibodies are applicable. Again, whether the mAbs are beneficial than the polyclonal antibodies is highly context based. For example, the application of mAbs in an agglutination test may be considered less beneficial than the polyclonal sera by virtue of the absence of antibodies to different epitopes on the antigen that would enable cross lining of the target antigen leading to agglutination. Although this disadvantage could be off set by the use of IgM isotype of mAbs that has a higher valency than IgG isotype. There could be cross reactions and non-specific agglutination by the use of polyclonal antibodies. Thus while application of mAbs are considered this should be largely driven by the context, availability of mAbs and alternate strategies available for that application. However, for therapeutic applications mAbs is a better choice since they are highly specific and can be engineered.

The broad areas of application of mAbs include:

- Diagnosis
- Therapy
- Imaging
- Research

Before starting mAbs production and characterization, the application of the mAb should be clear. First, decide whether a mAb is necessary or if a polyclonal antibody would suffice. Does the antibody need to recognize a native organism or to identify serological variants? In some assays, mAbs are not as sensitive as polyclonal antibodies for they can be strain or subtype specific. A mAb recognizes only a single epitope on a pathogen and antigenic variation of the target epitope can result in mAbs being unreactive to the serological variants. Polyclonal antibody recognizes multiple epitope on a pathogen. Hence, they can cross-recognize multiple strains of a pathogen through conserved surface epitopes, but conversely may not distinguish closely related strains.

Polyspecific antibody also contains a background of antibodies of the host animals. These irrelevant antibodies might create a high-background or unwanted reactivity for contaminants in antigen preparation used in the assay. In many cases, a monospecific polyclonal antibody is adequate and the best choices articularly when the immunogen is a highly purified or recombinant protein as they usually have low background reactivity. Production of mAbs requires:

- A greater investment of resources
- mAbs cost much more to develop, produce, validate and bulk produce
- mAbs can be made easily and reproducibly in large quantities without the lot variation
- mAbs are fully defined
- mAbs avoids undesirable cross-reactivity inherent in polyclonal preparations and
- High affinity mAbs can be derived easily from immune animals.

The lack of reliable myeloma partners has limited the hybridoma fusion technique in non-rodent species. Several laboratories have developed hybridoma techniques for non-rodent species such as rabbits, sheep, cattle and other species. The use of hybridoma fusions for these species mainly relies upon hetero-myeloma fusion partners and has not become widespread due to the low stability of the resultant clones.

9.2 Antigen Antibody Interactions–A Recap

Antibodies bind antigens using

- Hydrophobic forces
- Hydrogen bonds
- Van der Waals forces
- Electrostatic forces.

All of these bonds are reversible; antibodies *do not* bind antigens with *covalent bonds.*

Multiple bonding between the antigen and the antibody ensures that the antigen will be bound tightly to the antibody. Antibody affinity is the strength of the reaction between a single antigenic determinant and a single combining site on the antibody. It is the sum of the attractive and repulsive forces operating between the epitope and the paratope. Avidity is a measure of the overall strength of binding of an antigen with many epitopes and multivalent antibodies. Avidity is influenced by both the valence of the antibody and the antigen. Avidity is more than the sum of the individual affinities.

Specificity refers to the ability of an individual antibody combining site to react with only one antigenic determinant. The antigen-antibody reactions are highly specific. Antibodies can distinguish differences in the primary, secondary and tertiary structure of an antigen and also the isomeric forms of an antigen.

Cross reactivity refers to the ability of an individual antibody combining site to react with more than one antigenic determinant.

Cross reactions arise because the cross reacting antigen shares an epitope in common with the immunizing antigen or because it has an epitope which is structurally similar to one of the immunizing antigens (multispecificity).

The ease with which one can detect antigen-antibody reactions depends on their:

- ***Affinity*:** The higher the affinity of the antibody for the antigen, the more stable will be the interaction and it can be easily detected.
- ***Avidity*:** Reactions between multivalent antigens and multivalent antibodies are more stable and thus easier to detect.
- ***Antigen–antibody ratio*:** The ratio between the antigen and antibody influences the size of the complex and thus the detection of complexes
- ***Physical form of the antigen*:** If the antigen is a particulate agglutination of the antigen by the antibody occurs. If the antigen is soluble the precipitation of the antigen occurs following formation of large insoluble immune complexes.

9.3 Application of mAbs in Diagnosis

mAbs offer a well characterized homogenous serologic reagent specific for a particular epitope on an antigen. The advantages of using mAbs in diagnosis include the following:

- Enhances the sensitivity and specificity of existing diagnostic assays
- Consistent and reliable source of reagents
- Decrease diagnostic reaction times

- Can be made specific for multiple serotypes in cocktail configuration
- Amenable to various combinations such as mAb–polyclonal antibody combinations
- Choose specific isotypes relevant to the assay such as IgM for latex agglutination assays
- Can be engineered.

The disadvantages of using mAbs in diagnostic assays are:

- Costly and time consuming to produce and characterize
- Have a narrow range of reactivity
- Have unfavorable affinity characteristics
- Display problems due to homogeneity such as sensitivity to inactivation
- mAbs against weak immunogens/haptens are still difficult to obtain.

9.4 mAbs in Immunoassays

The immunoassay is an analytical method, quantitative or qualitative which uses antibodies as reagents to quantitate specific analytes. Immunoassays rely absolutely on specificity and affinity of interaction between epitope and paratope. They offer something completely different (Table 9.1) from the polymerase chain reaction (PCR). Both these techniques rely on interaction between two complementary sequences, linked to signal generation. Both can also involve an amplification step and can be either qualitative or quantitative. Both these technologies provide complementary information.

Table 9.1: Comparison of Immunoassays and PCR

Immunoassays	*PCR*
Provided information on protein	Provided information on mRNA
Detects conformation and sequence	Detects only sequence
Fully quantitative	Semi quantitative (real time PCRs can be quantitative)
Can also be applicable to non-protein entities	Only for nucleic acids
Can also be applicable for haptens such as steroid and thyroid hormones	Not applicable
Many assay formats available	Limited assay formats
May or may not correlate with mRNA levels	Higher mRNA levels do not necessarily mean higher protein levels
Neutralization of biological activity based assays possible	Not possible

Immunoassay's have applications in

- Human, veterinary and agricultural markets
- Environmental

- Food
- Industrial
- Therapeutic drug monitoring
- Drug abuse screening
- Water quality
- Pharmaceutical
- Clinical samples include serum, urine, blood, saliva, semen, discharges, washings, tissue extracts etc
- Environmental or agriculture samples may include water, soil extracts, plant extracts, animal products/tissues-blood, urine, milk, meat, food or industrial processes and effluents.

The critical reagents in immunoassays are antigens/antibodies.

Antibodies can be:

- Polyclonal antibodies
- mAbs
- Recombinant antibodies
- Poly mAbs
- Mono specific serum.

Antigens can be:

- Whole antigen
- Purified sub units
- Recombinant antigens expressed in:
    - Prokaryotic vectors
    - Baculo virus vectors
    - Yeast vectors
    - Eukaryotic vectors

Selection of the appropriate reagent is based on application, time and money. The binding between an antigen and antibody can be detected by the following labels:

- Radiolabel (RIA)
- Enzyme (EIA)
- Fluorescence (FIA)
- Luminescence
- Electrochemical
- Visual
    - Colloidal gold
    - Colored latex.

Antibodies or antigens are attached to a solid phase that may be either

- Plastic wells, tubes, capillaries
- Membranes
- Latex particles
- Magnetic particles.

The solid phase used to separate bound from free assay conjugate (label). Precipitation is a classic demonstration of antibody-antigen interaction. Antibody and soluble antigen aggregate to form a visible precipitate. Antibody must be bivalent (Fabs does not work efficiently). Antigen must be multivalent. Precipitation can also be seen in gels. Antibody and antigen diffuse toward each other and precipitate where there is equivalence. Variants of precipitation in gels include:

- Radial immunodiffusion
- Double diffusion
- Immunoelectrophoresis.

Agglutination is the reaction between antibody and particulate antigen. Presence of excess antibody can inhibit agglutination (prozone effect). For agglutination to occur, antibodies should cross link the antigen (epitopes on the antigen). Some antibodies bind but do not agglutinate. This is also dependent on the epitope density or availability.

Serum can be titered with bacterial agglutination reactions. Dilutions (Fig. 9.1) of serum are tested (usually two-fold). For example, if 1:256 dilution shows agglutination but 1:512 does not, the titer is 256. Titers can be monitored over time. Antisera are also used to type bacteria (against surface antigens, flagellar antigens, etc.) such as *E. coli* O157:H7.

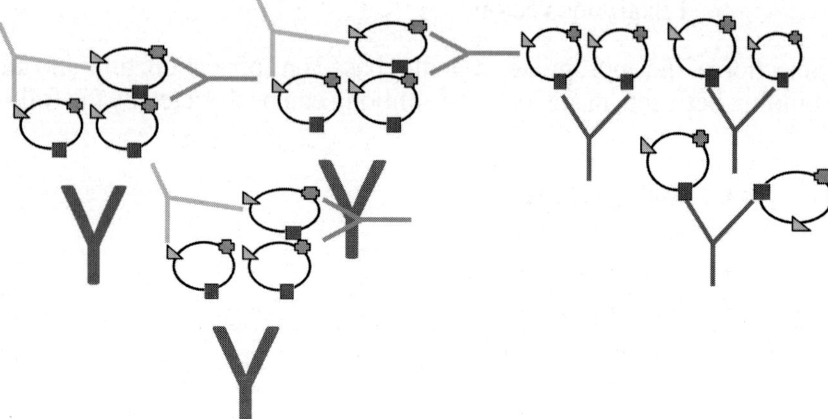

Fig. 9.1: Agglutination by polyclonal serum and mAbs.

9.4.1 Passive agglutination

Soluble antigens do not agglutinante. But if you attach them onto a particulate matrix such as latex bead or RBC it would undergo agglutination reaction. The presence of antibodies can also be detected and quantified using agglutination inhibition reactions.

9.4.2 ELISA

One of the common immunoassays using mAbs is the ELISA. The types of ELISA are described in Chapter 3. Here we would describe the application of mAbs using ELISA with specific examples. A typical ELISA (indirect) protocol is given below

- Dilute the protein (antigen) to be coated at a concentration of 2–10 ìg/ml in phosphate buffered saline or carbonate-bicarbonate buffer and add 100 ìl of this solution per well
- Incubate for 18–20 hr at 4°C or 1 hr at 37°C
- Block unoccupied binding sites with a blocking agent (200–300 ìl/well) using a blocking buffer
- Use plate immediately or store at 4°C with a desiccant
- Perform the assay by adding sample (antibody/serum) to be tested (50–100 ìl/well) and incubate for 1 or more hours
- Wash using PBS with 0.05% Tween-20
- Add enzyme-antibody conjugate (100–200 ìl/well) diluted in blocking buffer and incubate for 1 hour
- Wash again
- Add substrate
- Detect.

In the direct detection methods, the labeled primary antibody reacts directly with the antigen. However, direct detection is not widely used in ELISAs as in immuno histochemical staining of tissues and cells. This is a quick methodology, because only one antibody is used and the cross reactivity of secondary antibody is eliminated. The disadvantage of this detection includes reduction of immunoreactivity of the primary antibody as a result of labeling and such labeling is time-consuming and expensive. The signal amplification also would be minimal thereby reducing the sensitivity of detection.

In the indirect, two step method, first, a primary antibody is incubated with the antigen. This is followed by incubation with a labeled secondary antibody that recognizes the primary antibody. The advantages of indirect detection include:

- Labeled secondary antibodies are commercially available
- Primary antibodies made in one species to different antigens can be used with the same labeled anti-species secondary antibody

- Since the primary antibody is not labeled, maximum immuno reactivity is retained
- Increased sensitivity as each primary antibody can bind to many labeled secondary antibody, allowing for signal amplification
- Different visualization reporter molecules can be used with the same primary antibody.

The disadvantages of indirect detection include

- Cross-reactivity may occur with the secondary antibody
- An extra incubation step is required.

The goals in developing an ELISA assay are:

- To achieve the best signal: noise ratio
- To measure the analyte over a large dynamic range
- To have a robust, reproducible assay.

The signal (optical density in ELISAs) generated by a sample containing analyte, relative to the signal of the same sample without analyte, is the signal: noise ratio. As the signal: noise ratio increases, the assay becomes better at measuring small amounts of antigen.

The ideal concentrations of each assay reagent must be established empirically to have the ideal signal: noise ratio using the checkerboard titration. In a checkerboard titration the primary antibody is serially diluted across the plate, and the enzyme-labeled secondary antibody is serially diluted down the plate. This permits analysis of different concentrations of the two reagents in each well to obtain the best signal: noise ratio.

The most common ELISA method for detection of antigen in the sample is the sandwich or immunocapture ELISA. Here the analyte to be measured is bound between two antibodies–the capture antibody and the detection antibody. Either monoclonal or polyclonal antibodies may be used as the capture and detection antibodies in sandwich ELISA systems.

A polyclonal is often preferred as the capture antibody to pull down as much of the antigen as possible. Then an mAb is used as the detecting antibody to provide specificity. It has to be ensured that the capture and detection antibodies must recognize two non-overlapping epitopes. Even after the capture of the antigen by the capture antibody, the epitope recognized by the detection antibody must be available for binding. A ‘matched’ pair of capture and detection antibodies is a set that do not interfere with one another and can bind simultaneously. The specificity gained by using mAbs for both the capture and detecting antibody must be considered based on the availability and the cost and time required for producing two non-overlapping mAbs.

A 'self-sandwich' ELISA assay, in which the same antibody is used for the capture and detection, can result in limited sensitivity and lowered dynamic range of the assay. Antibody detection in the sera of affected animals is preferably done using indirect ELISA using a single serum dilution or a competitive ELISA. Indirect ELISA is easy to perform and is widely used for assessing vaccinal responses to antigens especially in poultry. Several commercial kits are available with software support to create a profile of the antibody titers in the flock. Its diagnostic value is limited although a 'fair' idea may be obtained using the differences in vaccinal and infection titers.

It is also desirable to use the kits from the same manufacturer rather than from different manufacturers' as comparison may not be foolproof. However, the profile of the antibody titer variation may still be considered.

There is no involvement of mAbs in such an ELISA system since antigen coated and blocked plates are used and serum at a single dilution is added following by anti-species conjugate and substrate. The ELISA ODs obtained are converted into predicted titers using a regression equation calculated based on correlation between single serum dilution OD values and the end point titer values determined by serial dilutions of several hundreds of samples compared during the evolution of the kits.

Competitive assays are preferred using either a labeled mAb especially for antibody profiling in exotic species of animals or birds like for example presence of antibodies to avian influenza (AI) in wild birds or to detect antibodies to specific epitopes on the antigen to be detected. To use an indirect ELISA for determining antibody titers against AI in wild birds, anti-species conjugate of that species of bird may be needed. Using say anti-chicken enzyme conjugates may or may not work depending on the amount of cross-reaction between chicken and that particular species of bird.

Another context where competitive ELISA is highly useful is when antibodies against a particular protective epitope are needed to be measured so that these titers correlate well with neutralization titers. For example, for measuring antibody responses to rabies virus, antibodies to the glycoprotein of the virus that plays a role in the entry of the virus into the nerve cells are important to prevent the entry of the virus. It is well known that once the virus enters the nerve cells death is inevitable.

Using an indirect ELISA with say purified whole virus antigen coated plates, it may be possible to detect antibodies directed against all the viral proteins, which may or may not correlate with protection. However, by using a mAb directed against the glycoprotein of rabies virus in a competitive ELISA format, indirectly antibodies against the epitope to which the mAb binds only, is measured because the rest of the antibodies though present may not interfere or compete with the binding of the mAbs.

Competitive ELISA with antigen labeled is often used when the antigen is small and has only one epitope, or antibody-binding site. Unlabeled antigen (to be detected) and the labeled antigen compete for binding to the capture antibody (mAb) and a decrease in signal indicates the presence of the antigen in the sample. The microplates for these ELISAs should have a minimum protein-binding capacity of 400 ng/cm^2 and a coefficient of variation of the protein binding below 5%.

While coating an ELISA plate the coating solution should be free of detergents as they compete for binding and cause low and/or uneven binding. For competitive ELISA assays, a lower coating concentration of antigen has to be chosen to ensure that the antibody is the limiting factor. Or else, mAbs as well as the antibody being detected in the sample would bind independently with out resulting in competition and lowered binding of the mAbs leading to no reduction in OD and (mis) classifying the sample as negative or having no antibodies.

A typical starting concentration of the antigen protein is 2–10 ìg/ml. Excessive concentrations of coating protein also leads to less binding that is called as the hook effect. Smaller molecules such as peptides and many drugs require chemically activated microplates such as maleic anhydride activated or maleimide activated plates for attachment. The maleic anhydride group reacts with primary amines (lysine, N-terminus) and the maleimide reacts with sulphahydryl groups (–SH, reduced cysteine residues), forming a covalent bond. During coating for ELISA, antigen is bound to the plate by passive adsorption. Some of the problems with such binding are:

- Improper orientation
- Denaturation
- Poor immobilization efficiency and
- Binding of contaminants along with the target molecule.

Antibodies attached to the ELISA plate through the Fc region using protein A, G, or A/G coated plates, orients them properly and preserves their antigen binding capability. Peptides and other small molecules, which are typically, difficult to immobilize, can also be biotinylated and attached to a Streptavidin or NeutrAvidin coated plate with high efficiency. In an ELISA, the unoccupied sites on the surface of the well have to be blocked to reduce the amount of nonspecific binding of proteins during subsequent steps in the assay. The preferred blocking system for each assay has to be determined empirically.

The ideal blocking buffer will bind to all potential sites of nonspecific interaction, eliminating background altogether, without altering or masking the epitope for antibody binding. For alkaline phosphatase conjugate, a blocking buffer in tris buffered saline should be selected because PBS interferes with alkaline phosphatase.

Washing steps are necessary to remove unbound reagents and reduce background, thereby increasing the signal: noise ratio. Insufficient washing will cause high background, while excessive washing may result in decreased sensitivity caused by elution of the antibody and/or antigen from the well. Washing is performed in a physiologic buffer such as PBS with 0.05% Tween-20 that is added to remove nonspecifically bound material.

Both polyclonal and mAbs work well in ELISA as primary antibodies. Polyclonal antibodies are less expensive and less time-consuming to produce and often have a high affinity for the antigen. mAbs have high specificity, purity and consistency that result in lower background. Crude antibody preparations such as serum or ascites fluid can be used or they can be affinity-purified using the immobilized antigen, depending on the requirements and sensitivities needed.

The choice of secondary antibody depends upon the species of animal from which the primary antibody is used. For example, if the primary antibody is a mouse mAb the secondary antibody must be an anti-mouse antibody obtained from a host other than the mouse. The host species of the secondary antibody will not affect the experiment. However, secondary antibodies can be prepared in different host species and, if a secondary antibody prepared in a particular species causes high background in a particular assay, another host species may be tried.

The secondary antibody can also be pre-adsorbed to serum proteins from other species to remove those antibodies that have the potential to cross-react with serum proteins, including antibodies. Antibodies for ELISA are typically used as dilution ranges of $^1/_{100}$–$^1/_{500000}$ from 1 mg/ml stock solution. The optimal dilution of a given antibody with a particular detection system must be determined experimentally using checker board titrations.

The bound enzyme (indicating the presence of analyte) converts that substrate to a detectable product. The intensity of the signal produced in the presence of the substrate should correlate with the concentration of the primary antibody and the respective antigen. Enzyme-labeled reagents can be detected using chromogenic, chemifluorescent or chemiluminescent substrates. The antibody dilutions will vary with the detection system employed. The secondary antibody enzyme conjugates can be affinity purified to avoid any potential cross reactions but such antibodies may be expensive. F(ab')2 fragments of antibodies are also available and are especially useful in assays in which binding between the Fc portions of antibodies and Fc receptor bearing cells must be eliminated such as in flow cytometry. The application of mAbs in various contexts of diagnosis and characterization of pathogens is listed with specific examples.

9.5 Performance Characteristics of Immunoassays

The performance characteristics of immunoassays are governed by the following:

Analytical sensitivity–of the assay is the smallest detectable amount of the analyte in question. It can be assessed by the end-point dilution analysis, which indicates the dilution of serum in which antibody is no longer detectable.

Analytical specificity–is the degree to which the assay does not cross react with other analytes. A test with low specificity, providing the sensitivity is high, can be used as a 'screening test' in situations where a large number of samples have to be screened and where there is a 'confirmatory test' that has high specificity.

Diagnostic sensitivity (D-Sn)–is the proportion of known infected reference animals that test positive in the assay; infected animals that test negative are considered false-negative.

Diagnostic specificity (D-Sp)–is the proportion of uninfected reference animals that test negative in the assay; uninfected reference animals that test positive are considered false-positive. It is desirable to include at least 300 reference samples from known-infected animals, and about 1000 samples from known-uninfected animals should be included to determine initial estimates of D-Sn and D-Sp, respectively.

Precision is a measure of dispersion of results for a repeatedly tested sample. Repeatability and reproducibility are estimates of precision.

Repeatability is the agreement between replicates within and between runs of the assays that is intra plate and inter plate variations.

Reproducibility is the amount of agreement between results of the same samples tested in different laboratories.

Accuracy is the amount of agreement between a test value and the expected value for an analyte in a standard sample of known activity. The results of tests can be classified as true positive (TP) or true negative (TN) if they are in agreement with those of the gold standard (or other standard of comparison). Alternatively, they are classified as false positive (FP) or false negative (FN) if they disagree with the standard.

Diagnostic sensitivity is calculated as TP/(TP + FN)

Diagnostic specificity is TN/(TN + FP); both these results are expressed as percentages. These calculations are done with the help of a 2 × 2 contingency table.

For example, comparison between the results of PCR and ACELISA on samples collected from EDS-infected chickens and used directly technique (on tissues) Dhinakar Raj *et al.* (2003).

Test	*PCR positive*	*PCR negative*	*Total*
AC ELISA positive	6 (a)	0 (c)	6
AC ELISA negative	1 (b)	53 (d)	54
Total	7	53	60

Sensitivity – a/(a + b) = $^{6}/_{7}$ × 100 = 85.7%
Specificity = c/(c + d) = $^{53}/_{53}$ × 100 = 100%
Accuracy = (a +d)/ (a + b + c + d) = $^{59}/_{60}$ × 100 = 98.3%.

Affinity is a thermodynamic expression of the binding energy of a paratope of an antibody to an epitope of an antigen. Affinity constants can vary from below 10^5 liters/mol to 10^{12} liters/mol. An antigen-antibody complex with an affinity constant of 10^{10} liters/mol has a 1000-fold greater affinity than one with an affinity constant of 10^7 liters/mol. High-affinity Abs:

- Will bind more Ag in a shorter incubation time
- Can be used at a higher dilution.

9.6 Application of mAbs in Antigenic Characterization of Viruses

Antigenic profile using a well-defined panel of mAbs is an important criterion for characterization of viruses. The characterized viruses can be given an 'antigenic finger print', which might allow differentiation of various isolates of same virus.

Peste des petits ruminants (PPR) is an acute contagious, infectious febrile disease of small ruminants characterized by erosive and necrotizing stomatitis, enteritis and severe broncho pneumonia followed by death in some cases. The causative agent, PPR virus (PPRV) belongs to the genus morbillivirus under the family Paramyxoviridae. Antigenically, the virus is closely related to rinderpest virus, canine distemper virus and measles virus.

For prophylaxis of PPR in India two vaccines are available using two different isolates, PPRV-Sungri/96 and PRV-AR/87, one originating from the Northern and the other from the Southern part of India. In order to differentiate these 2 vaccine strains, the viruses were antigenically characterized in an indirect ELISA test using a panel of 18 mAbs against various proteins of the virus.

It was reported that a majority of mAbs against nucleocapsid protein of PPRV had higher affinity to PPRV-Sungri/96 compared to PPRV-AR/87. The mAbs to matrix protein (MAbs 4D16, 4H4, 4H9) showed more or less equal affinity to both vaccine viruses while those to haemagglutinin (4B11), phosphoprotein (4A18) and uncharacterized had slightly higher affinity to PPRV-AR/87. This demonstrated that both viruses are antigenically close with a high antigenic correlation of r = 0.823. (Singh *et al.*, 2010).

9.7 Application of mAbs in Detection of Antibodies

A rapid c-ELISA was used for the diagnosis and surveillance of PPR. This assay detects antibodies in the serum samples of small ruminants to PPRV by quantifying the amount of mAb, P-3H12 after 30 min of incubation of a serum-mAb conjugate mixture on plates coated with a PPRV recombinant nucleocapsid protein. The threshold of percent inhibition (PI) was determined to be <50 on the basis of the mean PI plus 3 standard deviations for sera from PPRV-negative ruminants. The relative specificity and sensitivity of the c-ELISA were 98.5% and 93.4% respectively. The c-ELISA sensitively detected PPRV antibodies as early as 6 to 13 days post infection from infected goats (Kang-Seuk Choi *et al.* 2005).

9.7.1 A case study–development of a cELISA for PPRV antibody detection

mAbs against the PPRV whole virus was produced and characterized by methods outlined in the respective chapters. For application of the mAbs developed for development of a cELISA for detection of antibodies to PPRV, the following steps were followed:

- Selection of mAbs suitable to the test system
- Fixing optimal dilutions of mAbs and test serum
- Establishing a base line cutoff value
- Comparison of its performance characteristics with the 'gold' standard serum neutralization test.

9.7.1.1 *Selection of mAbs*

The produced mAbs were titrated by adding dilutions of 1:10, 50, 100, 500, 1000, 5000 and 10000 to antigen coated plates and running an indirect ELISA. The mAb that gave higher ODs (X2A5) even at higher dilutions were used. Then for further testing, three dilutions of the mAbs, corresponding to 100%, 75% and 50% of the plateau (saturation) OD on the titration curve were tested in cELISA (Fig. 9.2).

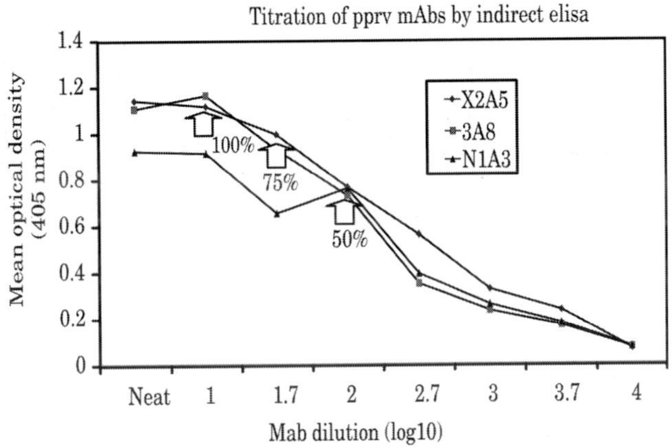

Fig. 9.2: Titration of PPRB mAbs by indirect ELISA.

9.7.1.2 *Fixing of optimal dilutions of mAbs and test serum*

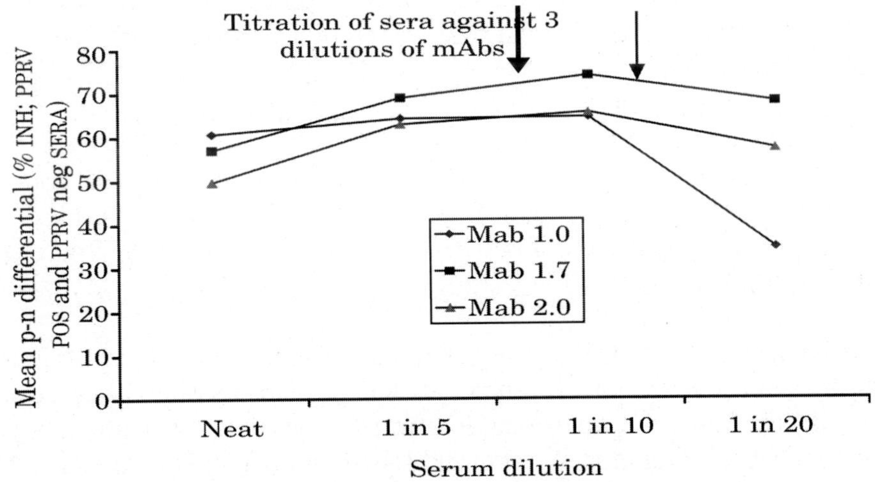

Fig. 9.3: Titration of sera against three dilutions of mAbs.

The criteria used for selection of the optimal dilutions of serum and mAbs were the positive negative differential. The PN differential is calculated by the difference in the percent inhibition (PI) values in cELISA of known PPR positive (SN positive) and known PPR negative (SN negative) serum samples. The chosen dilutions of the serum and results are shown in Figure below.

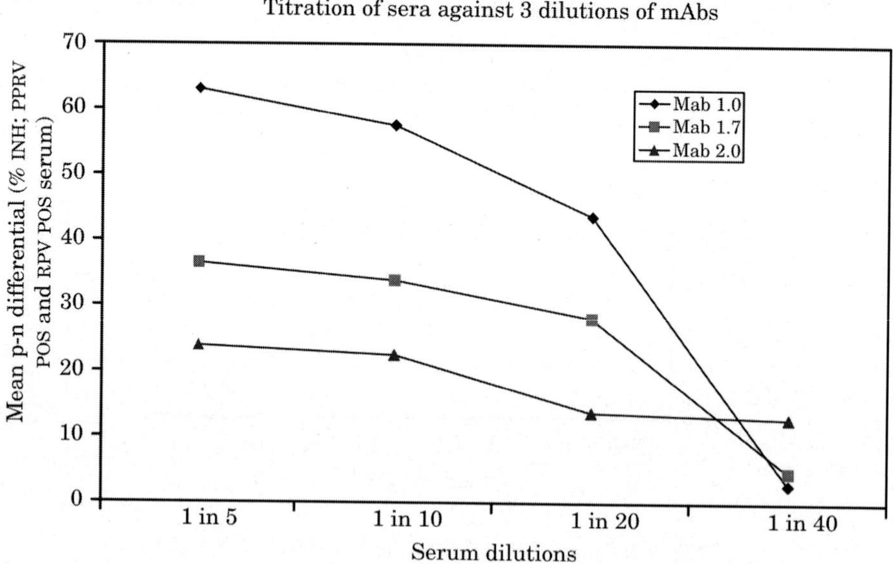

Fig. 9.4: Titration of sera against three dilutions of mAbs.

It was seen that a 1:10 dilution of serum and 1:50 dilution of mAbs was able to clearly differentiate the positive and negative serum samples, as evidenced by the highest PN differential.

The same experiment was repeated with PPRV negative but rinderpest (RP) virus positive serum and a double negative serum. This revealed that the optimal dilutions were shifted to 1:5 dilution of serum and 1:10 dilution of mAbs (Fig. 9.4). (Rinderpest is a closely related virus to PPRV and lot of cross reactivity is normally seen with polyclonal sera).

To counter check, both dilutions (1:10 dilution of the serum and 1:50 dilution of mAbs, and 1:5 dilution of serum and 1:10 dilution of mAbs were checked using sera collected from sheep and goats at different times post vaccination. It was clearly seen that 1:5 dilution of serum and 1:10 dilution of mAbs gave adequate differentiation of post-vaccinal antibody titers and hence these dilutions were chosen for further testing (Fig. 9.5).

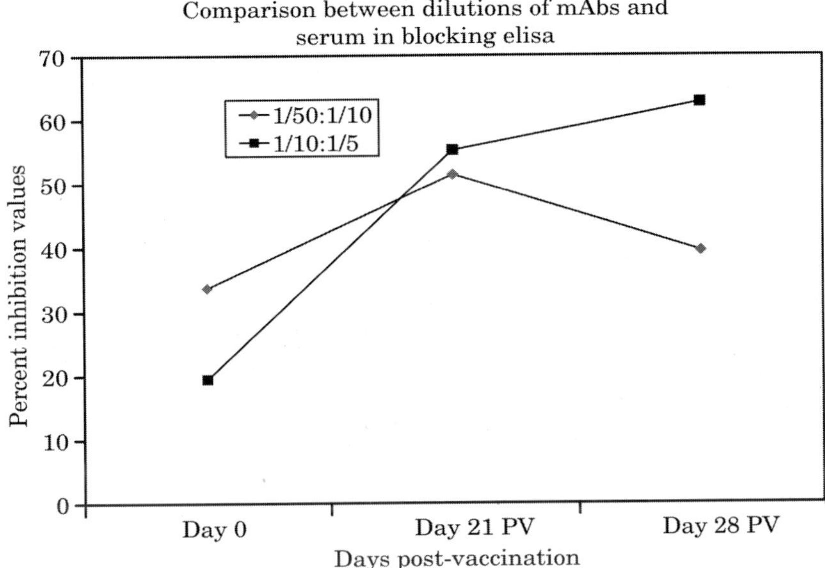

Fig. 9.5: Comparison of mAb and serum dilutions with PPRV vaccinated serum.

9.7.1.3 *Establishing a base line cutoff value*

The PI values in the cELISA of 103 serum samples known to be negative to antibodies to PPRV in the SN tests were calculated and the mean and standard deviations were used to arrive at the base line cut off value. The numbers of negative sera samples with the different PI values are shown in Fig. 9.6. The mean PI value of the negative samples was 22.55765 with a standard deviation of 7.942. Using 2.7 times the SD as a base line value, a PI of 44 was chosen, as a base line cut off. All samples having a PI value of above 44 are taken as positive for PPRV antibodies specifically.

This cut off is a 'man made' value estimate based on the distribution of the negative OD values of the samples tested by the user. In case instead of 103 negative samples tested in this example, 1003 samples had been tested, then the mean negative OD value and the SD would have been different and hence the base line cut off value to discriminate positive and negative ODs would also have been different. Then one could argue that a sample that has been declared positive based on 44% PI as cut off could also turn out to be negative if 50% cut off was used. That is why it is said that this is a continual process and for establishment of such a cut off value many thousands of negative samples need to be tested, not only a few hundreds.

If a sample has a PI value of 45% it can not be treated as positive neither a sample with a PI of 43% is treated as negative. In such cases these samples must be treated as suspicious and the samples may be tested again by collection of serum after a week or 10 days so that by this time the serum antibody levels could have risen giving a better demarcation of the PIs.

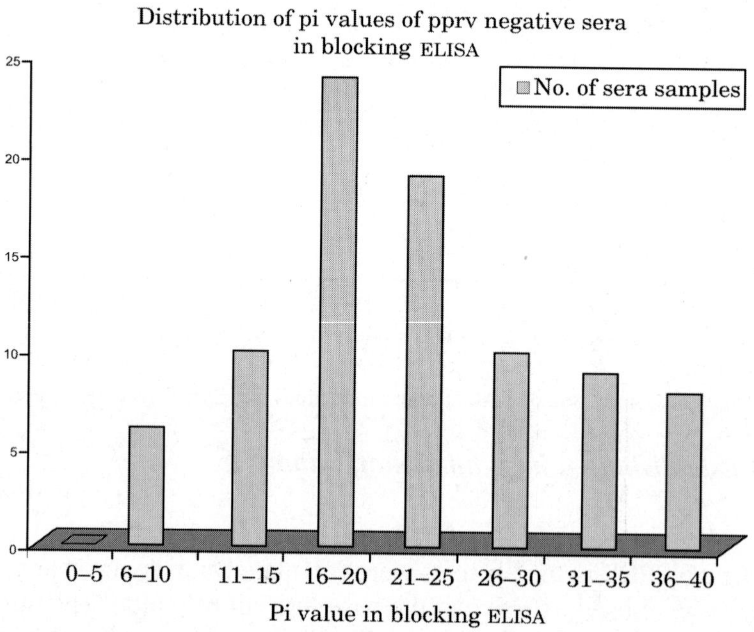

Fig. 9.6: Distribution of PI values of PPRV negative sera to establishment of cutoff.

If the base line cutoff is fixed higher, the specificity of the test could be increased but the sensitivity could be lower and vice versa. So depending on the requirement this can be prioritized. If an endemic disease if being diagnosed, then specificity can be the priority while for an exotic disease sensitivity could be the priority. However, the ideal assay should be both sensitive and specific.

9.7.1.4 *Comparison of its performance characteristics with the gold standard serum neutralization test*

A total of 156 sera samples were compared using both the cELISA and SN tests. The sensitivity, specificity and kappa value for these samples are shown in Table 9.2.

Table 9.2: Comparison of performance characteristics of cELISA and SN tests for detection of PPRV antibodies in sheep and goat sera

SN test	*cELISA*		*Total*	*DSp*	*DSn*	*Accuracy*
	Positive	*Negative*				
Positive	38	13	51	98.1%	74.5%	90.38%
Negative	2	103	105			
Total	40	116	156			

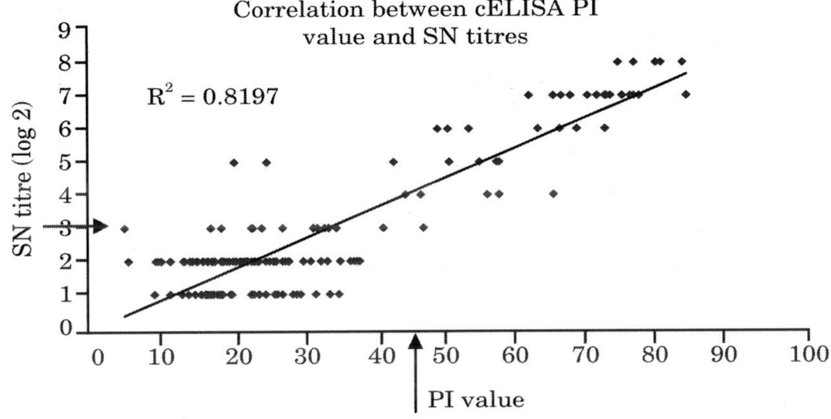

Fig. 9.7: Correlation between cELISA PI value and SN titres.

The correlation between the cELISA PI value and the log_2 SN titres, the gold standard test show a correlation coefficient of 0.8197. This is a fairly good correlation meaning that these 2 values are in agreement. This is the methodology for developing any assay using mAbs and comparing the same with an existing gold standard test to validate the developed assay.

9.8 Application of mAbs in Detection of Antigen (Virus Protein)

A sandwich or antigen capture ELISA using polyclonal sera to capture the antigen from clinical samples and a PPR virus specific mAb (clone 4G6) to an epitope on the nucleocapsid protein as the detecting mAb has been developed. The test is specific to PPR as it failed to detect rinderpest vaccine virus (RBOK strain).

Another similar test available commercially uses mAb against the PPRV as coating antibody and a biotinylated mAb as the detector antibody. This test has been extensively used for diagnosis of PPRV outbreaks throughout India (Singh *et al.*, 2004).

9.9 Application of mAbs in Detection of Antigen (Virus Protein) Based Quality Control of Vaccine

mAbs can also be used for assessing the quality (potency) of the live attenuated vaccine preparations based on positivity or titres obtained in antigen capture ELISA (AC-ELISA). The conventional quality control test for live attenuated vaccines would include titration in appropriate cell cultures such as Vero cells for PPRV titre in vaccine batches. This would take at least 6-8 days to determine the quality and dose of vaccine. In a study, freeze-dried PPRV vaccine batches were tested simultaneously by both virus titration and AC-ELISA to correlate the titre of the vaccine virus with reactivity in AC-ELISA. The vaccine batches with titre more than 10^3 $TCID_{50}$/ml gave positive results in AC-ELISA and the correlation coefficient between the virus titration and AC-ELISA reactivity was 0.96. Thus AC-ELISA was found to be a preliminary useful technique for the quality control of PPR vaccines. (Saravanan *et al.,* 2008).

9.10 Application of mAbs in Detection of Antibody/antigen to Viruses having Multiple Serotypes

Bluetongue virus (BTV) is the prototype member of the genus Orbivirus in the family Reoviridae. The ten dsRNA segments encode five structural proteins (VP1-VP5) and three non-structural proteins (NS1-NS3). The genome is contained within a core particle consisting primarily of VP3 and VP7, which is in turn encased in an outer capsid consisting of VP2 and VP5. VP2 is responsible for attachment of BTV to mammalian cells and contains epitopes responsible for virus neutralization and serotype specificity. To date, 24 serotypes of BTV (BTV-1 to BTV-24) have been identified by serum neutralization assays (SNT).

Blue tongue is non-contagious disease transmitted by Culicoides biting midges and the virus is considered able to infect all species of ruminants, although clinical disease is limited to mostly sheep. Clinical signs include fever, hyperaemia, coronitis, oedema, erosions and ulcerations of the dermis. In severe cases death may occur in 8–10 days. The application of mAbs in BTV diagnosis or BTV-specific antibody detection is interesting. The choice of the protein specificity of the mAbs is critical. mAbs against the serotypically conserved VP7, the group specific antigen, are used to detect antibodies to BTV (Table 9.3) in sheep sera using c-ELISA bases methods irrespective of the serotype of the virus involved.

Use of mAbs against the serotype-specific VP2 may or may not react with BTV of other serotypes, but would be useful to detect BTV of a particular serotype. Another animal virus with several serotypes is the foot-and-mouth disease (FMD) virus, a member of the genus Aphthovirus. The diagnosis of FMD should also be coupled with typing of the virus as this information is needed for vaccine updating. Serotype-specific and non-specific mAbs developed against different FMD virus vaccine strains are extensively used to study any possible antigenic variations during vaccine production and in typing ELISA. A typical FMD typing ELISA is based on the principle of AC-ELISA using a mAb cross reactive with all FMD virus serotypes/polyclonal serum as the coating antibody and the serotype-specific mAbs as the detector antibody. Appropriate known serotypes of the reference strains are also used and based on the ELISA reactivity of the samples with the mAbs, the serotype can be determined (Seki *et al.*, 2009).

Table 9.3: Commercially Available BTV ELISA for Detection of BTV Antibodies

cELISA kit	*Available from*
BDSL	http://www.BDSL2000.com
VMRD	http://www.vmrd.com
ID-Vet	http://www.id-vet.com
Pourquier	http://www.institut-pourquier.fr
Ingenasa	http://www.ingenasa.es
IZS	http://www.izs.it

9.11 Application of mAbs in differentiation of Vaccinated from Infected Animals (DIVA)

One of the several available methods for DIVA is to detect antibodies to the non-structural proteins of the virus that would occur only in infected animals and not in animals vaccinated with inactivated whole vision as vaccine antigen (without the presence of non-structural proteins). Based on this, the detection of FMD virus non-structural protein 3D antibodies using a cELISA has been used as an indirect indicator of FMDV infection. A cELISA was developed using the recombinant FMDV-3D as an antigen and the mAb F32–44 (Yang *et al.*, 2007).

Another facet of application of the mAbs against the non-structural protein of FMD virus is the use of these mAbs to remove any contaminating non-structural proteins from the vaccine preparation with out reducing the efficacy of the vaccine so that their inadvertent presence would not interfere in DIVA using detection of antibodies to non-structural proteins in infected animals.

Such a study involved the mAb, 3BIgG, against the prokaryotically expressed FMD virus non-structural protein. These mAbs were conjugated to the epoxy-activated sepharose 6BFF. Following incubation with the inactivated FMDV the sepharose was removed by centrifugation. The non-structural protein depleted vaccine potency was not reduced but this vaccine would be less interfering in DIVA based on non-structural antibody detection (Dong *et al.*, 2010).

9.12 Application of mAbs in *in vivo* Depletion of T Cells

In vivo depletion of human lymphocyte populations is performed to eliminate harmful responses such as graft rejection or auto-reactivities. Selective inhibition of certain unwanted immune responses by depletion of specific lymphocyte populations was made possible with mAbs against specific cellular markers. The target cells are depleted either through a complement dependent mechanism for which complement-binding antibody isotypes like IgG2a, IgM are needed or by phagocytosis or induction of apoptosis if non complement-binding isotype (IgG1) mAb is used. However the latter effect is delayed to several days. In ruminants, depletion of CD4 T cells has been achieved using mouse mAbs by the inoculation of the calves with 4 doses of 4 mg of anti-CD4 mAbs on days 0, 2, 4 and 7.

The depletion of CD4 and CD8 T cell populations in the host animal serves as a good model to dissect the role of these specific cell types in the pathogenesis and immune responses of certain diseases (Naessens *et al.,* 1998). A few other techniques that are used for detection of infectious pathogens using mAbs include:

- Immunohistochemical staining
- Immuno-electron microscope
- Fluorescent antibody test or Confocal microscopy
- Western immunoblot
- Flow cytometry.

9.13 Application of mAbs in Aflatoxin Detection

Aflatoxins are highly toxic mycotoxins produced by some *Aspergillus* species namely *Aspergillus flavus*, *Aspergillus parasiticus* and the rare *Aspergillus nomius* during the growth on foods and feeds. The major aflatoxins of concern are AFB1, *B*2, *G*1 and *G*2. Aflatoxin *M*1 is a major metabolite of aflatoxin *B*1 and is often found primarily in animal tissues and fluids.

Owing to the weak antigenicity and the low molecular weight of aflatoxin *B*1, it must be coupled to carrier protein (BSA) in order to elicit an immune response. Antibodies produced against a hapten-carrier antigen result in antibodies against for the hapten, the carrier and also for various mixtures of these molecules.

mAbs cross-reactive with four major aflatoxins were obtained using a two-step screening procedure. The first step was an indirect ELISA followed by a modified indirect cELISA in which the aflatoxins *B*1, *B*2, *G*1 and *G*2 were all used as competitors that resulted in eight hybridomas that secreted antibodies with good cross-reactivity and high affinity to four aflatoxins (Zhanga *et al.,* 2009).

9.14 mAbs to Identify Receptors for Molecules

mAbs are useful to bind the specific protein from a heterogenous mixture and this complex can be used to immobilize the receptor for the target protein. Using this technique, the receptor for leukotoxin of *Mannheimia haemolytica* has been identified a β2 integrin. The anti-leukotoxin mAbs are coupled to the sepharose beads in an immunoaffinity column that would bind the leukotoxin. Then the leukotoxin susceptible cells (ruminant leucocytes) are passed through the column that would bind to the toxins through its receptor. The mAbs to be used should be non-neutralizing so that the neutralizing epitope of the toxin is still available to bind to the receptor.

The eluted proteins from the column are run on SDS-PAGE and blotted onto PVDF membranes and used in N-terminal sequencing. This proved that the receptor binding to the leukotoxin is the β2 integrin. (Lawrence *et al.,* 2008).

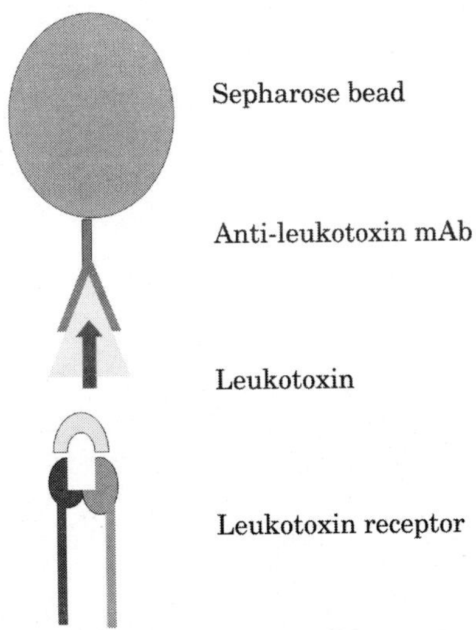

Fig. 9.8: Immunoaffnity purification of receptor for leukotoxin using mAbs.

9.15 mAbs in interferon quantification and diagnosis of *Mycobacterial* diseases

The standard method for diagnosis of tuberculosis (TB) in cattle is by the single intra dermal tuberculin (SID) test that involves detection of the delayed type hypersensitivity reaction elicited by the intra dermal inoculation of bovine tuberculin purified protein derivative (PPD) and assessed after 72 hr. The moderate sensitivity of this test coupled with low specificity due to significant cross-reactivity with a typical mycobacteria, proved stumbling blocks in the accurate identification of infected animals. In 1985, the interferon-gamma (IFN-γ) assay was developed which involved the overnight culture of whole blood with PBS (nil antigen control), bovine PPD or avian PPD, followed the next day by quantification of IFN-γ in the separated plasma samples using the IFN-c specific ELISA. *M. bovis* infection is indicated when bovine PPD stimulates more IFN-γ than both avian PPD and the nil antigen control. This assay was developed into a commercial kit by CSL Animal Health, Australia, and is sold under the trade name BOVIGAM™. This diagnostic method was possible due to mAbs available against IFN-γ (Fig. 9.9). The assay method is based on AC ELISA where in one mAb against IFN-γ is used as the coating antibody, plasma samples as source of IFN–γ followed by another mAb coupled against IFN-γ coupled to either biotin or directly to enzyme. In case of biotin-coupled mAb, this step should be followed by streptavidin enzyme conjugate and substrate.

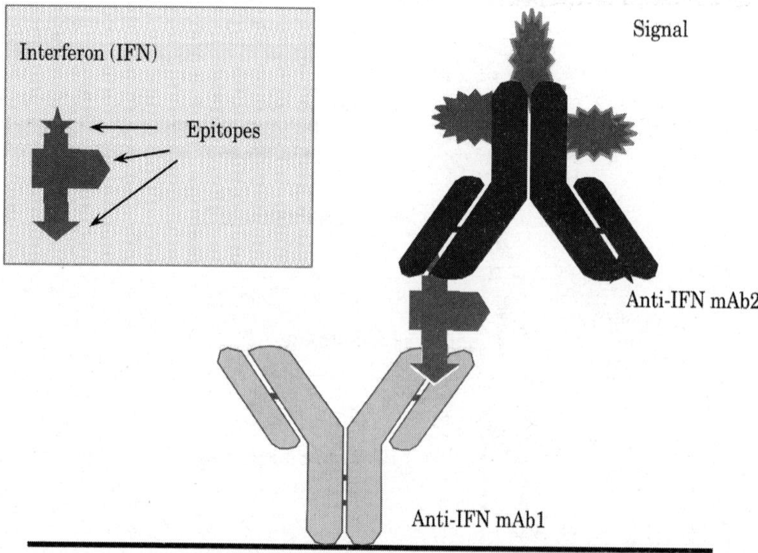

Fig. 9.9: IC-ELISA for the detection and quantification of IFN gamma for diagnosis of tuberculosis.

Although cytokine detection using sandwich ELISA is robust and sensitive, they require multiple washing steps, are timeconsuming and do not allow real-time detection. Presently cytokine molecules are detected using impedimetric or surface plasmon resonance (SPR)-based sensors. Glass slides are imprinted with anti-CD4 Abs, enclosed inside a flow chamber and exposed to RBC-depleted human blood. After affinity selection, CD4 T-cells are activated *in situ* to secrete cytokines followed by detection using a SPR chip containing Ab layer for detection of IFN-γ. Surface plasmons are collective oscillations of electrons on metallic surface with the optical frequency. The mAb is immobilized on gold sensor surface and the corresponding antigen in the flow would bind changing the refractive index. This change is detected by changed angle of surface plasmon resonance.

9.15.1 Elispot

Instead of measuring the cytokines produced, the cytokine producing cells are counted as a measure of T-cell activation. In this technique called ELISPOT, the secreted cytokines are directly captured by the anti-cytokine mAb coated (Fig. 9.10) on the ELISPOT plate, which would avoid

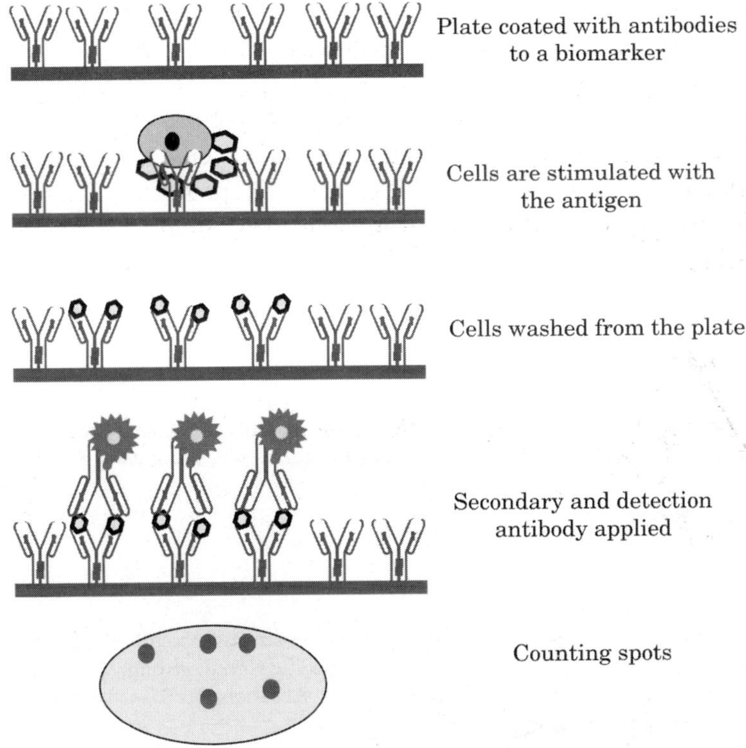

Fig. 9.10: Principle of ELISPOT.

- Diffusion or dilution of cytokine in the supernatant
- Degradation of cytokine by proteases
- Binding to soluble cytokine receptors probably present in the sample.

Advantages

- Detects functional T-cells
- High sensitivity
- Automation.

Disadvantages

- Does not allow the phenotype of T-cells producing the cytokine
- Does not allow sort or purification of the cytokine producing cells.

In ELISPOT assays, the PVDF membrane inside the wells of a 96-well plate is coated with primary antibody (anti-cytokine mAb). Next, the PBMCs are grown on this membrane so that the secreted cytokine of interest will bind to the antibody. This is then detected using a labeled secondary antibody. The cytokine protein will be seen in the vicinity of that secreting cells as a spot of colour. Each spot represents the foot print of the original cytokine secreting cell. The membranes are then scanned using software that quantifies the number and percentage of cells secreting the cytokine protein. ELISPOT measuring two cytokine producing cells simultaneously are also available so also fluorospot that uses fluorescent based detection (Fig. 9.11).

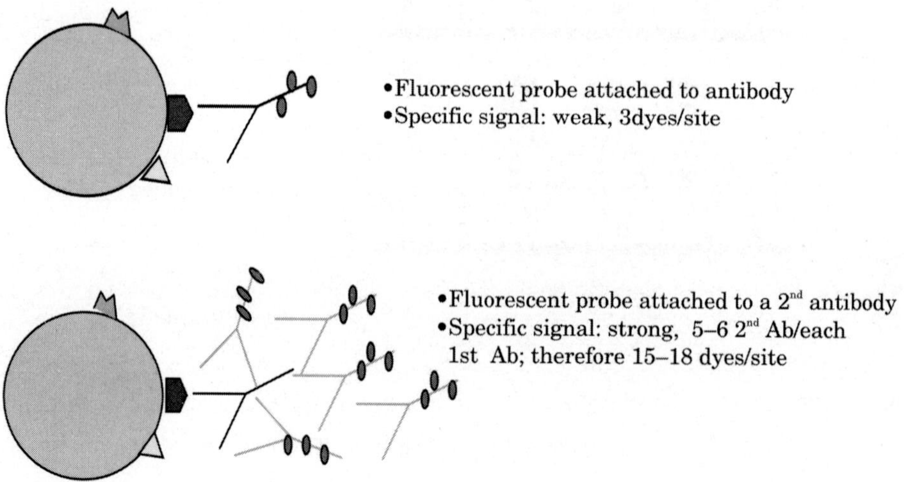

Fig. 9.11: Direct and indirect fluorescent antibody staining that is used in flow cytometry.

9.16 mAbs in Immunophenotyping

The lymphocyte subclasses can not be determined using phenotypic means since these cells are not phenotypically different. The cells identified in a blood smear include neutrophils, basophils, eosinophils, monocytes and lymphocytes. The subclasses of lymphocytes such as T-helper or T-cytotoxic cells can only be identified using mAbs against cell-specific markers such as CD, CD8 etc (Fig. 9.12). The advent of mAb technology complemented growth in immunology in these areas.

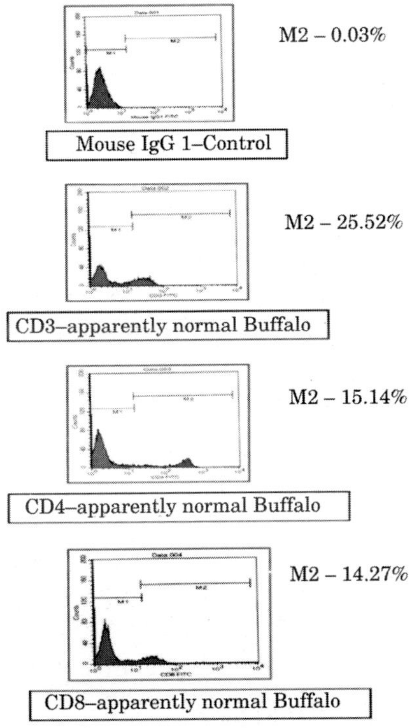

Fig. 9.12: Single parameter histogram of peripheral blood mononuclear cells from a representative apparently normal buffalo analyzed by flow cytometry with mAbs against bovine lymphocyte differentiation antigens (Raj *et al.*, 2007).

Table 9.4: Mean (±SD) Percentages of Lymphocyte subpopulations present in the Peripheral Blood, Spleen and Lymph nodes of Apparently Healthy adult Buffaloes

mAbs	*Specificity*	*Peripheral blood*	*Spleen*	*Lymph node*
PT85A MHC	MHC class I	89.4 ± 7.0	92.1 ± 4.0	98.7 ± 1.0
TH14A	MHC class II (DR)	28.9 ± 1.6	21.3 ± 7.5	Not done
TH81A5	MHC class II (DQ)	19.2 ± 1.7	20.0 ± 1.3	Not done
H42A	MHC class II (DP?)	28.2 ± 2.6	17.4 ± 3.5	21.2 ± 2.3
MM1A	CD3	33.5 ± 8.3	40.1 ± 18.0	53.5 ± 8.4
CH138A	CD4	14.2 ± 1.6	10.1 ± 1.6	38.1 ± 3.6
CACT80C	CD8	13.1 ± 1.3	11.2 ± 1.4	21.0 ± 5.3
GB21A	Gamma delta TCR	2.1 ± 0.6	12.4 ± 2.4	7.8 ± 2.5
B7A1	WC1-N1	1.0 ± 0.2	1.0 ± d0.6	17.5 ± 7.9
BAQ4A	WC1-N2	1.1 ± 0.6	2.3 ± 0.2	2.0 ± 0.6

9.17 Application of mAbs in measuring Immunoglobulin levels

Total immunoglobulin (Ig) levels are conventionally measured using the single radial immuno diffusion technique (SRID) or the Mancini's method using anti-isotype specific antibodies produced in a foreign species followed by adsorption to remove cross-reacting antibodies. Although the use of mAbs would overcome these difficulties and would be more specific, since they recognize single epitopes they do not cross-link antigens sufficiently to form insoluble precipitates which are required in the SRID test.

If mAbs are prepared against Ig classes or subclasses, these can be used in a sandwich ELISA format to determine the levels of Igs in any fluid or sample (Table 9.5). Development of mAbs specific for bovine IgG1 (DAS 17), IgG2 (DAS 2), IgM (DAS 6), IgA (DAS 7) and the light chain (DAS 9) has been described previously (Srikumaran *et al.*, 1987). These mAbs were found to cross-react with the corresponding buffalo Igs in radioimmunoassays (Raj *et al.*, 2003); and were used as ascites fluids.

IgG1, IgG2 and total Igs present in the samples tested were quantified using bovine Ig isotype-specific Mabs and purified monoclonal bovine Ig isotypes as standards, in a sandwich ELISA. The ELISA plates were coated with the appropriate isotype-specific mAb at a concentration of 1 mg per ml at 4 °C overnight. Following washing, the plates were blocked with 2% gelatin for 1 h at 37°C. After washing, the samples and standards were added, and incubated for 1 h at 37°C. After washing, peroxidase conjugated anti-bovine Ig antibodies (whole molecules) were added and incubated for another hour at 37°C, followed by three washes and addition of the substrate (0.022% of 2,2'-azino bis (3-ethyl) benz-thiazoline-6-sulphonic acid, ABTS, in sodium citrate buffer pH 4.2 containing 0.015% of hydrogen peroxide). The reaction was stopped with 0.1 M hydrofluoric acid after 10 minutes of incubation at room temperature and optical density was read at 405 nm. Standard curves were generated using the purified bovine standards and regression equation was established. Using the equation, the values of Ig isotypes present in the samples were determined.

Table 9.5: Buffalo Immunoglobulin Concentrations Estimated using Bovine Class Specific Antibodies in a Sandwich ELISA Method

Immunoglobulins in	*IgG1 (mg/ml)*	*IgG2 (mg/ml)*	*Ig (mg/ml)*
Buffalo serum	14.68 ± 1.75	12.59 ± 1.08	32.95± 5.90
T-gel wash	0.35 ± 0.37	0.42 ± 0.29	0.82 ± 0.19
T-gel eluate	13.66 ± 2.63	11.15 ± 1.91	24.73 ± 4.16
Recovery	93.1%	88.6%	75.8%

9.18 mAbs and Stem Cells

Stem cells are unspecialized precursor cells that are capable of self-renewal and to differentiate into other cell types. Stem cells are essential for development and repair of tissues. Stem cells are comprised two general types, somatic (fetal or adult) or embryonic. Embryonic stem cells (ESs) originate from the inner cell mass of a blastocyst, are considered pluripotent, capable of transforming into cells of all three somatic germ layers (ectoderm, mesoderm and endoderm) as well into germ cells. In contrast, adult stem cells are considered to be multipotent giving rise to only cell types of one particular lineage.

Although the pluripotent state of ES cells is defined functionally, many molecular markers have also been used to characterize it. Pluripotent ES cells are characterized by high level expression of Oct-3/4, a member of the POU transcription factors, and Nanog. In addition, undifferentiated primate ES cells and human ES cells express SSEA-3 and SSEA-4, but not SSEA-1. Undifferentiated mouse ES cells express SSEA-1 but do not express SSEA-3 or SSEA-4. Undifferentiated human ES cells also express a very high level of alkaline phosphatase enzyme.

Thus a panel of antibodies is used to characterize these cells. They include mAbs against alkaline phosphatase, SSEA-1 and SSEA–4 for use in flow cytometry or immunochemistry. Some of the available mAbs against stem cell markers include CD34, CD38, CD90, CD117/c-Kit, CD123, CD133, CD144, CD324 (E-Cadherin), CD338/ABCG2, CD150, CD309, CD324 and so on. The list is ever increasing.

9.19 mAbs in Pregnancy Diagnosis

In humans, the presence of human chorionic gonadotropin (hCG) in the urine of the females is indicative of pregnancy. A qualitative detection is sufficient for this purpose and lateral flow based home testing strips are available based on the capture or sandwich ELISA method. A mAb against hCG is coupled to coloured latex or colloidal gold and impregnated on the conjugate matrix pads. Another mAb2 or polyclonal antibodies (uncoupled) is immobilized on the NC membranes. When the hCG is present in the urine sample, this is captured by the mAb1 coupled to gold and moves laterally to meet the mAb2 immobilized on the membrane and form a complex (sandwich) which produces a 'coloured line' there. This line is produced by the collection of the gold particles in a narrow zone. A control line is used to ensure that the test is working, based on the anti-mouse antibodies immobilized that would bind to the mouse mAb1 coupled to gold. Thus the appearance of 2 lines shows that the sample is positive, and appearance of one line shows that the sample is negative. If no line appears then the test has not worked.

However, in animals, hCG is not present and only progesterone levels in serum or milk is used as an indicator of pregnancy. But quantitative estimation is required since the progesterone levels are lower in non-pregnant state which increases during pregnancy. Further, the window of difference is also very narrow, about 3 ng in non-pregnant animals and about 10 ng in pregnant condition. The increase in levels of progesterone may also occur in other conditions such as persistent corpus luteum. Thus the situation is little complicated in animal. Not only do you require a highly sensitive test but also the specificity of the test would be compromised by other pathological conditions.

Progesterone is a steroide hormone with a molecular weight of 314 daltons and is secreted during pregnancy. In cattle, the progesterone level reaches a peak on the 21st and 22nd day of pregnancy. Hence, the levels are estimated using the competitive ELISA format is shown in Fig. 9.13.

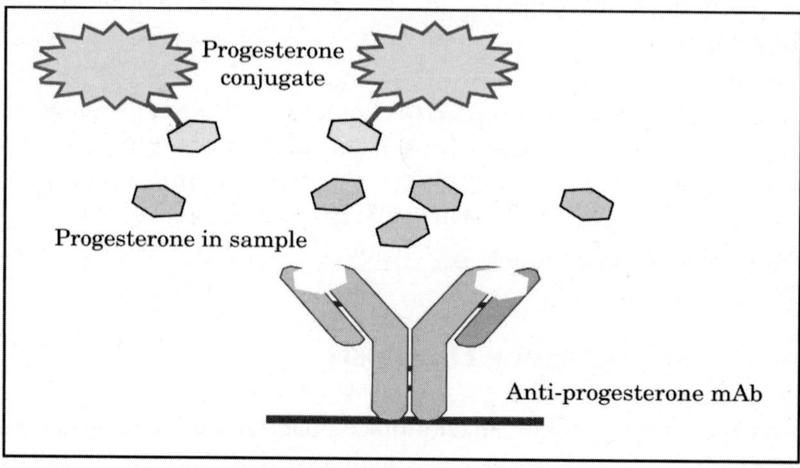

Fig. 9.13: ELISA for the detection.

The same competitive format can also be used in the lateral flow assay. The progesterone mAb labeled with gold is impregnated on the colloidal matrix. Progesterone is imprinted on the NC membrane. Now the progesterone present in the sample would compete with the progesterone imprinted on the NC membrane for the anti-progesterone mAbs thereby preventing or reducing its binding to the progesterone on the membrane. If there is no progesterone in the sample all of the gold coupled progesterone mAbs would bind to the progesterone on the NC membrane producing a coloured line. Thus there would be no colour if the sample contains progesterone (Fig. 9.14) that is it is positive. In this case, appearance of 2 lines indicates that the sample is negative.

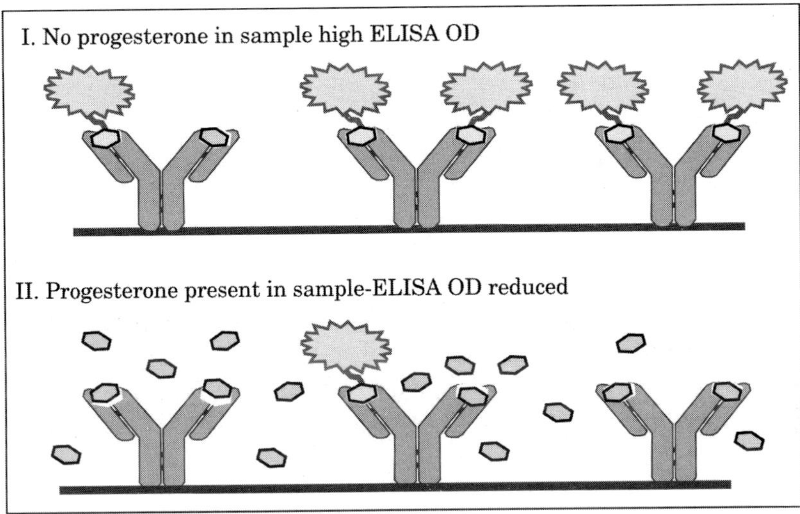

Fig. 9.14: Competitive ELISA for estimation of progesterone.

9.20 Anti-idiotype mAbs as Vaccines

Anti-idiotypic antibodies whose paratope is homologous to portions of the immunogenic protein of infectious organisms functionally mimic these epitopes and induce protective immune responses. mAbs against the rinderpest virus specific H protein (Ab1) is secreted by the clone designated A12A9. mAbs produced against this mAb1 (A12A9) were designated Ab2 of clone D9D8. This is the anti-idiotype mAb which would mimic the original antigen, the H protein on the virus. Ab3 produced in rats using D9D8 Ab2 as an immunogen reacted with the antigen H and hence is similar to Ab1. Thus Ab2 is an antigen mimic and this anti-idiotypic antibody competed with H protein of the virus for binding to idiotypic antibody in a dose-dependent manner.

From this anti-idiotypic mAb2 clone, D9D8, cytoplasmic RNA was extracted, reverse transcription and polymerase chain reactions were performed to amplify the variable regions of the heavy (VH) and light (VL) chains and cloned in prokaryotic and eukaryotic vectors. When recombinant plasmids containing VH and VL genes were injected into femoral muscle of Balb/c mice either alone or with boosters of purified Ab2 or recombinant VH or VL proteins, antibodies specific for H protein were detected by indirect ELISA in the sera of inoculated mice. This proves that not only the anti-idiotype mAb (Ab2) but also the DNA from the heavy and light chain of the immunoglobulin from the Ab2 secreting hybridoma can act as a DNA vaccine. The recombinant antibody producing DNA can work as a vaccine in the complete absence of the antigen Vani *et al.* (2007).

9.21 mAbs in Bacterial and Parasitic Diseases

mAbs are useful, as in the case of viruses, for diagnosis and characterization of other micro organisms, including bacteria and parasites. The contexts in which mAbs are applicable as listed above are also applicable for bacterial and parasitic disease diagnosis, pathogen characterization, passive immunotherapy and serology. cELISA has also been used for detecting antibodies to *Brucella* using mAbs against a common epitope of smooth lipopolysaccharide (S-LPS).

mAbs have been produced that can cross react with all members of the genus *Leptospira* and also specific to pathogenic serovars alone. These mAbs have been used for detection of *Leptospira* antigen in urine samples by ELISA based methods. mAbs against the major outer membrane protein LipL32 of the pathogenic *Leptospira* spp were shown to neutralize *Leptospira*-mediated human red blood cell lysis *in vitro* and protect hamsters from lethal infection.

M. tuberculosis 16 kDa protein (also called Acr antigen) is a major membrane associated protein, whose expression is increased in organisms growing inside infected macrophages. Blocking of the Acr antigen with mAbs interferes with the intracellular growth of the bacteria and limits their cell-to-cell dissemination.

mAbs against core LPS of *Campylobacter fetus* subspecies has been used for detection of the organism using sandwich ELISA. All samples positive on ELISA screening with this mAb were subsequently tested with serotype specific mAbs to recognize serotype A- and/or serotype B-specific *C. fetus* subspecies LPS epitopes.

Cryptosporidium parvum is a major cause of diarrhoea in humans and calves and can persistently infect immuno compromised hosts. Neutralizing mAbs against the apical complex and surface antigens CSL, GP25-200, and P23 could passively immunize against cryptosporidiosis. mAbs against CSL could significantly reduce *C. parvum* infections. mAbs against conoid of *Eimeria acervulina* sporozoites significantly inhibited sporozoite invasion of CD8 T-cells. mAbs against the *Eimeria* microneme protein 2, that plays a role in parasite adhesion to the host cell to initiate the invasion process are useful tools for the investigation and characterization microneme-related proteins in *Eimeria* species and to study their pathogenesis.

9.22 mAbs in Immunochemistry

Immunohistochemistry (IHC) is the demonstration of Ag in tissue sections using Abs. The reporter system can be a coloured product visible by light microscopy or a fluorescent stained product visible with ultraviolet light. The antigens used for preparation of antibodies for use in IHC include either purified proteins of synthetic peptides as follows:

Purified proteins	*Peptides*
Sequence May or may not be known	Known amino acid sequences
Protein folding	Linear
Post translational modification	No modifications
Protein purification difficult	Highly pure
Contaminating protein more antigenic	Contaminating proteins not present

The antibodies also can be either polyclonal of mAbs. The immunologic promiscuity of polyclonal Abs is both advantageous and disadvantageous. It renders more possibilities of detecting an Ag but there is a possibility of cross reactivity. The main advantage of mAbs is their higher specificity. The following information on the antibody characteristics need to be known for efficient use of the antibody in IHC:

- Presentation of the Ab–affinity purified, whole serum, supernatant, ascites etc
- Ig isotype
- Protein concentration
- Species reactivity,
- Cellular localization,
- Application (*e.g*., immunoprecipitation, western blotting, ELISA, Flow cytometry
- Images of the immunoreaction.

Fixation

Fixation of tissues is necessary to:

- Adequately preserve cellular components
- Prevent autolysis
- Facilitate immunostaining.

There are two types of fixatives, coagulating and non-coagulating fixatives. Formaldehyde is the gold standard of fixatives for IHC. The basic mechanism of fixation is by formation of addition products between formalin and uncharged reactive amino groups (–NH or NH_2) that forms cross-links. This could change the conformation of biomolecules that may interfere with the recognition by Abs.

Coagulating fixatives such as ethanol precipitates proteins by breaking hydrogen bonds in the absence of protein cross-linking. Removal of water with ethanol destabilizes protein hydrophobic bonding and the protein gets unfolded.

Antigen retrieval

Antigen retrieval methods reverse changes produced during fixation. The most common antigen retrieval methods include

- Enzymatic-trypsin, proteinase K, pronase, ficin and pepsin
- Heat based retrieval.

Endogenous peroxidase activity

Peroxidase activity naturally present in red blood cells, granulocytes and neurons can also react with DAB to produce a brown product. This is removed by the pretreatment of tissue sections with a diluted solution (0.003–3%) of H_2O_2 in methanol. Since the use of methanol might detach frozen sections from the glass slide endogenous peroxidase activity can also be suppressed by using 0.3% H_2O_2 in 0.1% sodium azide.

Endogenous alkaline phosphatase

Two isoenzymes of AP in mammalian tissues can produce back ground staining; the nonintestinal form is easily inhibited by 1 mM levamisol (L-tetramisole), whereas the intestinal isoform is blocked with 1% acetic acid mAbs are extensively used to localize the antigens using IHC (Fig. 9.15).

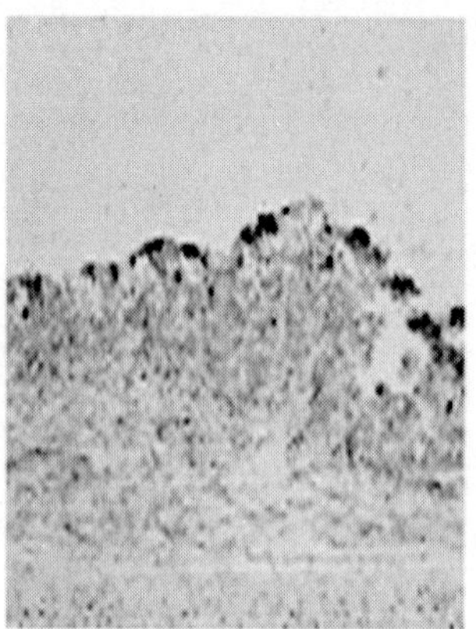

Application of mAbs in detecting virus antigen in tracheal epithelial cells by IHC

Fig. 9.15: IHC for viral antigen detection.

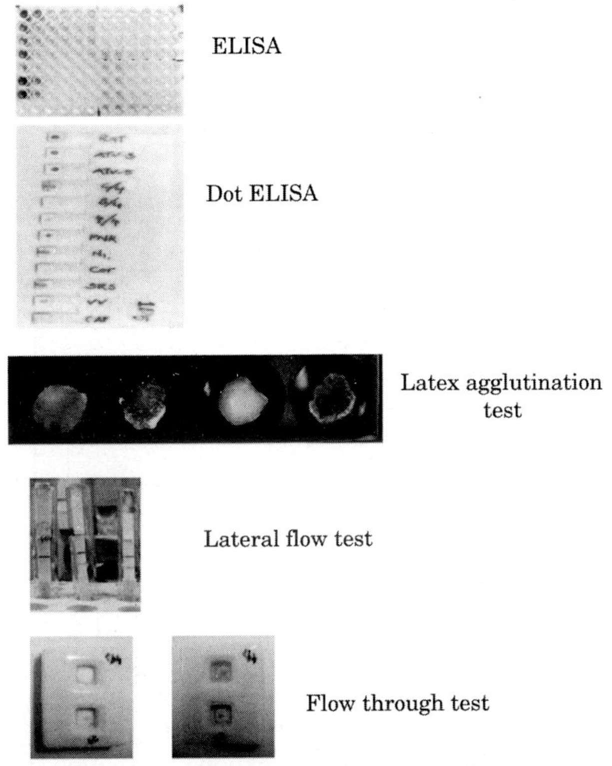

Fig. 9.16: Formats of diagnostic assays using mAbs.

9.23 mAbs in Immunoaffinity Purification

mAbs can be used either to purify a target antigen from a heterogenous mixture or to remove a contamination protein from a mixture. In the former case, the protein of interest has to be eluted while in the latter case the flow through would contain the protein of interest (the bound protein is the one to be removed). This method is used to purify mAbs from cell culture fluids, which would have bovine Igs as contamination proteins from the FCS, by the use of anti-mouse Ig coupled columns.

mAbs can also be coupled to columns and used to purify the antigen from a mixture. In fact, this technique is used for capturing the antigen in AC-ELISA or sandwich ELISA in which the coating mAb bound to the ELISA plate captures the antigen from the sample, which is then detected by the detecting mAb (Fig. 9.16 and 9.17). This is equivalent to purification of the antigen in the ELISA well. However, for this step, the AC-ELISA is the same as indirect ELISA. The coupling method for coupling mAbs should be mild and reversible so that the biological activity of antibodies would be retained and also allowing for their proper orientation. The mAb coupling methods includes:

- Random direct coupling via lysine amino groups
- Coupling via carbohydrate side-chains
- Coupling via free hinge region SH groups in partially reduced Fab' fragments
- Indirect coupling and orientation via protein A or G

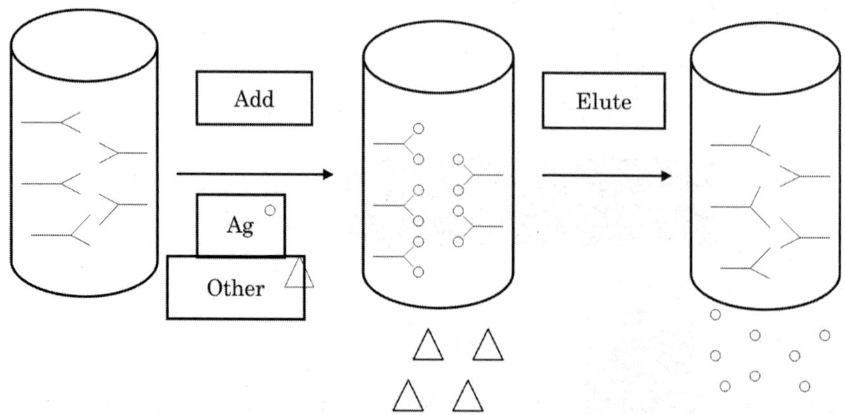

Fig. 9.17: Purification of antigen (protein) using mAbs.

mAbs have been immobilised on Sepharose 4B and used to isolate fully cytolytic C9 from human plasma. A 1200-fold purification was obtained with yield of 30–40%. A special class of mAbs, called as the polyol-responsive mAbs have been used preferably for immunoaffinity chromatography because the elution conditions required a very mild with a combination of a nonchaotropic salt and a low molecular weight polyhydroxylated compound (polyol) (Nancy *et al.*, 2009).

9.24 Application of mAbs as Therapeutics

One of the main applications of mAbs is for therapy (Table 9.6). However, this does not apply a lot to animal sciences as it does to human medicine. The antibody itself is not responsible for killing of the target or cancer cells. But it identifies the target specifically so that other effector mechanisms of the body's immune system can lead the attack. The two defense mechanisms used by the immune system are complement mediated cytotoxicity (CMC) and antibody dependent cellular cytotoxicity (ADCC). CMC is a process where a cascade of events such as complement activation directly leads to target cell lysis or causes recruitment of other immune system cells to the location for effector cell function. ADCC involves the recognition of the antibody marked target cells by immune cells that directly lead to target cell death. mAbs used as therapeutics have the following mechanism of action:

- Direct cytotoxicity through ADCC, complement-dependent cytotoxicity or induction of target cell apoptosis
- Immuno conjugates–mAbs act as delivery vehicles for radioisotopes, cytotoxic molecules such as diphtheria toxin or biological agents like interferon
- mAbs either block or stimulate a particular cell membrane receptor molecules (*e.g.* growth factor signal receptor) or ligand (vascular endothelial growth factor, VEGF).

To denote the different constructs of mAb, the suffixes:

- Umab (human) (*e.g.* panitumumab),
- Momab (murine) (*e.g.* tositumomab),
- Ximab (Chimeric) (*e.g.* cetuximab) and
- Zumab (humanized) (*e.g.* trastuzumab).

Murine mAbs have a short half-life, are inefficient at eliciting effector functions and are highly immunogenic. However, the development of chimeric and humanized mAbs, which are less immunogenic, have longer half-lives and are efficient in eliciting effector functions have heralded the success of therapeutic mAbs. Chimeric antibodies typically have a half-life of 4–15 days, humanized from 3 to 24 days, and recombinant human antibodies11–24 days.

The mode of action of antibodies *in vivo* is highly dependent on the antibody isotype. Mouse IgG2a, IgG2b and IgG2c are the most potent in mediating ADCC while IgG2a and IgG2b efficiently activate the complement cascade. In humans, IgG1 and IgG3 are the most effective in mediating ADCC and CDC. The mouse equivalent to human IgG1 is IgG2a, not IgG1.

FcgRs bind to human and mouse IgG in the CH2 domain near the hinge region. In humans, six FcgR family members are present which include FcgRI (CD64), FcgRII a, b, c (CD32 a,b,c) and FcgRIII a, b (CD16 a,b). In mouse, the human equivalents of FcgRI, FcgRIIb and FcgRIIIa only have been described.

Most of the licensed mAbs are unconjugated products of the humanized IgG1 class. IgG2 and IgG4 have unique physicochemical properties. Human IgG2 antibodies can form covalent dimers *in vivo*. IgG4 antibody forms molecules with one heavy chain and one light chain that lack inter-heavy chain disulphide thereby it can also form a hybrid molecule with dual antigen specificity by combining with a similar molecule of another IgG4.

Vascular endothelial growth factor (VEGF) is the most potent angiogenic factor that exerts its effect through binding to VEGF receptors present on endothelial cells and angioblasts. The dependency of malignant tumors on angiogenesis makes VEGF or its receptor as potential therapeutic targets. Bevacizumab is a humanized mAb against VEGF that prevents VEGF from binding to the receptor and thus prevents subsequent stimulation of intracellular signal transduction pathways.

Epidermal growth factor receptor (EGFR) or *HER1* when bound to its ligand such as EGF, transforming growth factor-α, epiregulin, amphiregulin leads to stimulation of several intracellular signal transduction pathways, ultimately resulting in cell proliferation and inhibition of apoptosis. Two anti-EGFR mAbs are currently available for the treatment of tumours. Cetuximab is a chimeric immunoglobulin G1 antibody, and panitumumab is a fully human immunoglobulin G2 antibody (Jing and Zhenping 2010).

Table 9.6: mAbs Approved for Therapeutic use

Generic name	*Trade name*	*Antibody*	*Antigen*	*Indication*
Muromomab	Orthoclone	murine IgG2a	CD3	Allograft rejection in renal transplant
Abciximab	Reopro	chimeric Fab	GPIIb/IIIa receptor	Prevention of cardiac ischemic complications
Rituximab	Rituxan	chimeric IgG1κ	CD20	Non-Hodgkin's Lymphoma, chronic lymphocytic leukemia and rheumatoid arthritis
Daclizumab	Zenapax	humanized	IL-2Rα IgG1κ	Prophylaxis of acute organ rejection in renal transplants
Basiliximab	Simulect	chimeric IgG1κ	IL-2Rα	Prophylaxis of acute organ rejection in renal transplantation
Palivizumab	Synagis	humanized IgG1κ	RSV F protein	Respiratory syncytial virus infection
Infliximab	Remicade	chimeric IgG1κ	TNFα	Crohn's disease and rheumatoid arthritis
Trastuzumab	Herceptin	humanized IgG1κ	Her2	Breast cancer
Alemtuzumab	Campath	humanized IgG1κ	CD52	B-cell chronic lymphocytic leukemia
Ibritumomab Tiuxetan	Zevalin	Y90-murine IgG1κ	CD20	B-cell non-Hodgkin's lymphoma
Adalimumab	Humira	human IgG1κ	TNFá	Rheumatoid arthritis and Crohn's disease
Omalizumab	Xolair	humanized IgG1κ	IgE	Moderate to severe persistent asthma
Tositumomab	Bexxar	I^{131}-murine IgG2aλ	CD20	Non-Hodgkin's lymphoma
Cetuximab	Erbitux	chimeric IgG1κ	EGFR	Head and Neck cancer, colorectal cancer

Table 9.6: (*Contd...*)

Table 9.6: (*Contd...*)

Generic name	*Trade name*	*Antibody*	*Antigen*	*Indication*
Bevacizumab	Avastin	humanized IgG1κ	VEGF-A	Various solid tumors
Natalizumab	Tysabri	humanized IgG4κ	α4-integrin	Multiple sclerosis and Crohn's disease
Ranibizumab	Lucentis	humanized Fab	VEGF-A	Age-related macular degeneration
Panitumumab	Vectibix	human IgG2κ	EGFR	Metastatic colorectal carcinoma
Eculizumab	Soliris	humanized IgG2/4κ	C5	Paroxysmal nocturnal hemoglobinuria
Certolizumab pegol	Cimzia	Peglated humanized Fab	TNFα	Crohn's disease and rheumatoid arthritis
Golimumab	Simponi	human IgG1κ	TNFα	Rheumatoid arthritis, psoriatic arthritis and ankylosing spondylitis
Canakinumab	Ilaris	human IgG1κ	IL-1β	Cryopyrin-associated periodic syndromes
Ustekinumab	Stelara	human IgG1κ	IL-12/IL23	Plaque psoriasis
Ofatumumab	Arzerra	human IgG1κ	CD20	Chronic lymphocytic leukemia
Tocilizumab	Actemra	humanized IgG1κ	IL-6R	Rheumatoid arthritis
Denosumab	Prolia	human IgG2κ	RANK ligand	Postmenopausal women with risk of osteoporosis
Catumaxomab	Removab	murine/rat hybrid IgG	EpCAM and CD3	Intraperitoneal treatment of malignant ascites
Edrecolomab	Panorex	murine IgG2a	EpCAM	Colon cancer
I^{131}-TNT	Cotara	I^{131}-chimeric IgG1	DNA	Lung cancer
Nimotuzumab	Theracim	humanized IgG1	EGFR	Nasopharyngeal carcinomas and head and neck tumours

TNF alpha, an inflammatory cytokine maintains the inflammatory response against infections. TNF- alpha is present in both soluble and transmembrane forms and is produced by a wide variety of cells, including macrophages, natural killer cells, granulocytes, fibroblasts and T cells. There are two types of TNF receptors, TNFR 1 and TNFR2 which are found in all cells except the red blood cells. mAbs against TNF- alpha blocks cell activation, cell proliferation, cytokine and chemokine production and the formation and maintenance of granulomas. TNF-alpha inhibitors are used in the treatment of rheumatologic diseases. There are currently four TNF-alpha inhibitors approved for use:

- adalimumab
- infliximab

- certolizumab pegol and
- etanercept.

9.24.1 Antilymphocyte antibodies used in treatment of malignancies

Alemtuzumab–fully humanized IgG1 against CD52 and is used in the treatment of B-cell chronic lymphocytic leukemia, T-cell prolymphocytic leukemia, and non-Hodgkin's lymphoma.

Ibritumomab tiuxetan–^{90}Y-ibritumomab tiuxetan is a chimeric molecule composed of ibritumomab, a murine anti-CD20 IgG2a mAb, conjugated to tiuxetan, a chelator that attaches to ^{90}Y.

Rituximab–chimeric human-mouse IgG1 anti- CD20 mAb used in the treatment of non- Hodgkin's lymphoma and other B-cell malignancies.

Tositumomab–^{131}I-tositumomab is a radiolabeled murine IgG2a mAb against CD20 used in the treatment of non-Hodgkin's lymphoma and other B-cell malignancies.

9.24.2 Anti-myeloid receptor antibody

Gemtuzumab–a fully humanized anti-CD33 IgG4 mAb conjugated with the cytotoxic antibiotic calicheamicin that is indicated for the treatment of CD33-positive acute myelogenous leukemia.

9.24.3 Antiangiogenesis antibodies

Bevacizumab–Bevacizumab is a recombinant humanized IgG1 mAb against human VEGF that is used in the treatment of advanced colorectal cancer, non-small-cell lung cancer, and breast cancer.

9.24.4 ErbB (EGFR) receptor antibodies

Cetuximab–a chimeric murine-human IgG1 mAb against ErbB1 that is useful in colorectal and head-and-neck cancer.

Panitumumab–human IgG2 mAb against ErbB1 used in the treatment of advanced colorectal cancer.

Trastuzumab–humanized recombinant mAb against HER2, which is over expressed by certain types of breast tumors.

9.24.5 Graft-versus-host disease and transplant rejection mAbs

Basiliximab–chimeric murine-human IgG1 mAb against the alpha chain of the IL-2 receptor (IL-2R alpha or CD25), is indicated in the prevention of rejection of renal transplants

Daclizumab–recombinant humanized IgG1 anti-CD25 mAb that affects activated T cells through the IL-2R alpha chain and is indicated in the prevention of rejection in renal transplant recipients.

Muromonab–OKT3 is a murine IgG2 mAb against CD3 indicated for acute rejection in solid organ transplant recipients.

9.24.6 mAbs for cardiovascular disease

Abciximab–Fab' fragment of a chimeric human-mouse mAb against the glycoprotein IIb/IIIa receptor, which is responsible for platelet aggregation and is indicated as an adjunct in the treatment of acute coronary syndrome.

9.24.7 mAbs for neurologic disease

Natalizumab–humanized recombinant IgG4 mAb that binds to the $\alpha 4\beta 1$ (very late activating antigen 4) and$\alpha 4\beta 7$ integrins, indicated for the treatment of relapsing multiple sclerosis.

9.24.8 mAbs for pulmonary disease

Omalizumab–chimeric humanized IgG1 mAb that binds human IgE, is indicated for the treatment of asthma.

Palivizumab–humanized mAb of IgG1 against an epitope in the A antigenic site of the F protein of RSV and is indicated for the prevention of RSV infections.

9.25 Engineering Fc region of the mAbs

The Fc part of the mAb drives the effector function of the antibody following specific recognition of the epitope by the Fab. These effector functions can also be engineered through the following methods

- Introduction of specific amino acid changes to the Fc region of the mAb to facilitate enhanced binding to the Fc receptors resulting in enhanced ADCC.

- Modification of the branching sugar attached to asparagine 297, located close to the FcγR-binding interface of IgG
- Alteration of the binding of mAbs to the neonatal Fc receptor (FcRn) in order to modify the serum half-life of the mAb.

9.26 Antibody Drug Conjugates

Antibody-drug conjugates (ADCs) combine the specificity of mAbs with the potency of cytotoxic molecules, thereby taking advantage of both components. There are 3 key components of an ADC: the mAb, the drug and the linker. Ideally, the mAb will specifically bind to an antigen that is expressed only on tumor cells but not on normal tissues. This specificity allows the utilization of drugs that otherwise would be too toxic for clinical application without this targeted therapy. The linkers used for the conjugation of the drug to the mAb should provide conditional stability, so that drug release occurs after tumor binding, rather than in circulation. Some of the drugs used in ADCs include:

- Auristatins
- Maytansines
- Calicheamicins.

Auristatins and maytasines both exert their cytotoxic effects by binding to tubulin, causing G2/M cell cycle arrest, and subsequently leading to apoptosis. Calicheamicin is a DNA strand cleaving agent. These drugs are very potent but will indiscriminately destroy both healthy and diseased tissue by stopping mitosis and hence can not be used without targeting.

The first and only ADC licensed for clinical use is Gemtuzumab Ozogamicin (Mylotarg; Wyeth) which was approved by the FDA in 2000 is for the treatment of relapsed acute myelocytic leukemia in adults. The drug payload in this ADC is N-acetyl-g-calicheamicin.

Human epidermal growth factor receptor 2 (HER2) is a 185 kDa protein with an intracellular tyrosine kinase domain and an extra cellular ligand binding domain. HER2 plays an important role in cell growth, survival and differentiation. HER2 over expression leads to malignant transformation and is directly associated with poor clinical outcomes in breast, ovarian, gastric, prostate cancers. The development of anti-HER2 antibody called trastuzumab (Herceptin™) has revolutionized the treatment of breast cancer.

Although trastuzumab has been used extensively for cancer therapy, its therapeutic efficacy is limited only in patients who manifest +3 level of HER2 over expression. To improve its efficacy, an ADC, Trastuzumab-DM1, trastuzumab coupled with maytansinoid which is a derivative of the antimitotic drug maytansine.

Catumaxomab (Removab, Fresenius Biotech GmbH, Germany) is a trifunctional antibody (trAb) that binds to three different cell types: tumor cells, T-cells, and accessory cells. It has antigen-binding specificities for epithelial cell adhesion molecule (EpCAM) on tumor cells and also for the CD3 antigen on T-cells. Catumaxomab also binds to type I, IIa, and III Fcc receptors on accessory cells such as macrophages, dendritic cells and natural killer cells through its Fc part.

The anti-tumor activity of catumaxomab results from T-cell-mediated lysis, ADCC and phagocytosis via activation of FccR-positive accessory cells. Since April 2009, catumaxomab has been approved in the European Union for the intraperitoneal treatment of malignant ascites (MA) in patients with EpCAM-positive carcinomas where standard therapy is not available or no longer feasible.

Catumaxomab is the first trAb and the first drug worldwide to be approved specifically for the treatment of MA. It is also in clinical trials for a number of other indications including ovarian and gastric cancer.

Although there are about 26 mAbs approved by the US Food and Drug Administration (FDA) for therapeutic use, solid tumors are relatively resistant to intact antibody-based therapies as only a small amount of mAbs accumulate in the tumor tissue. To improve tumor penetration the following approaches are used.

- Novel antibody formats, such as the single-chain Fv (scFv; 25–30 kDa)
- 'PEGylation' - covalent conjugation of small recombinant antibody with poly ethylene glycol to increase the molecular mass and the hydrodynamic radius
- Genetic fusion of antibody fragments to albumin or albumin-binding proteins
- Bispecific antibodies to recruit serum IgG that provides the Fc-associated effector functions and prolongs residence time in serum
- Multimerization to increase the functional affinity (avidity) of antibody fragments.

The monovalent recombinant antibodies (*i.e.* scFvs, Fabs or single-domains) are converted into multivalent formats to:

- Increase the functional affinity
- Decrease dissociation rates
- Enhance biodistribution.

Multimeric antibodies have been grouped into:

- IgG-like (orthodox)
- Non-IgG-like (heterodox) formats.

Orthodox formatting strategies engineer antibodies that mimic the structure of IgG, creating mostly monospecific bivalent antibodies.

The heterodox format includes all engineered antibodies that do not imitate the original IgG structure. Different strategies are used to multimerize antibody fragments.

Bispecific T cell engager (BITE) is a bispecific single-chain antibody consisting of two scFv antibody fragments, joined via a flexible linker, that are directed against a surface antigen on target cells and CD3 on T cells.

Molecular constructs to generate stable, trimeric scFv has been developed based on the bacterial barnase–barstar module. The ribonuclease barnase (12 kDa) and its inhibitor barstar (10 kDa) form a very tight complex in which the N- and C-termini are accessible for fusion. Similarly a scFv is fused to a tumor necrosis factor (TNF) that forms a homotrimeric structure which retains both TNFa activity and the ability to bind antigen recognized by the scFv.

9.27 Radioimmunotherapy for infectious diseases using mAbs

Alternate therapy for infectious diseases are needed for the following reasons:

- Highly resistant microorganisms
- Immuno suppressed individuals
- Dearth of new anti-microbial drugs.

Radioimmunotherapy (RIT) originally used for cancer treatment is now being used with organism-specific mAbs, as a novel therapy for treatment of infectious diseases. For example, murine cryptococcosis has been treated with a mAb to *Cryptococcus neoformans* capsular glucurono xylomannan labeled with Bismuth-213 or Rhenium-188.

9.28 Single Domain Antibodies

In some species such as camels and llamas even a single variable antibody domain could bind to antigen with high affinities that are called heavy chain antibodies

(HcAbs). While the antigen-binding paratope of the conventional antibodies is formed by the variable domains of heavy and light chains (VH and VL), those of the HcAbs is formed only by the heavy chain variable domain, which is designated VHH in camelid and variable domain of the shark new antigen receptor (VNAR) in shark IgNARs. Camelid HcAbs come in two variants, distinguished on the basis of the lengths of their hinge region and designated as long and short-hinge isotypes.

Similarly single domain antibody (dAb) based on a single human antibody variable domain, VH or VL, has been generated with high affinity and specificity. To date, three antibody Fab fragments have been approved for clinical applications, including abciximab (Reopro®, anti-GPIIb/IIIa receptor), ranibizumab (Lucentis®, anti-VEGF) and certolizumab pegol (Cimzia®, anti-tumor necrosis factor α, TNFα).

9.29 Affibody

Affibody molecules are a class of engineered affinity proteins with potential applications in therapeutic, imaging and diagnostic areas. Affibody molecules are 6.5 kDa single domain proteins with high affinity and specificity to any given protein target. They are a viable alternative to antibodies and represent an emerging class of affinity ligands. Affibody molecules were originally derived from the B-domain in the immunoglobulin-binding region of staphylococcal protein A. The B-domain is a relatively short cysteine-free peptide of 58 amino acids that is folded into a three-helical bundle structure. The B-domain was mutated at key positions to enhance the chemical stability and the resulting engineered variant was denoted the Z-domain. Affibodies are based on the Z domain scaffold than can bind to any given target. Affibody molecules with specific binding to proteins such as insulin, fibrinogen, transferrin, tumor necrosis factor-alpha, IL-8, gp120, CD28, human serum albumin, IgA, IgE, IgM, HER2 and EGFR have been generated.

9.30 Ribosome Display Technology

Ribosome display is used for the selection and evolution of scFvs. It starts with *in vitro* transcription and translation of the template gene library to give rise to the scFv–ribosome–mRNA ternary complexes. The scFv displayed on the ternary complex, is selected by binding to an immobilized ligand and captured on a solid surface. Bound ternary complexes are eluted from the surface by either destroying the complex (*e.g.* with EDTA) or by competitive elution with free ligands. The eluted mRNA from the recovered complexes is subjected to reverse transcription-PCR to obtain DNA which can be used in the next round of selection. Compared with phage display technologies, ribosome display is a powerful alternative with an advantage to optimize antibodies *in vitro*.

9.31 mAbs in Imaging

Molecular imaging is the ability to visualize, characterize, and measure processes on molecular and cellular levels non-invasively in living systems. Noninvasive molecular imaging approaches include:

- Nuclear resonance imaging
- Optical resonance imaging
- Magnetic resonance imaging
- Computed tomography
- Ultrasound
- Photo acoustic imaging.

These techniques require accumulation of a signal delivered by a probe at the target site. mAbs fulfill this criterion by virtue of their high specificity but their long circulation time in blood makes them unsuitable as imaging probes.

Fast clearing fragments, such as scFv with a single antigen-binding site (monovalent) demonstrated low accumulation in tumors. Using scFv as building blocks, production of larger, bivalent fragments, such as scFv dimers (diabodies, 50 kDa) and scFv fusion proteins (80 kDa minibodies and 105 kDa scFv-Fc), resulted in higher tumor accumulation because of their longer residence time in blood. Imaging studies with these fragments after radiolabeling have demonstrated excellent, high-contrast images in gamma cameras and positron emission tomography scanners.

Antibody fragments conjugated to fluorescence (near infrared dyes), bioluminescence (luciferases), and quantum dots have been applied with optical imaging and iron oxides nanoparticles for magnetic resonance imaging.

For diagnostic imaging, only a handful of mAbs have been approved in the United States for single-photon emission computed tomography (SPECT) imaging. Some of them include:

Arcitumomab- ^{99m}Tc-labeled Fab' fragment of the anti-CEA IgG1 murine mAb IMMU-4 and is indicated for detection of advanced colorectal cancer.

Technitium fanolesomab- ^{99m}Tc-fanolesumab is a murine anti-CD15 IgM mAb labeled with ^{99m}Tc which indicated for imaging of acute appendicitis. However, the drug was withdrawn from the market in 2005.

Capromab pendetide-indium-111-radiolabeled murine mAb (7E11-C5.3) covalently joined to a linker-chelator molecule directed against human prostate-specific membrane antigen and is used in the detection of recurrence of prostate cancer.

Nofetumomab-^{99m}Tc-nofetumomab merpentan is the Fab' fragment of the IgG2 murine antibody NR-LU-10 against carcinoma associated glycoprotein antigen radioconjugated with ^{99m}Tc and is indicated in lung cancer.

Because these imaging agents are murine mAbs, repeated use in humans is not advisable. This can be overcome by the use of humanized mAbs, only one is available in the market which is Votumumab* (HumaSPECT, (Intracel Corp., Rockville, MD)) human IgG3 against altered cytokeratins.

Rheumatoid arthritis (RA) is a chronic inflammatory autoimmune disease of unknown aetiology that leads to progressive joint destruction, functional disability and extra articular complications. The clinical management of RA targets pro-inflammatory cytokines (*e.g.*, TNF-α, IL-1 and IL-6) and membrane-bound receptors (*e.g.*, CD3 and CD4). A pre-therapy scintigraphic approach identifies the presence of the relevant receptors involved in the pathophysiology of the disease directly by means of the specific radiolabelled mAb that will eventually be used for treatment. Some of the mAbs used for molecular imaging of RA are

Anti-TNF á mAbs for RA

- Infliximab (Remicade) Centocor, Inc., ^{99m}Tc labeled chimeric IgG1
- Adalimumab (Humira) Abbott Labs, ^{99m}Tc labeled fully human IgG1.

Other targets include CD3, CD20, CD4 and E-selectin

- Rituximab (Rituxan/Mabthera) Genentech/Roche - ^{99m}Tc labeled chimeric IgG1 against CD20
- MAX.16H5– ^{99m}Tc labeled murine IgG1 against CD4
- 1.2B6–Murine IgG1 ^{111}in against E-selectin
- OKT–3 (Muromonab) Ortho Pharma ^{99m}Tc labeled murine IgG2 against CD3.

9.32 Intrabodies

Intrabodies are intracellular antibodies (intrabodies) targeted to specific subcellular compartments by fusion to specific signal peptides where it binds its cognate target.

The advantages of intrabodies are

- High specificity
- Long half life
- Inhibition of post translational modification
- Complement siRNA knock down approach.

If a mAb is available against a specific target, a single chain Fv intrabody is made fused to specific signal peptides for targeting to specific subcellular compartments. Intracellular antibodies that are expressed and retained inside the endoplasmatic reticulum are called as ER-intrabodies. They are used to block translocation of secreted and cell surface molecules from the ER to the cell surface thereby resulting in functional inhibition of the target protein. An ER intrabody to toll like receptor 2, was generated from a mAb against human and murine TLR2 (Kirschning *et al.,* 2010).

9.33 Fc Fusion Proteins

Fc fusion proteins are molecules in which the immunoglobulin Fc region is fused genetically to a receptor, ligand, enzyme or peptide. Fc fusion proteins are alternatives to mAb based therapeutics. Most biologically active proteins or peptides have fast renal clearance and hence a short half life. The advantages of genetically coupling the Fc region of the antibody to the peptide/protein are:

- Increase in the serum half life of the fusion protein
- Prevention of endosomal degradation due to the pH dependent binding to the neonatal Fc receptor (FcRn)
- Improves solubility and stability of the protein.
- Facilitates protein-A affinity purification.

Soluble receptor-Fc fusion proteins act as antagonists to block receptor–ligand interaction or as agonists to stimulate receptor functions. The original Fc fusion protein was the immunoadhesin, which consisted of fusion of IgG Fc region with the ligand binding region of CD4 molecule that could specifically inhibit CD4 activity. Four Fc fusion proteins have been approved by FDA as therapeutic drugs.

Etanercept (Enbrel1) is composed of fusion between the 75 kDa soluble extra cellular domain (ECD) of the TNF-α receptor II (TNFR II) and the Fc domain of human IgG1. This neutralizes both the membrane bound and soluble forms of

TNF-α thereby reducing the concentrations of serum inflammatory cytokines, hence indicated for rheumatoid arthritis.

Alefacept (Amevive1) is composed of a fusion between the ECD of lymphocyte function-associated antigen 3 (LFA-3) and the Fc domain of human IgG1. This is used in patients with moderate-to-severe plaque psoriasis. LFA is the co-receptor for CD2 on T cells or NK cells. By binding to CD2 on these T cells, alefacept effectively inhibits T cell activation.

Abatacept (Orencia1), consisting of the ECD of human cytotoxic T lymphocyte associated molecule-4 (CTLA-4) fused to the Fc domain, blocks the interactions between CD80 or CD86 on APCs and CD28 on T cells. This is also indicated for RA.

Atacicept contains ECD of the transmembrane activator and CAML interacting (TACI) molecule fused to the Fc domain of human IgG. It blocks maturation and development of B cells and hence used in several autoimmune diseases.

Mimetibody™ are fusion constructs wherein bioactive peptides are genetically linked to an Fc region of an antibody. A Mimetibody, CNTO 528, contains a 20 amino acid erythropoietin mimetic peptide that can bind and activate the erythropoietin receptor.

9.34 Alternate Hosts for mAb Production

mAbs can also be produced in rabbits, chickens and other hosts by conventional, phage display technology or cloning methods. Rabbit polyclonal antibodies generally tend to have higher affinity and titres than mouse antibodies. However, rabbit mAbs were not possible to be produced because plasmacytomas are not formed in rabbits and rabbit B cells are difficult to transform *in vitro* with viruses. The mouse-rabbit hetero hybridomas generated are highly unstable and do not secrete antibodies continuously. However, the generation of c-*myc*/v-*abl* transgenic rabbits led to the production of rabbit plasmacytoma cell lines that served as fusion partners for stable rabbit mAb production. Rabbit mAbs are produced like the mouse mAbs fusing the immunized spleen cells with B cell line, 240E-W2 with PEG-4000 followed by selection with HAT. In IHC, rabbit mAbs permit higher working dilutions and in some instances optimal staining can be obtained even without antigen retrieval.

The procedure for the preparation of scFv mAbs by the chicken phage display technique is briefly described. 15 Inbred chickens are immunized intraperitoneally (i.p.) with antigen with adjuvant at least 3–4 times with 2–3 weeks interval between each injection. Four days after the final injection, spleen cells are isolated from immunized chickens and RNA extracted from them, immunoglobulin variable region (VH and VL) genes are amplified and a scFv phage library is constructed. The phage-display scFv library is panned against the antigen coated on to ELISA plates. Recombinant chicken IgY are generated using the VH and VL genes from phage displayed chicken antibodies using plasmid vectors for construction of the light and heavy chains, respectively. Constructed plasmid DNAs were transfected in to recipient cells. Like hybridomas, these transfected cells can be selected, screened and cloned as stable transfectomas that secrete a monoclonal antibody.

Cloned calves expressing human chromosome coding for human antibodies (transchromosomic calves) is also possible for production of human polyclonal antibodies by bovines immunized with human antigens. Bovine cells containing the human chromosomes were fused with cow's eggs and the resultant embryos were transferred into recipient cows to produce cloned, transchromosomic calves. The human chromosome fragment was retained in the calves and human antibody proteins were detected in the blood of newborn calves. This study was published in Nature Biotechnology entitled "Cloned Transchromosomic Calves Producing Human Immunoglobulin" (Kuroiwa. *et al.*, 2002).

CHAPTER 10

ANTIBODY ENGINEERING

10.1 Introduction

Antibodies are made up of light and heavy chains each consisting of domains of about 110 amino acids. Antigen specificity is conferred by the variable domains of the heavy (V_H) and light (V_L) chains. The specificity of the antibodies are determined by six complementary determining regions (CDRs), three in V_H and $V_{L.}$

They form hyper variable loops that come together in three dimensions to form the antigen binding site. Antibodies achieve diversity due to variations in the amino acid sequences of the CDRs. The framework regions can also influence the conformation of the hypervariable loop indirectly.

10.2 Antibody Genetics

B-cell has the ability to produce a vast variety of different antibody specificities (amino acid sequences in the CDRs) by gene rearrangement, combinatorial diversity, imprecise joining and mutations. Immunoglobulin light chain has a large number of variable (V) and junctional (J) segments and one constant (C) segment. During maturation of B-cell, loci are rearranged with one of the V segments combining with one J segment then the VJ gene segment is apposed to the C segment. The heavy chain locus also consists of D segment and multiple constant regions. Rearrangement of V (D) J segments together with combination of heavy and light chains contribute to the diversity of antibody.

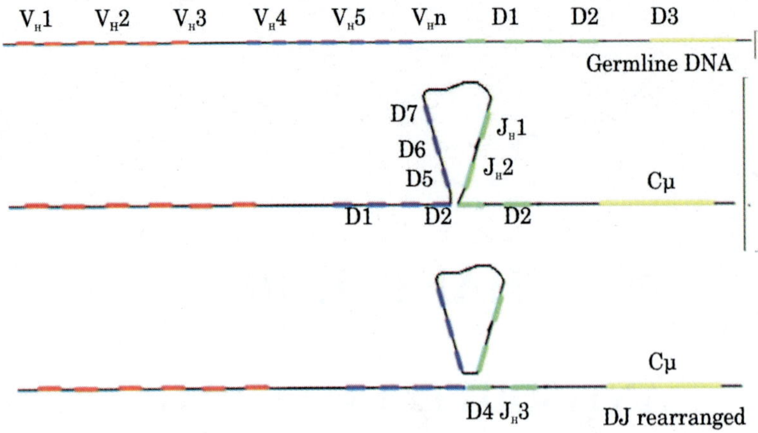

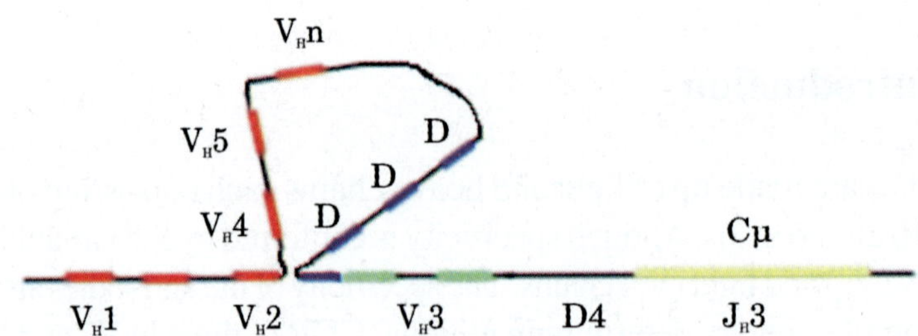

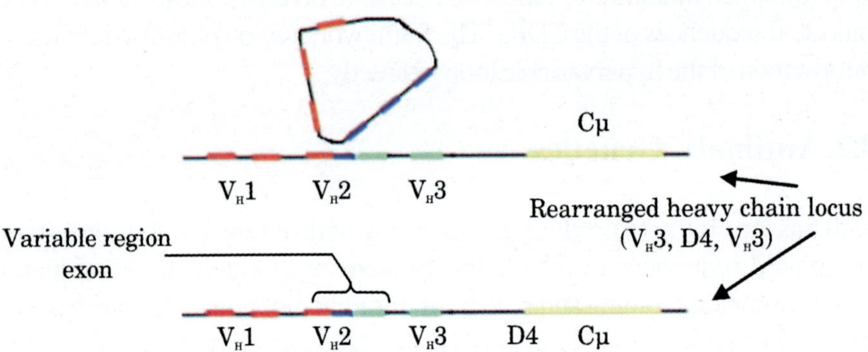

Fig. 10.1: Gene rearrangement in the heavy chain locus.

Similar gene rearrangement occurs for the light chain but with out the diversity region (D). Only VJ rearrangement occurs, followed by apposition to the C region.

The antibody (epitope) specificity is endowed due to the particular gene rearrangement that has occurred in a particular B cell, much prior to the exposure to the antigen. The purpose of immunization is to increase the frequency of the B cells than are capable of reacting with the different epitopes of the antigen. During mAb production, if these B cells fuse with the myeloma cells, we end up with production of mAbs of the desired specificity. The initial mAb production done in mice suffered with the following limitations when applied for therapy in humans.

- The mouse Fc portion of mAbs interacted variably with the human cellular Fc receptors which is required to accomplish the effector functions
- The serum half life of mouse mAbs were low
- The mouse mAbs were recognized as foreign by the human immune system and they developed human anti-mouse antibodies (HAMA). The HAMA responses can be anti-isotypic and anti-idiotypic. The HAMA precludes repeated treatment with mouse mAbs since this could be ineffective or lead to anaphylaxis and shock.

The above problems can be obviated by:

- Combining the variable region of the mouse mAbs with the constant region of the human antibody (Chimeric antibodies)
- Combining only the six CDRs of the murine mAbs with the other part of the antibody from human source (Humanized antibodies).
- Production of completely humanized antibodies.

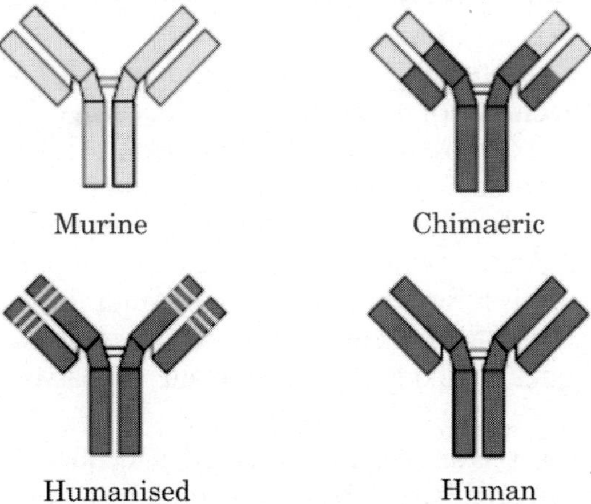

Fig. 10.2: Chimeric and humanized antibodies.

10.3 Humanized Antibodies

Immunologically, the best alternative to therapeutic murine mAb is a human mAb. Preparation of totally human mAbs has the following limitations.

- Ethical issues prevent the direct immunization of humans with most biologic agents and one cannot readily harvest cells from human spleens
- Absence of a good human myeloma fusion partner that does not lose chromosomes with continued growth in cell culture.

An alternative approach is to immortalize B cells by formation of lymphoblastoid cell lines involving infection with Epstein Barr virus (EBV), a B-lymphotropic herpes virus. Once transformed, EBV-infected B-cell lines tend to grow in clumps, release virus, and secrete low levels of antibody, primarily of the IgM isotype. They also require repetitive cloning which is labor intensive.

Another approach to overcome the immunogenicity problems associated with murine mAbs is to re-engineer the antibody to make it 'human-like'. This involves the incorporation of the heavy (H)- and light (L)-chain variable (V) regions of a given murine mAb into an expression plasmid (for example, pJH2-24-95B1) that contains the constant (Cμ) region of human IgM. Upon transfection of cells, the resulting plasmid construct expresses a human-murine hybrid (chimeric) IgM molecule that retains the specificity of the "parent" murine MAb but reacts like human IgM.

10.3.1 Veneering and hyperchimerization of antibodies

The antigenicity of a protein is primarily dependent on the nature of its surface. Hence the immunogenicity of mAbs could be reduced by replacing the exposed residues which differ from those usually found in humans. This judicious replacement of exterior residues would have little, or no, effect on the interior domains, or on the inter domain contacts. Thus, ligand binding properties would be unaffected as a consequence of alterations which are limited to the variable region framework residues. The process is referred to as veneering since only the outer surface of the antibody is altered. The procedure for veneering makes use of the available sequence data for human antibody variable domains available in various databases.

Hyperchimerization is an alternative method of identifying residues outside of the CDR regions that are likely to be involved in the reconstitution of binding activity. In this method, the human sequences are compared with murine variable region sequences and the one with highest homology is selected as the acceptor framework. The different residues are replaced by the more commonly occurring human residues.

Antibodies are proteins and all the methodologies applicable for recombinant protein expression can be used for expressing the antibodies as recombinant proteins. The conventional antibodies have heavy and light chains as independent polypeptide chains that get 'assembled' to form the mature antibody with a particular epitope specificity and CDRs from heavy and light chains constitute the antigen combining site. However, this situation may not be ideal for expression strategies since it does not allow construct to be coded by a single gene.

Hence the smallest portion of the antibodies that can still combine with the epitope on the antigen is the CDRs on heavy and light chains and if they are combined in to a single polypeptide chain using a peptide linker, it is called a single chain fragment variable (scFv) or single chain antibody. If it is stabilized by a disulphide bond it is called a disulphide stabilized fragment variable (dsFv). The advantages are:

Size is dramatically reduced compared to a full antibody that makes it more accessible. It allows expression by a single sequence of nucleotides (gene) coding for the sequence of the amino acids that make the desired combining antigen combining site. Further reduction in size is achieved by the use of single domain antibodies (sdAb or nanobody) that consists of single monomeric variable domain (CDRs only from the heavy chain and no light chain contribution). Some species of animals like camels and llamas and sharks possess only single domain antibodies in nature. The sizes of these antibodies are as follows:

Conventional antibody = 2 heavy chain + 2 light chains = ~ 150–160 kDa
Fab fragment = One light chain and half of heavy chain = ~ 50 kDa
Single chain fragment variable=CDRs from light and heavy chain=~25 kDa
Single domain antibodies = CDRs from heavy chain = ~ 12–15 kDa

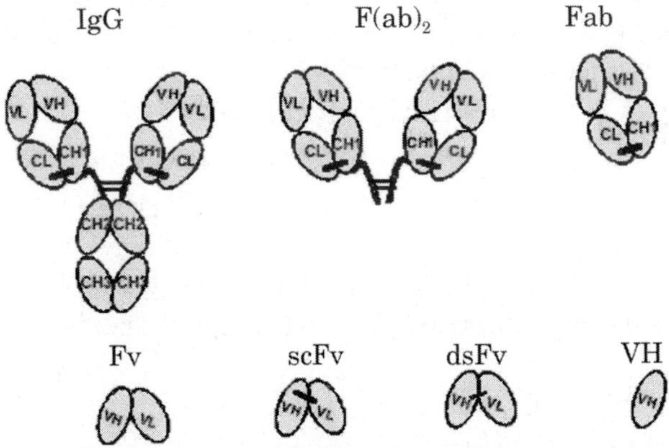

Fig. 10.3: Structure of immunoglobulin G (IgG) and its antigen binding segments. IgG–whole molecule; $F(ab)_2$ Fragment antigen binding (both segments); Fab–Fragment antigen binding; Fv–variable fragment; scFV–single chain Fv fragment; dsFv–disulphide-stabilized variable fragment; VH–Variable Heavy chain fragment.

There are various components/fragments of IgG that contribute to the overall function of IgGs (Fig. 10.3). Expression of one or more of these fragments requires strategies that are consistent with their structural and functional properties. Various Ig fragments are usually generated using different proteolytic enzymes (enzymes that clip proteins after or before specific amino acid residues) and are readily purified from intact IgGs. The Fab portion of IgG is critical for antigen specific effects while the Fc portions facilitates a variety of signaling effects that result in activation of cells via Fc receptors. Hence, depending on the primary need for the antibody fragments, the cloning strategies should incorporate sequences for expression of one or more subunits of the various IgG fragments.

The generation of an entire antibody molecule requires: (i) co-ordinate synthesis of its various fragments; (ii) appropriate folding and secondary structure formation; (iii) accumulation of functional antibodies in sufficient amounts for harvesting. These requirements limited the use of conventional bacterial expression systems since expression of smaller fragments such as Fv fragments (Fig 10.3) resulted in non-covalent interactions altering the stability and thereby the purification steps involved in obtaining the functionally active Fv fragments. But at the same time, single chain Fv (scFv) fragments where the V_H and V_L domain are linked by a flexible peptide linker of 15–20 amino acids were found to be stable. The following strategy is applicable to engineer and purification of scFv fragments:

- Immunize or infect mice with antigen/agent of choice
- Isolate B cells from spleen or use hybridomas specific to antigen of choice
- Isolate mRNA
- Synthesize first strand of cDNA with random hexamers
- PCR amplification of cDNA (second strand) of individual V_H and VL_L chains using degenerate primers engineered to have a linker sequence and sites for restriction enzyme digestion
- Overlap PCR to join V_H and V_L fragments
- Digest PCR fragments with appropriate restriction enzymes consistent with the engineered sites
- Clone PCR products in to expression vectors of choice
- Transform *E. coli* strains compatible for over expression of scFv fragments
- Screen for clones expressing scFv fragments specific to the antigen of interest
- Screen for reactivity with antigen or specific epitope
- Purify scFv fragments using conventional affinity chromatography exploiting the engineered tags (6x histidine or FLAG tags).

Expression can be performed in prokaryotic and eukaryotic systems to generate mAbs or their fragments with defined biological functions.

The strategies are multiple depending on the needs such as (i) ease of manufacture; (ii) reduced contaminants and enhanced bio-safety considerations; (iii) increased concentrations of mAbs; (iv) ease of generating clinically applicable preparations; (v) proper configuration for antigen recognition and neutralization; (vi) native biological properties/features such as post-translational modifications (N-linked glycosylation) and (vii) reduced side effects due to lack of cross-species properties (such as murine antibodies for humans).

10.4 Prokaryotic Systems

Advantages

1. Ease of use. Large volumes of bacterial cultures (*e.g. E. coli*) over expressing recombinant antibody fragments can be processed in batches using large fermentors.
2. Rapid enrichment of the over-expressed antibody fragments from the whole bacterial cells.
3. Availability of well-characterized plasmids, phages employing routine molecular biology techniques to over express antibody fragments.
4. Established good laboratory practices for rapid, commercial grade antibody fragments.

Disadvantages

1. Improper folding of the antibody fragments due to a variety of constraints.
2. Potential for low yields of proteins due to incompatibility of eukaryotic codon usage in bacterial systems.
3. Lack of appropriate post-translational modifications such as glycosylation of select residues leading to reduced or inconsistent neutralization properties.
4. Lack of biological functions such as interactions with the Fc receptors.
5. Need for toxicity evaluations due to select bacterial components such as lipopolysaccharide or endotoxins.

10.5 Eukaryotic Systems

Advantages

1. Proper protein folding as needed for clinical applications in humans and animals due to concerted actions of chaperones and other.

2. Accumulation in sufficient quantities in select intra-and extra- cellular locales such as in roots, tubers and leaves as observed with expression of antibodies in plants.
3. Appropriate post-translational modifications due to trafficking of the antibody fragments through eukaryotic sub-cellular organelles such as endoplasmic reticulum and Golgi apparatus.
4. Stable maintenance of plasmids expressing antibody fragments in select cell lines and transgenic plants for continued propagation over several generations.
5. Established procedure for large-scale manufacture of fragments from mammalian cells similar to large scale human and animal vaccine production.

Disadvantages

1. Limited concentrations of the antibody fragments.
2. Contamination issues with mammalian host cells, potential for co-precipitation of intact and helper virus particles.
3. Contamination with immunogenic mammalian host-cell proteins
4. Need for use of stable plasmid vectors that may carry viral origins of replication and other components that are restricted for clinical applications due to bio-safety considerations.

The considerations of appropriate prokaryotic or eukaryotic hosts are predominantly determined by eventual use of the antibodies generated. There are no significant bio-safety associated risks of using these methodologies for antibody fragments used for diagnostic purposes. The needs for good and safe laboratories practices may preclude use of some these strategies described below for clinical applications.

10.6 Recombinant Expression of Antibody Fragments

As shown in Fig 10.3, the structure of the IgG molecule is complex and its functions resulting in tools useful for diagnostic or therapeutic purposes is dependent on the following:

- Interactions of multiple subunits
- Variations in the DNA sequence contributing to the specificity to various antigens
- Proper structural arrangements of these fragments (such as formation of disulphide bridges and other salt bridges).

While there is a large body of information available on the structure function correlates of IgG molecule, several aspects of these correlates have to be taken into consideration for generation of antibody fragments via recombinant DNA technology. For reasons of clarity, we will focus on the recombinant expression of the minimal regions of IgG single chain Fv fragments that will facilitate its use for diagnostic or therapeutic purposes. A brief outline of the procedure involved is outline in Fig 10. 2.

10.6.1 Isolation of mRNA from spleen cells or hybridomas

In order to clone functional IgG genes to express single chain Fv fragments hybridomas known to express Mabs of a particular isotype or specificity, if available, should it would facilitate rapid preferential isolation of mRNA specific to fragments that are monoclonal and desired isotype. In most cases, it is not possible to have hybriodmas of the required specificity, under these circumstances, spleen cells from natural or experimentally infected animals can be used to isolate mRNA. While it is possible to obtain mRNA from B cells with multiple specificities, it is essential to incorporate strategies that will aid in the differentiation and selection of those mRNA (or cDNA) encoding for IgG fragments.

Isolate RNA 1 to 5×10^6 hybridomas or B cells. This can be achieved with a variety of methods such as use of Trizol, RNABee and other phenol-based RNA extraction formulations that facilitate rapid isolation of intact RNA in sufficient quantities.

Use Trizol or RNA Bee at a specific concentration of 1ml of reagent to $1–2 \times 10^5$ cells (or as recommended by the manufacturer). It is essential to add enough amounts of these reagents so as to facilitate rapid isolation of total RNA free of RNAses that will denature the RNA and limit the synthesis of cDNA. If sufficient amount of these reagents are not used the functions of RNAses may not be sufficiently inactivated leading poor quality and/or quantity of RNA. These RNA isolation procedures are well established and should not pose problems to isolate considerable yields of RNA of good quality to facilitate cDNA synthesis. Several commercial kits utilizing the presence of polyA tails in mRNA.

There are several commercial kits available for isolation of mRNA with polyA tails employing non-phenolic isolation reagents resulting in yields approximating 1 to 10 µg of mRNA. These kits employ methods for rapid lysis of cells and portioning of the nucleic acids and proteins. The polyA tail at the end of mRNA is then used for the preferential enrichment of the mRNA by the capacity to bind to oligo-dT-cellulose columns that are usually provided with the kit or can be prepared separately. The complementarity of the polyA tail to a stretch of Ts linked to cellulose will provide for the affinity purification of mRNA. The loading capacity of the oligo-dT columns plays a critical role in the purity of the mRNA and conventionally total RNA from 1 to 5 million cells will provide 1–10 μg of mRNA. If the larger yields of mRNA is needed multiple extractions using oligo-dT columns should be carried out.

If spleen cells from mice (or rat) immunized with a given antigen or from experimentally or naturally infected animals are used as the source of RNA, the splenic tissue should be dispersed in HBSS (or other tissue culture medium such as RPMI or DMEM could be used) using a sterile sieve (similar to that used for generation of hybridomas). The connective tissue and other tissue debris can be separated by slow speed centrifugation for 15 to 30 sec. at less than 200 × g. It is feasible to obtain the total RNA and subsequently enrich for mRNA from spleen cells.

Alternatively, the B cells can be preferentially purified using magnetic beads conjugated with antibodies specific to B cells. This procedure provides an additional enrichment of mRNA needed for the generation of cDNA specific to the antibody fragments (scFv). Approximately 5×10^7 B cells are obtained form a single mouse spleen and the efficiency of the isolation of total mRNA should determine the number of spleens required for successful generation of engineered scFv fragments.

10.6.2 Generation of cDNA

Precipitate the total mRNA from hybridomas or spleen cells with 2.5 volumes of chilled ethanol (–20ºC), 10 μl of glycogen (10mg /ml, serves as a carrier) and one tenth volume of 2.5M/pH5.0 potassium acetate (facilitates precipitation of RNA as a salt). If needed the mRNA can be stored in ethanol at –20ºC for up to a month. It is highly recommended that the extracted RNA is converted to cDNA as soon as possible. The precipitated RNA is collected by centrifugation and at 16000 × g at 4ºC for 30 min. A microcentrifuge could be used for this purpose with precautions to clean the centrifuge of RNAs if it is routinely used for DNA extractions. After washing with chilled 90% ethanol to remove any contaminants, the RNA pellet is dried and resuspended in RNAs-free (diethylpyrocarbonate (DEPC)–treated ddH_2O) water and the concentration of RNA is then determined spectrophotometrically at 260nm. The ratios of 260/280 will help to decide if the quality of the RNA is sufficient for further processing. A portion of RNA is stored at this stage for use as a control to determine the levels of DNA contamination. Approximately 0.1 to 0.5 μg of RNA and 1–2 μl of random hexamer primers in a final volume of 50 μl of reaction mix to generate the first strand of cDNA. The procedure involves use of template (cDNA) random hexamers for priming, reverse transcriptase to convert RNA to first strand of cDNA and a reaction mix containing all the needed constituents such as dNTPs in appropriate buffers to complete the reactions.

The precise conditions vary depending on the vendor used for obtaining the reagents needed for generating the cDNA, while the general principle is to rapidly convert RNA to the first strand of cDNA. The first strand of cDNA can then be used as the template with degenerate primers to obtain the PCR products specific to V_L and $_{VH}$ chains that are specific to the antigen or a particular epitope on an antigen of interest.

10.6.3 Primer design for PCR amplification of V_L and V_H using the first-strand cDNA as the template

The following features have to be captured during the design of the primers:

1. Sequence variability of the V_H and V_L fragments
2. Sequence needed for connecting V_H and V_L fragments
3. Stabilization sequence $(Gly_4Ser)_4$ to facilitate stability of the expressed V_H-V_L fragments as single chains
4. Sequences that facilitate anchoring of the degenerate primers in the constant region of the IgG genes
5. Required restriction enzyme sites to clone these fragments in to plasmids, phage DNA and other cloning systems for expression in prokaryotic and eukaryotic expression hosts.

The design of primers should include the following guidelines

- Engineer restriction enzymes sites based on final destination expression plasmid
- Engineer linker sequences at appropriate ends of V_H and V_L amplicons
- Engineer FLAG tag or 6x histidine–specific sequences
- Engineer overlap sequence on appropriate ends of V_H and V_L amplicons for overlap PCR and fragment assembly
- Incorporate degeneracy as needed for obtaining the variable region sequences.

An example for the rational design of primers is provided here but this strategy should be modified depending on the source of cDNA used from either cloned hybridomas or from total B cells from spleens from infected or immunized mice (or other sources).

10.6.4 Assembly of the PCR fragments

In the following example the assembly of PCR fragments is directed in such a way that it will facilitate the cloning of mouse scFv fragments (Fig.10.4).

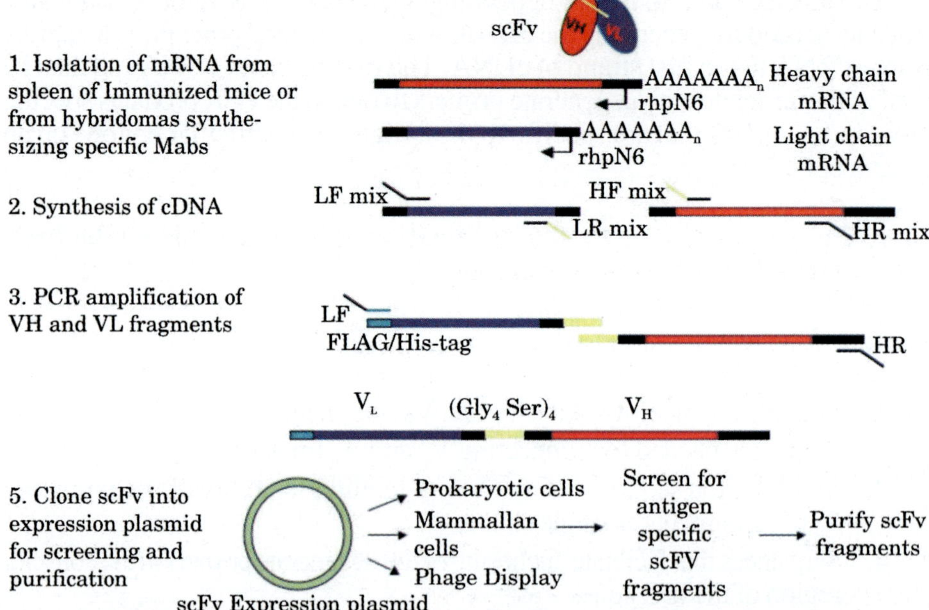

Fig. 10.4: Schematic representation of the steps to engineer scFv fragments

- Orientation of the PCR fragments: It is critical to design the primers such that the orientation of PCR fragments generated is consistent with the engineering of functional scFv fragments. The orientation of the segments are as indicated-V_L-$(Gly_4S)_4$-V_H-into plasmid vectors that can be used for expression in *E. coli*, mammalian cells or in phage display systems. There are several vectors that can be used providing distinct advantages such origins of replication, selectable antibiotic markers, restriction enzymes sites for subsequent deletion of select tags and expression of specific proteins essential for use of phage display systems.
- Generate forward and reverse primers with varied levels of degeneracy for the V_L and V_H chains.
- The reverse primers to amplify V_L also have an engineered restriction enzyme site and the sequence coding for a tag such as either FLAG tag or 6X Histidine tag. The levels of degeneracy should vary from 2 to 16 depending on the sequence that need to be amplified.
- One reverse primer specific to specific to the mouse λ gene that contains additional sequences similar to the reverse primers of VL regions.
- The forward primers to V_L regions has the sequence specific for encoding the $(Gly_4$-$Ser)_4$ linker and a limited set of degeneracy.
- The reverse primers to amplify V_H are also engineered similar to reverse primers of the V_L region in terms of the degeneracy but with the sequence specific to $(Gly_4$-$Ser)_4$ linker.

- The forward primer for the V_H region is generated similar to that of the forward primer for V_L region with limited degeneracy and with engineered restriction sites to facilitate the eventual cloning of the fused V_L-$(Gly_4S)_4$-V_H into compatible restriction sites in plasmids or phage DNA for expression.
- The first step of the two-step PCR amplification strategy of the generation of individual V_L and V_H PCR products using conventional PCR reagents. The individual products are then used as templates for the second step of the two-step PCR amplification strategy. The presence of the sequence overlap at the appropriate ends of these PCR products will facilitate the "fusion" of the V_L and V_H products using primers that are specific to the VL and VH PCR products. At the end of this step of the procedure, both the V_L and V_H amplicons will be a part of a single amplicon with the linker sequence between the two fragments and with all the features incorporated in the designed primers such as the required restriction enzyme sites and FLAG or 6X-Histidine tags.
- The PCR products corresponding to V_L-$(Gly_4S)_4$-V_H regions is digested with the appropriate restriction enzymes flanking the required regions and the digested products are separated on 1% agarose gel. The PCR products are gel purified, concentrated and cleaned using PCR cleaning cartridges and used to clone into vectors capable of expression of the cloned fragments either in *E. coli*, mammalian cells or as phages with compatible restriction enzyme sites. Usually the vector to insert ratio is between 3:2 and can be varied to obtain an equitable distribution of all the amplicons representing the products of various degenerate primers. Approximately 20 to 50 ng of insert can be used in the ligation reaction which is carried out at 15ÚC overnight in the presence of 1unit of ligase in reaction volume of 10 µl with 1X concentration of reaction buffer. In most cases, the conditions described from the vendor for T4 DNA ligase should be used as a guide to obtain maximal transformation efficiency.

10.6.5 Transformation of *E. coli*

Several strains of commercially available laboratory strains of *E. coli* can be used. Electrocompetent cells are prepared by reseeding an overnight culture in 1liter of LB at a dilution of 1:100 and incubated at 37ÚC with shaking until the cell grows to density of 0.5 (OD_{600}). The cells are chilled on ice for 15 to 30 min and washed with 1L of chilled autoclaved ddH_2O. The cells are pelleted at 4000 ×g for 15 min and washed again with 500 ml of chilled autoclaved ddH_2O. The pellet is washed once again in 20 ml of 10% glycerol (v/v in water). The final pellet is re-suspended in 2 to 3 ml of 10%glycerol with a final concentration of 3×10^{10} cells/ml. The electrocompetent cells may be stored at –80°C in aliquots of 40 µl per tube until used.

10.6.5.1 *Electro transformation of E. coli*

When electroporation is used as a method of transformation of *E. coli*, it is essential to ensure that the DNA used is free of any salt. The presence of salt even at low levels would result in little or no transformation efficiency. The ligated DNA from step 9 is precipitated for at least 2 hours in ½ volume of 7.5 M ammonium acetate/ 2.5 volumes of ethanol and the centrifuged at 11000×g for 10 min and the pellet is washed with 70% ethanol to remove salt. It is helpful to add 1–2 µl of tRNA (20 mg/ml) to the DNA ligation reaction to serve as a carrier as the levels of nucleic acid present is low. It is advisable to wash the DNA pellet twice in 70% ethanol to minimize the levels of salt even though this procedure may lead to loss of DNA in the precipitates. The DNA pellet is dried and dissolved in 5 µl of ddH_2O and 1 to 2 µl of this sample is used to electrotransform *E. coli* using gene pulser Xcell Electroporation System (Bio-Rad Laboratories). There are other models that can be used for this purpose. Each electroporator require use of specific plastic cuvettes which can hold defined volumes of cells. Sterile, single use Gene Pulser cuvettes with 0.2 cm electrode gap are routinely used as it requires less than 50 µl of cells. The electrocompetent cells mixed with the DNA to be transformed is placed in the cuvette and subjected to pulse of 12kV/cm with time constant of 4 to 5 m/sec. This can be achieved by setting the gene pulser at 25 µF (capacitance), 2.5 kV (voltage) and Pulse controller unit to 200 Ω. It is routine to observe lower or no transformation efficiency if the time constants are lower than 4 presumably due to the presence of salts in the DNA preparation or if the bacterial cells are not sufficiently washed. At times if the contaminant salts are at sufficiently high concentration, there would be an 'arc' leading to complete loss of transformation efficiency. Electrotransformation procedure is highly efficient and easy to execute with the only limitation that an electroporator is an essential piece of equipment needed for this procedure. If an electroporator is not available, it is possible to use *E. coli* cells amenable for transformation by heat shock at 42°C albeit at low levels of transformation efficiency.

10.6.5.2 *Selection of transformants*

Immediately following electrotransforamtion, the cells are resuspended in 500 µl of medium rich in glucose (SOC medium) and incubated at 37°C for 1hr to allow for cells to recover and after which 50 to 100 µl of cells need to be plated on LB agar plates supplemented with appropriate antibiotics conferred by the vector used in the ligation reaction. The plates should be incubated overnight at 37°C and colonies visible on the plates should be propagated in liquid LB medium containing the same antibiotics in 96 well plates. Dispense 100 to 200 µl of LB plus antibiotic into each well and inoculate each well with individual colony from the LB plates. It is essential to pick as many colonies as possible into 96 well plates as it will eventually facilitate rapid screening for scFv that can react with the antigen/s of choice. If the numbers of colonies are too few, it is critical to redo the ligation or transformation. Following incubation of the plates at 37ºC overnight they can be frozen with the addition of 20 µl of glycerol to each well as a cryopreservant. The plates can be gently agitated to mix the glycerol and plates can be stored at –80 ºC for several months. It is a good practice to duplicate the plates if repeated freeze thawing is expected to occur during the screening process. A few random colonies should also be checked for presence of plasmid with insert of appropriate size and if there is a greater percentage of colonies without insert, it is essential to recheck the ligation procedure. Since the cloning procedure utilizes double digests, the chances of self ligation of the vector without insert is minimal.

10.6.5.3 *Screening of transformants*

Since there is a potential for every single bacterial colony selected to encode for a different V_L-$(Gly_4S)_4$-V_H region due to the degeneracy of the primers used, it is essential that a robost screening methodology is readily available for screening of transformants. Several techniques can be used to undertake a high throughput screening (if the cDNA is from spleen cells from animals immunized with a bacterial pathogen and no selective pressure applied for isolation of specific B cells) to identify V_L-$(Gly_4S)_4$-V_H region of interest that interact with the antigen or even epitope of choice.

10.6.5.4 *Colony hybridization*

A routine procedure to screen for colonies with V_L-$(Gly_4S)_4$-V_H regions of interest is to grow templates of the clones frozen in 96 well plates in new plates where the LB growth medium is supplemented with appropriate antibiotics and 1mM IPTG to drive the expression of V_L-$(Gly_4S)_4$-V_H regions under the control of IPTG inducible promoters. The induction should done by incubating the plates at 37ÚC for 2 to 4 hr at which time a few microliters of the culture can be spotted to nylon membrane or coated as antigen on to ELISA plates. The membranes or plates are incubated with specific biotinylated antigens or peptides of interest and after appropriate washing steps the blots or plates are developed with streptavidin conjugated with HRPO followed by incubation with appropriate substrate. Either colorimetric detection reagent or the more chemiluminescence based systems followed by conventional autoradiography. It is possible that the above procedure results in extensive background, which can be minimized by standardization using *E. coli* expressing the empty vector (serving as the negative control). It is also feasible to lyse cells from wells induced with IPTG employing mild detergents followed by incubation of 50 to 100 µl of lysates from the each well as coating antigen on ELISA plates. The plates are then treated with biotinylated antigen/s or peptides and developed using streptavidin conjugated with HRPO or other chromogenic substrates. A good negative control (lysates from *E. coli* containing the empty vector) and positive control (antisera from immunized mice used for obtaining the spleen cells) should be included to validate the specificity of the assays. Once putative clones are identified, it is essential to perform an immunoblot assay where the antigen/s of interest is separated on SDS-PAGE gel and transferred to PVDF membrane and probed with the lysates from the putative bacterial clones that are tentatively positive for synthesis of antigen-specific V_L-$(Gly_4S)_4$-V_H. The presence of FLAG tag or 5X Histidine tag present on V_L-$(Gly_4S)_4$-V_H can be exploited for detection of the binding using anti-FLAG tag or anti His-tag antibodies conjugated to HRPO or alkaline phosphatase. The blots can be developed using conventional chromogenic substrates or ECL specific to the conjugated enzymes. These are well-established procedures and can be carried out using laboratory equipment and reagents needed for immunoblot analysis or ELISA.

10.6.5.5 *Phagemids*

If the PCR products encoding for scFv molecules were cloned into pBluescript II phagemid vectors (plasmids with phage origin of replication; Stratagene), it is possible to select for colonies via both Blue/White(without insert/with insert) and screen for the presence of V_L-$(Gly_4S)_4$-V_H regions using procedures similar to colony blot analysis Since the degenerate primers used should result in different amplicons, the specificity of V_L-$(Gly_4S)_4$-V_H regions has to be ascertained by using procedure described for colony blots employing antigens that are labeled with biotin and using streptavidin conjugated to chromogenic substrates for determining the colonies positive for reactivity with the antigen of choice. A major advantage of using this system is the capability of generating pBluescript II phagemids as single-stranded DNA, which is amenable for performing sequencing and site-directed mutagenesis. This latter strategy will help in procedures to enhance the reactivity of the scFv fragments for antigens of choice.

10.6.5.6 *Expression in mammalian host cells*

A variety cell lines are available to express plasmids containing origins of replication compatible with maintenance and propagation in mammalian cells where the expression of scFv fragments are under the control of promoters functional in eukaryotic cells. A major advantage of the use of mammalian cells is streamlined processing for purification of antibodies without complications from components of prokaryotic cells such as endotoxin. Moreover, if proper conformation and folding of the engineered antibodies are critical parameters of its functionality, it is much easier to obtain those conformations in homologus systems.

10.6.5.7 *Purification of engineered scFv fragments of interest*

Once the scFv fragments specific to antigen of choice have been identified, it is possible to use the 6X-histidine tag or FLAG tag to purify these fragments employing affinity columns with matrices that are capable of binding to 6X-histidine (Nickel affinity columns) or those that are coupled with antibodies against FLAG tag. The total lysates of prokaryotic or eukaryotic expression hosts are used in the purification process as described in *Chapter 11* for purification of recombinant proteins. The fragments can be analyzed for additional binding and neutralization properties and used as needed.

It should be borne in mind that the generation of cDNA specific to the antigen binding domains of antibodies is dependent on the degeneracy of the primers and hence a robost, rapid method to identify the scFv fragments specific to the antigen of interest is a critical step in the utility of this methodology. There are a few additional steps that can be taken to minimize the lack of specificity of the cDNA synthesis by using hybridomas that have been characterized to secrete a monoclonal antibody of specific isotype. It is critical to be cognizant of the fact that some of the hybridomas may produce additional non-specific antibodies, which may complicate the generation of scFv fragments. Compared to using the spleen cells as a source of polyclonal B cells, there is much greater chance of obtaining the scFv fragments with specific reactivity to the antigen of choice.

10.7 Therapeutic Antibodies

One of the major advantages of developing engineered antibodies is their use as therapeutic antibodies in human and veterinary medicine. Engineered antibodies provide the advantages of minimal cross-species specific issues. Engineered antibodies can be readily used for neutralization of toxins, bacterial or viral products, and neutralization of signaling molecules in cancer cells as well as in other disease conditions involving the cardiovascular and neurological systems.

The first clinical use of antibodies to neutralize the diptheria toxin was developed by von Behring in 1880s for which he was awarded the first Nobel Prize in Medicine in 1901. Since then a number of sera against viral and bacterial agents have been developed from humans and animals and used with varying degrees of success as prophylactic and therapeutic agents against a number of infectious diseases. The greater understanding of the immune mechanisms especially the formation of immune complexes and the reactivity of the host immune system to components of the heterologous antibodies has given rise to the need to develop antibodies without these side effects.

The advances in the methods in molecular biology, phage display systems and functional genomics have helped in the development of strategies to "humanize" antibodies to derive the beneficial effects of antibody mediated effects without the deleterious consequences of reactivity associated with heterologous antibodies. These developments have resulted in more than 30 different polyclonal and monoclonal antibodies approved by the Federal Drug Administration in 2008 (the agency that evaluates the efficacy of drugs before approval for clinical use) and this list of antibodies are continuing to expand at a rapid pace. These therapeutic antibodies have been used in the treatment of a variety of inflammatory diseases, cancers, neutralization of toxins following serious complications with infectious agents and in treatment of disorders of the cardiovascular and nervous systems for which surgical procedures are not readily available. Some of the FDA approved therapeutic mAbs are given in Table 10.1.

Table 10.1: Some of the FDA approved therapeutic mAbs

Product	*Specificity*	*Product type*	*Indication*
Orthoclone OKT3	CD3	Mouse	Transplant rejection
ReoPro	gpIIb/gpIIa	Chimeric Fab	Cardiovascular disease
ZenaPax	CD25	Humanized	Transplant rejection
Rituzan	CD20	Chimeric	Non Hodgkin lymphoma
Remicade	TNF alpha	Chimeric	Crohn disease, rheumatoid disease
Simulect	CD25	Chimeric	Transplant rejection
Synagis	RSV	Humanized	Respiratory syncytial virus
Herceptin	Her – 2	Humanized	Metastatic breast cancer
CroFab	Snake venom	Ovine Fab	Rattle snake antidote
DigiFab	Digoxin	Ovine Fab	Digioxin overdose
Mylotarg	CD33	Humanized	Acute myeloid leukemia
Campath	CD52	Humanized	Chronic lymphocytic leukemia
Zevalin	CD20	Mouse	Non Hodgkin lymphoma
Omalizumab	IgE	Humanized	Anti-allergic
Cetuximab	EGF receptor	Chimeric	Cancer
Bevacizumab	VEGF	Humanized	Cancer
Panitumumab	EGF receptor	Human	Cancer
Eculizumab	Anti complement 5	Humanized	Immunlogical

Alternate strategies are available for the production of fully human antibodies using transgenic technology. The steps involves in such a strategy are as follows:

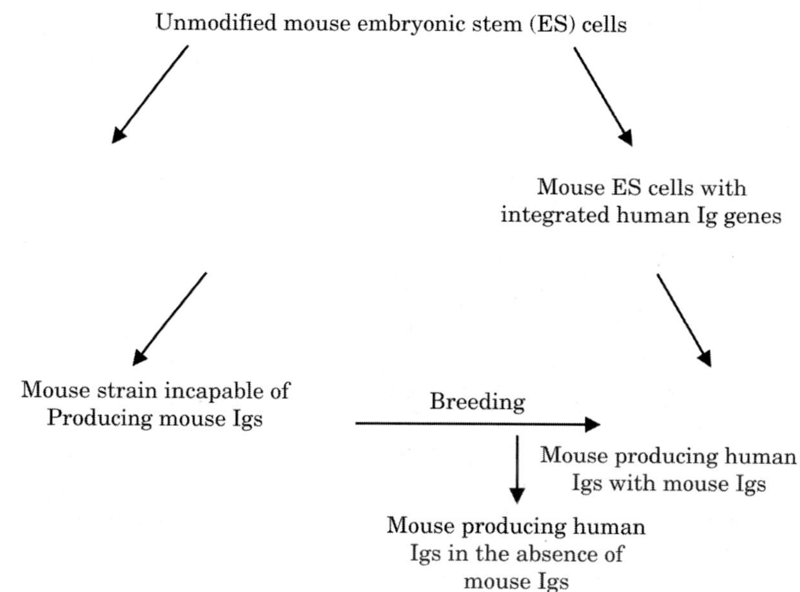
Unmodified mouse embryonic stem (ES) cells
Mouse ES cells with
integrated human Ig genes
Mouse strain incapable of
Producing mouse Igs
Breeding
Mouse producing human
Igs with mouse Igs
Mouse producing human
Igs in the absence of
mouse Igs

CHAPTER 11

ALTERNATIVES TO MONOCLONAL ANTIBODIES

11.1 Introduction

In recent years, techniques which allow production of mAbs without hybridomas or even animals used for providing lymphocytes or myeloma cells) have been developed. The antibody genes are isolated from lymphocytes of immunized animals and then cloned and expressed in bacteria, just like any other recombinant proteins. These antibodies produced in bacteria are screened for specificity to the antigen of interest. Thus, while hybridoma technology could immortalize antibody producing cells, recombinant phage technologies immortalizes genes responsible for antibody production. Other techniques such as computer graphics are also used to build specific antigen binding sites in antibodies.

11.2 Production of Recombinant Antibodies by Phage Display Technology

There are a wide variety of methods and tools now available for the generation of recombinant antibodies exploiting the versatility of the phage display technology. While it is beyond the scope of this textbook to capture these methods, a broad approach is described to lay the foundation for understanding the advantages and potential pitfalls of this system. The strategies described in the seminal work of Barbas *et al.* (1991) to assemble combinatorial antibody libraries on the surface of phages to generate what are called as phage antibodies or Phabs, would be used as the base methodology to elucidate ways to generate antibody reagents via alternate approaches that have properties similar to mAbs.

11.2.1 What are bacteriophages?

These are viruses that infect and replicate in bacterial cells. They have very minimal genomes that can be manipulated and they express specific proteins that facilitate interactions with proteins or receptors on bacterial cells. Those bacteria that express these receptors are susceptible to infection with phages. There are two types of bacteriophages: (i) lytic phages that lyse or kill the bacterial cells that they infect in a very precise fashion; (ii) lysogenic phages that infect bacterial cells and integrate into their genome and are stably carried for several generations.

11.2.2 Summary of steps involved in the generation of scFv using phage display system

1. Isolate mRNA from B cells from immunized or infected mice or use hybridomas secreting mAbs of known specificity
2. Convert to cDNA and PCR amplify using degenerate primers to capture the VH and VL chains repertoire
3. Clone PCR fragments into phagemid vector pComb 3
4. Infect compatible strains of *E. coli* with the phagemid. Infect with helper phage to obtain intact phage particles expressing V_H and V_L chains
5. Identify the phage particles of interest by panning using antigen or other substrates of interest
6. Convert phage DNA from particles of interest into plasmid DNA by restriction enzyme digestion and relegation.
7. Re-transform appropriate strains of *E. coli* for expression of soluble scFv specific to antigen of choice
8 Similar strategies can be used for expression of IgGs.

11.2.3 What is a phage display system?

A commonly used phage that replicates and has all the genetic elements to assemble fully formed particles in *Escherichia coli* is a filamentous bacteriophage such as M13 (Fig 11.1). This phage does not kill *E. coli* and has been the mainstay of phage display systems. A variety of these friendly phages have also been used to establish techniques for manipulating their genome to express peptides and proteins of interest. The phage particles expressing these peptides or proteins are then used to explore the functions of the peptides/proteins using a variety of assays. For example a bacterial protein (a ligand) may interact with a mammalian protein (a receptor) to initiate a series of molecular events such as facilitating bacterial infections. If the identity of the bacterial protein that is critical for infection is not known, phage-display systems could be used to help identify that protein. The entire genome of the bacteria can subjected to restriction enzyme digestion such that small DNA fragments can be cloned to a specific phage gene (resulting in a fusion protein) that would result in the expression of short peptides on the surface of phages. The phage particles (10^{10} to 10^{11} particles) each expressing a different peptide on the surface are allowed to bind to the purified receptor of interest from mammalian cells. The phage particles are "panned" over receptor coated plates to facilitate binding of phages expressing peptides specific to the bacterial protein that is known to facilitate the binding to the receptor on mammalian cells. The unbound phages (having sequences encoding for peptides not specific to the receptor) are washed, facilitating enrichment of phages expressing peptides specifically interacting with the receptor protein. After performing further rounds of 'panning' a highly enriched population of phages are used to infect *E. coli* cells. A number of different strategies are then employed to find the identity of the peptides binding to the receptor such as sequencing of single stranded DNA from individual phages or after conversion of the phage DNA to a circular plasmid (see below). While phage display systems are routinely used in identifications of ligand/receptor interactions, there are several advantages to exploit this system for expression of antibody fragments that retain reactivity to antigen/s of interest. The biggest advantage of the use of phage display system is the generation of a large repertoire of particles expressing peptides on the surface that can be exploited via high throughput assays (HTP assays) for rapid identification of proteins involved in the specific interactions. A large number of receptor/ligand interactions as well as other protein-protein interactions have been establish using these methods. Recently there is renewed interest to employ phage-based therapy to modulate defined regions/domain of proteins known to play a role in various pathogenic processes. For example phage particles directed at the Arg-Gly-Asp (RGD) domains of proteins to prevent adherence and movement (metastasis) of cancer cells over tissue matrices with variable levels of success.

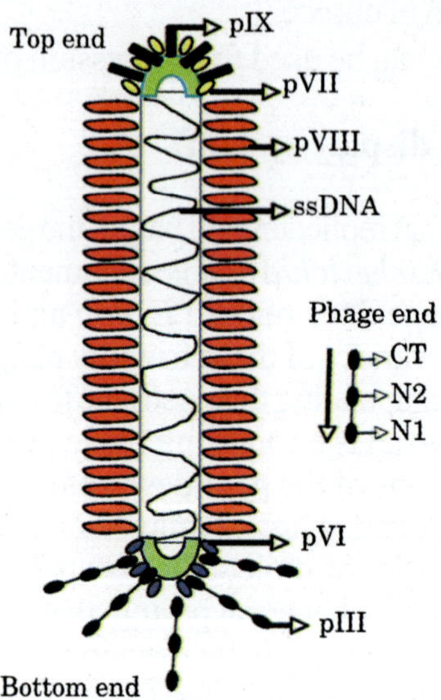

Fig.11.1: Schematic representation of a filamentous phage.

As the name indicates the phage has a filamentous shape with its single stranded DNA enclosed in a cylindrical coat. The vertical side of the coat is comprised of major coat protein pVIII. One end indicated as the top end of the particle consists of pVII and pIX and is the end that comes out of the bacterium first during the phage assembly. The bottom end of the phage comprises pIII and pVI. The incorporation of these minor coat proteins signal the termination of assembly of phage particles. pIII consists of 3 domains (N1, N2 and CT) linked by flexible linker regions. The interaction of the N2 domain with the F pilus present on certain strains of *E. coli* initiates the infection process. Once the phages come in contact with the F pilus of a bacterial cell, the N2 domain will dissociate and facilitate N1 to interact with another bacterial protein called TolA. After this step there will be transfer or translocation of phage DNA into the cytoplasm of the bacterial cell. The CT domain has been shown to be the structural stability of the phage and may participate in the formation of the entry pore needed for the injection of DNA from the phage into the bacterial cell.

11.2.4 What are phagemids?

Phage particles incapable of assembling into full particles due to truncation of their genome are called phagemids. The phagemids are routinely used to manipulate their genome to clone exogenous DNA fragments. The incomplete viral particles are fully capable of infecting their prokaryotic hosts but are incapable of forming complete viral particles. Therefore, it is essential to re-infect the prokaryotic cells originally infected with phagemids with a helper phage, which will in turn provide the requisite genetic material sufficient to completely assemble the phage particles. The strategy described in this chapter to generate scFv utilizes the phagemids. Which in the presence of a specific helper phage will be converted to an expression plasmid in *E. coli* which can then be induced to express scFv specific to antigen/ s of interest.

11.3 Manipulating Structural Proteins of Filamentous Phages for Antibody Libraries

It is critical to understand the role of various phage proteins in the structure, entry, assembly and release of the phage particles from its bacterial host in order to exploit phage-based methodologies for expression of antibodies. The filamentous phage particles commonly used in phage display technologies are 6.5 nm in width and about 1μm in length (Fig 11.2). Its genome consists of single stranded DNA within a cylindrical protein coat. Much of the coat made of the major coat protein pVIII. At the top end of the phage is the capped with around 5 copies of pVII and pIX. The top end of the phage emerges first following assembly from a bacterial cell. The minor coat proteins pIII and pVI that are present at the bottom end of the phage play an important role on the termination of the assembly of phage particles. The pIII also plays an important role in the binding to the F pilus on the bacterial cell–a critical interaction that initiates the infection of the host cell. The pIII has three domains that are linked by flexible linker modules. The phage initiates infection by the interaction of the N2 domain of the pIII with the F pilus, leading to the dissociation of the N1 and N2 domains. This facilitates the interaction of the N1 domain with the bacterial protein TolA. The final step in the infectious process is the translocation of the phage DNA into the cytoplasm of the bacterial cell through a pore. The CT domain plays an important role in maintaining the structural integrity of the phage particle as well as in the generation of the entry pore through the phage DNA translocates to the cytoplasm of the bacterial cell. Most phage display systems are driven by the physical linkage of the proteins expressed on the phage to its genotype. By cloning short segment of foreign DNA in to the genes encoding for these polypeptides, it is possible to express these proteins or peptides as fusion coat proteins. There are select advantages in using the gene coding of pIII or pVIII as they facilitate expression of these heterologous proteins on the surface of the phage. The filamentous phages with surface exposed proteins or peptides of interest can then be selected by "panning" over matrices coated with ligands or antigens of interest. In this way the genomic and phenotypic properties and the replication cycle of the filamentous phages in the bacterial cells are customized depending on the purpose of using phage display system such as for expression of antibodies, identification of protein-protein interactions or phage therapy.

11.3.1 Expression of antibodies using phage display system

The strategy used for generation of scFv fragments are described in detail in *Chapter 10*. The steps involved in the generation of cDNA using degenerate primers by PCR are essentially similar except the restriction enzymes sites engineered have to appropriate to the pComb 3 vector or its derivatives that will be used for the packaging of the fd phage. Once the PCR products for light and heavy chains are generated using degenerate primers as described in *Chapter 10*, the amplicons are digested with appropriate restriction enzymes and cloned into pComb 3 vector, which will result in an ampicillin resistant phagemid. The light and heavy chains are cloned sequentially as shown in Fig 11.2 and 11.3 at the appropriate restriction enzyme sites. The phagemids were transformed into *E. coli* XL-1 Blue cells (Stratagene) and grown in superbroth (30 g tryptone; 20 g yeast extract; 10 g Mops per liter; pH 7.0) at 37°C supplemented with appropriate antibiotics. Cultures were grown to a density OD600=0.4 at which time was infected with the helper phage VCSM13 at phage to cell ration of 20:1. The cultures are grown for another hour at 37°C prior to adding kanamycin conferred by the helper phage. The cultures were incubated for 16 hrs after which the phage particles were isolated from liquid culture by clearing the supernatant at least twice by centrifugation for 10 min at 4°C. The phage particles are precipitated with polyethylene glycol (3.3% PEG8000/0.4M NaCl) followed by re-centrifugation as described above. The phage pellet were re-suspended in TBS (50 mM Tris-

HCl pH 7.5/150 mM NaCl) and stored at 4°C. It is also possible to obtain phage particles can be purified by scrapping form agar plates and employing the above procedure to purify the particles.

Primer design

- Engineer restriction enzymes sites based on final destination expression plasmid
- Engineer linker sequence at appropriate ends of VL and VH amplicons
- Engineer FLAG tag or 6X- Histidine-specific sequence
- Engineer overlap sequence on appropriate ends of VL and VH amplicons for overlap PCR and fragment assembly
- Incorporate degeneracy as needed for obtaining the variable regions sequences.

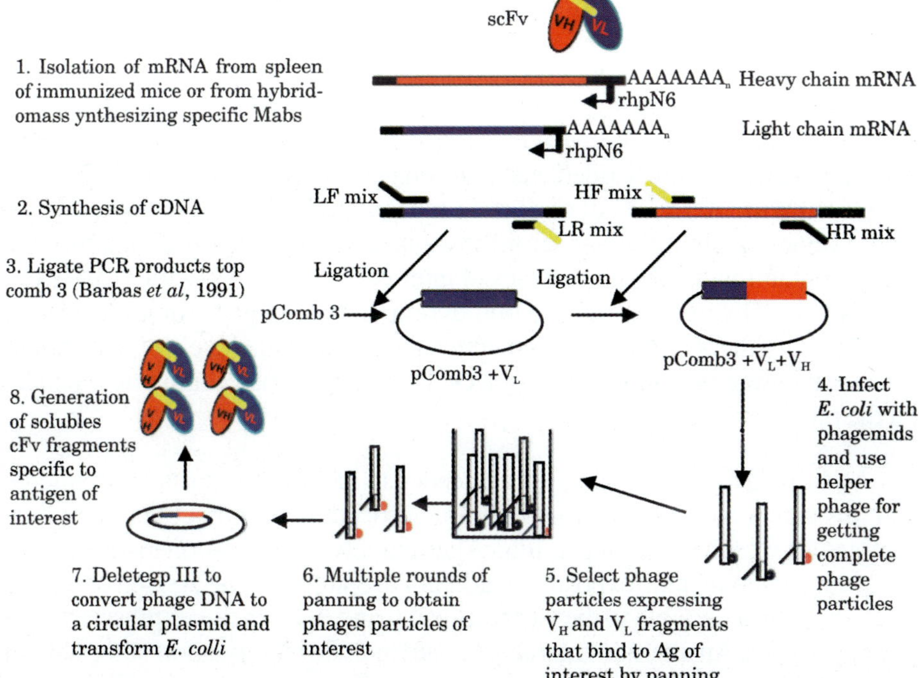

Fig. 11.2: Schematic representation of genertion of scFv fragments employing phage display system.

11.3.2 Affinity purification by phage particles expressing antibody of interest

Once the phage particles have been purified, it is essential to obtain or purify phage particles that express light and the heavy chain fragments that are specific to the antigen used in the generation of B cells. Alternatively, the phage display system can also be used as the method of generation of a large repertoire of antibody fragments that are capable of binding to different epitopes of the same antigen or against different antigens (if B cells used for the preparation of cDNA were isolated from experimentally or naturally infected animals). The affinity purification of the phage particles specific to the antigen of interest is a crucial step in the utility of this strategy. Since the construction of the phagemids and the superinfection with the helper phage is directed towards the expression of the variable heavy and light chains as fusion proteins on the surface of the phage, it is essential to isolate or pan these positive phages form those expressing chains not specific to the antigen of choice.

A simple procedure to allow the phages expressing variable heavy and light chain to attach to the antigen (1–2 mg/ml) coated on the ELISA plates in 0.1 M bicarbonate coating buffer at pH 8.6 in a volume of 25 to 50 µl at 4ºC overnight. After blocking the unbound sites using non-fat dry milk in phosphate buffered saline at 37 ºC for 1 hr, the phage particles in a volume of 50 to 100 µl obtained as described above are allowed to bind to the antigen of interest for 2 hr at 37ºC. The phage particles not expressing antibody chains specific to the epiotpes present on the antigen are washed by using a wash buffer with mild detergents. The wells are washed up to 10 times with TBS/Tween (50 mM Tris-HCl pH7.5/ 150 mM NaCl/0.05% Tween) over a period of 1 hr at room temperature. After washing the wells with distilled water, the phage particles still bound to the wells are eluted with 50 to 100 µl of elution buffer (0.1M HCl adjusted to pH 2.2 with glycine containing bovine serum albumin at a concentration of 1mg/ml). The eluate containing the phage particles of interest is neutralized with 3 to 6 µl of 2 M Tris base. The initial input and output ratio of the phage particles need to be titrated using the XL-1Blue *E. coli* cells to determine the levels of enrichment for each panning step and counter-selected with appropriate antibiotics encoded on the phages.

Additional rounds of panning are needed to identify the particles of interest and this can be done employing the same procedure and by collecting phage samples after each round of panning. Alternatively, modification to the panning procedure could include exposure of additional epitope on the antigen of interest that may be inaccessible to the variable heavy and light chains expressed on the phage particles. An alternative strategy could include biotinylation of the antigen which then can be incubated antibodies bound to streptavidin. The biotin-streptavidin interaction is highly specific and this interaction can be exploited to expose additional epitopes on the antigen that may be accessible to the antibody regions expressed on the phages. A variety of such subtle modifications to the base experimental procedure could facilitate rapid and reliable identification of phage particles expressing the variable heavy and light chains combinations. It should be borne in mind that the appropriate combination of the light and heavy chains on the phage particles is critical to binding and the repertoire of these combinations screened from a large number of phage particles ~10^{11} facilitates the screening process and in conjunction with a multiple panning steps it is technically feasible to obtain phage particles of interest very rapidly. Once the specific phage particles have been identified it is essential to convert the genome of the phage to a circular plasmid that will facilitate the expression of the antibody fragments as soluble proteins (Fig. 11.3). The pComb 3 phagemid described above for surface display can be readily manipulated by restriction enzyme digestion followed by DNA ligation that would result in a circular plasmid with a prokaryotic origin of replication capable of allowing this plasmid to be stably maintained in *E. coli*. The bacterial cells can then be induced with IPTG to express the antibody fragments that can be purified in accordance with the need for use of theses antibodies in diagnostic and therapeutic applications.

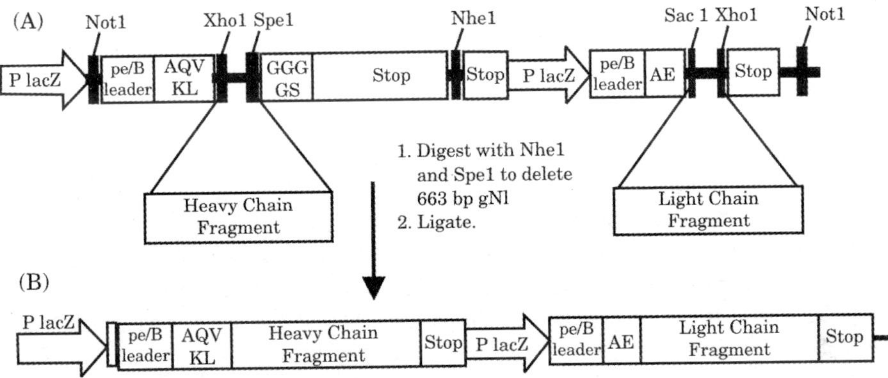

Fig.11.3: Phagemid vector for surface display (A) and for expression of soluble scFv or Fab producing forms (B). The pComb 3 phagemid construction is as described in ref (1). The vector is designed for cloning of combinatorial Fab fragments and can be adapted for other scFv fragments by incorporating sequences that will facilitate a linker sequence as detailed in *Chapter 10*. The sequence between the Spe1 and Nhe 1 sites can be excised and re-ligated resulting in the removal of the pIII gene resulting in the formation of a construct that can be used for the soluble expression of scFv fragments. The constructs shown can be modified by engineering appropriate restriction enzyme sites on primers used for generation of DNA fragments used in the cloning procedure.

11.3.2.1 *Advantages of phage display system*

1. The ability to generate a large population of phages with various combinations of variable light and heavy chains facilitates rapid identification of phages with specificity for the antigen of interest.
2. Readily available tools to generate phagemids, phages and methods to produce large quantities of specific antibodies

3. Cost effective as the down stream processing methods are relatively inexpensive. Use of bacterial strains with targeted mutations in the lipopolysacharride genes allows for purification antibodies without the persistent problems of endotoxin contamination.
4. Ability to expand the antibody repertoire by identifying unique binders that are not readily recognizable by conventional methods of generating mAbs.
5. Affinity maturation by site-specific alterations. By selectively engineering changes to the sequence encoding for the variable heavy and light chains, it is possible to enhance the binding efficacy of the secreted antibody fragments.

11.3.2.2 *Limitations of phage display system*

1. It is possible that the correct combination of variable light and heavy chains are not selected
2. Lack of expression of the antibody fragments as a gIII fusion protein.
3. Lack of stability of the phages expressing antibody fragments
4. Lack of stability of scFv fragments or proper conformational forms of antibodies for functional analysis.

There have been significant advances in the phage display systems and a number of recent reviews are a good starting place to obtain the state of art methodologies that can be used to generate intact antibodies. The current advances in genomics and molecular biology have resulted in several strategies for rapid generation of antibody fragments that can be engineered as per the specifications essential for the ultimate use of these substances.

11.4 Production of Mono-specific Sera using Recombinantly Expressed Proteins

The production of mono-specific serum using recombinant proteins has been divided into two parts. The first part (see 11.3.1) focuses on the generation of recombinant proteins that can be used as antigens in a variety of immunization protocols. The same protocols can be used to generate antigens for diagnostic purposes as well as for characterizing Mabs for their specificity. The second part (see 11.3.2) focuses on the generation of mono-specific serum in experimental animals against these recombinant antigens.

11.4.1 Production of recombinant proteins

There are several advantages to overexpression and purification of recombinant proteins from *E. coli.*

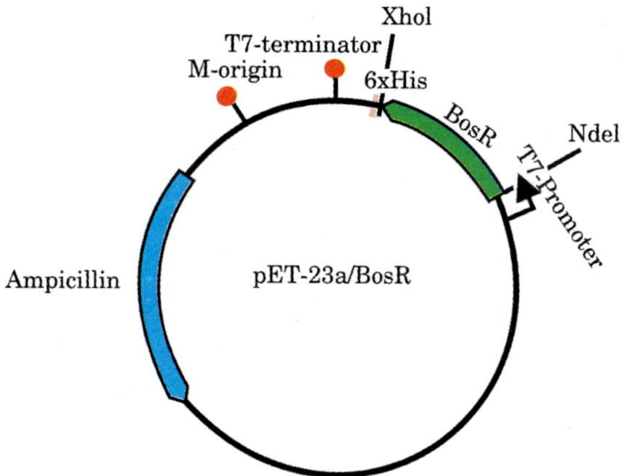

Fig. 11.4: mAp of the overexpression plasmid pET23a with a cloned bacterial gene BosR. Note: The presence of a strong prokaryotic promoter (T7) and a terminator, a prokaryotic origin of replication and a 6X-Hsitiidne tag at the C-terminus providing a means for purification of the recombinant proteins. While NdeI and XhoI are shown in this figure there are other cloning sites that provide a means to clone genes or cDNA fragments with compatible restriction enzyme sites. The 6X-Histidine tag can also be fused at the N-terminus and can be removed from the recombinant proteins by the use of select proteases that clip at a defined amino acid sequence between the N-or C-terminus a the recombinant proteins and the 6X-Histidine tag.

1. Ease of use, variety of plasmids and host strains
2. Streamline methods for enrichment and purification of recombinant proteins
3. Inexpensive scale-up procedures
4. Use of recombinant proteins as antigens for generation of Mab, use as antigens for screening and for diagnostic purposes
5. Generation of antibody fragments for reactivity with defined epitopes
6. Generation of truncated proteins for epitope mapping
7. Generation of therapeutic and diagnostic antibody fragments without endotoxin contamination
8. Recent development of engineered host *E. coli* strains to facilitate proper dimerization of antibody fragments
9. While these procedures require several cloning steps, the availability of standardized procedures facilitates rapid, large scale purification of specific recombinant proteins
10. A number of recombinant proteins from *E. coli* are routinely used for several such purposes.

The example used to illustrate the steps involved in the overexpression and purification (Fig. 11.4) are for a soluble bacterial protein and the procedure could be adapted for expression of any soluble protein. The strategy can also be used for generation of specific recombinant antigens for immunization purposes for the generation of mAbs, as a reliable and easy source of antigen for screening of mAbs and for analysis of the epitope specificities during the characterization of the mAbs. The advantages include ease of production of large quantities of recombinant proteins as well as truncated segments of a specific protein that could be used for the generation of epitope specific antibodies for diagnostic or therapeutic purposes. Moreover, similar strategies could be used to generate single chain Fv or variable heavy chain fragments of mAbs depending on the intended use of these mAbs.

11.5 Steps Involved in the Overexpression of Recombinant Proteins

11.5.1 Choice of overexpression plasmid

Care has to be taken in determining the features of the overexpression plasmid to be used. Some of these features include

a. Ease of propagation of the plasmid-origins of replication that facilitate propagation in prokaryotic and eukaryotic systems
b. Promoters capable of driving expression to high levels in both prokaryotic or eukaryotic hosts
c. Additional features such a 6X-histidine tag for facilitating affinity purification of the recombinant proteins; epitope tags such as V8 or Flag for immunodection of the purified antigen are to be considered depending on the nature of the ultimate use of the recombinant antigens
d. Restriction enzyme sites that will facilitate rapid cloning of a gene or DNA segment of interest.

11.5.2 Cloning of the gene of interest into an expression plasmid

As shown in Fig 11.4 the strategy includes use of overexpression plasmid pET23a which provides certain advantages such as a strong T7 promoter facilitating increased expression of the cloned gene, C-terminal 6X-Histidine tag, counter-selectable markers and ease of use in bacterial host cells that allow for accumulation and purification of proteins.

Amplify a gene of interest from bacterial, viral, parasitic organisms. In most cases it possible to amplify the gene of interest from the total genomic DNA and in other cases from the cDNA generated from the total RNA.

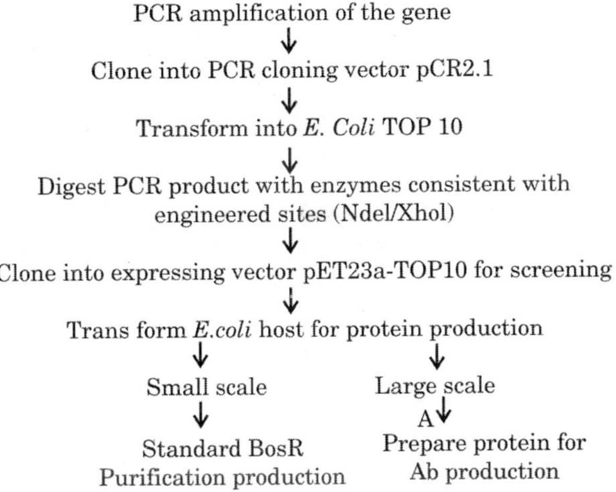

Fig. 11.5: Schematic representations of the steps involved in overexpression and purification of recombinant proteins. Note it is possible to directly clone the PCR products after digestion with appropriate enzymes consistent with the engineered sites as well as those present on the expression vector.

Fox example in order to overexpress a bacterial protein termed BosR from the spirochetal pathogen *Borrelia burgdorferi*-the causative agent of Lyme disease-the *bosR* gene was amplified using primers (short stretches of nucleic acids with sequence corresponding to the 5'and 3' end of the *bosR* gene. In most cases, the nucleotide and deduced amino acid sequences are readily available in databases open to the public for organisms whose genome has been sequenced. In some cases the investigators who have access to genome sequences that have not been deposited in public databases would readily provide the information on a case-by-case basis. In a large number of cases, especially for eukaryotic organisms, the cDNA sequence information would be accessible via a number of databases accessible to the public.

Primer 1 bos R-F- ACGCCATATGAACGACAACATAATA
Primer 2 bos R
ACGCCTGGAGGGATCCCCTAGGAACCAGAGATCC
TAAAGTGATTTCCTTGTTC

The engineered primers have sequences (underlined) that are recognized by the restriction enzymes Nde1 and Xho1 as well as 4 additional nucleotides at the 5' end to facilitate digestion with restriction enzymes directly on the PCR products to generate PCR products that could be cloned into the expression vector (pET23a) with compatible ends. The reverse primer, in this case, also encodes for thrombin cleavage site (nucleotides indicated in red). This will allow for the engineering of a thrombin cleavage site between the C-terminal residue of BosR and the 6X-Histidine tag which can be removed by proteolytic cleavage using purified thrombin during the elution stage of the purification of recombinant BosR (see below for details). The primer design should take into consideration the melting temperature of the target sequence, the percent AT versus GC. A good rule of the thumb is to avoid a stretch of Ts' at the 3'end and also complementary sequences that could lead to formation of primer-dimers. The PCR products that will presumably have the engineered restriction enzyme sites can be purified and cloned into pET23a with compatible ends and cloned using T4 DNA ligase.

The total genomic DNA template from prokaryotic sources used to generate the PCR products can be obtained using conventional DNA extraction procedures such as phenol-chloroform or non-phenolic compound based kits from Qiagen and other vendors can be used to the total DNA.

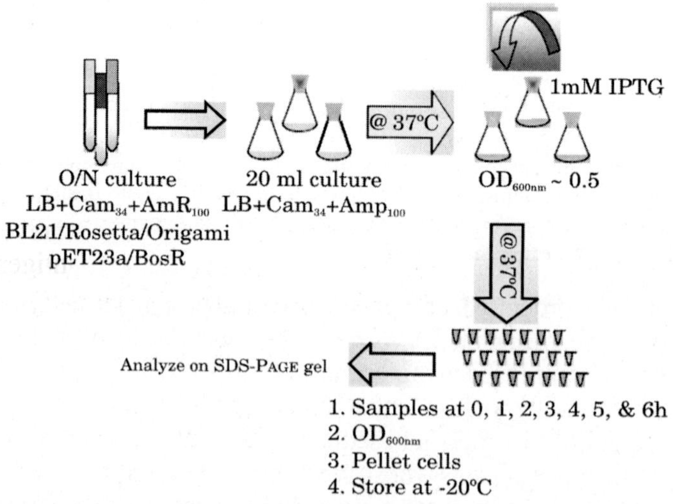

Fig. 11.6: Schematic representation of small scale induction of recombinant proteins. A variety of *E. coli* expression hosts such as BL21®, Rosetta®, Origami® etc can used. In addition to the antibiotic needed for the selection of the expression plasmid (ampicillin), additional antibiotics are to be supplemented to retain the mutations that confer select phenotype in these hosts such as normalized tRNAs and reduced misfolding of recombinant proteins.

In most cases a simple lysis buffer containing lysozyme, SDS in an appropriate buffer can be used to lyse bacterial cells followed by incubating the sample in boiling water for a minute. The samples can then be centrifuged to obtain a quick (though "dirty") DNA preparation that can be used as a template if the target genes are anywhere between 1 to 3kbs. If the size of the genes is greater than 3kb it may be critical to obtain the total genomic template DNA using phenol-chloroform or commercial non-phenolic compound based kits.

Since several overexpression plasmids carry origins of replication that result in low copy numbers per bacterial cell to avoid the potential for toxicity associated with the rapid expression of recombinant proteins, the cloned products should be transformed into *E. coli* strains such as TOP 10 to facilitate screening of colonies with the right insert in the overexpression vector.

Once a few colonies have been identified to carry the overexpression plasmid with the correct insert, it is important to sequence the cloned product to ensure that there are no inadvertent stop codons/alterations in the amino acid sequence due to infidelity in the PCR reactions. This particular issue is of great significance in the use of the above procedure for using recombinant proteins as immunogens for generating mAbs as a single amino acid change has the potential for altering the secondary and tertiary structures of the proteins leading to changes in the conformational epitopes that may be critical for inducing a B cell response that would eventually lead to isolation of 'interesting' hybridomas that recognize these epitopes.

The mAbs against conformational epitopes tend to be important tools for blocking the interactions of antigens with their target ligands and also tend to neutralize infectivity of viruses. Moreover, some of the antigens may have critical stretches that contribute to linear epitopes and it is essential that sequence verification of the cloned gene and the deduced amino acid sequence analysis will prevent any potential pitfalls (such as reduced or no reactivity of mAbs to native proteins) in the generation of mAbs or use of recombinant proteins as antigens either for screening of mAbs or as diagnostic tools.

11.5.3 Transformation of *E. coli* expression hosts

Several *E.coli* expression hosts are routinely used depending on the intended use of the recombinant antigens. The selection of the expression host is again dependent on the subsequent use of the recombinant antigen and the methodology used for the purification. If the recombinant proteins are to be used a routine diagnostic antigen where the amount of the protein that can be purified is critical, conventional *E. coli* strains that facilitate expression of T7 driven genes can be used. In some cases such as use of recombinant proteins as enzymes or for identification of maAs that react with conformational epitopes, it is critical to facilitate proper or native folding of the proteins. While it always possible for recombinant proteins expressed in large amount to form what are known as inclusion bodies, the proper folding of proteins can be controlled by the use of engineered *E. coli* strains that facilitate folding driven primarily by the amino acid sequence of the expressed protein.

It is also possible that several recombinant proteins are generated from sequences whose codon usage is vastly different from that of the native codon usage of *E. coli*. Under these circumstances there could significant problems in the overexpression of the recombinant proteins and this could be partly circumvented by the use of strains of *E. coli* that have normalized tRNAs that facilitate expressions independent of the native codon usage of *E. coli*. Therefore, the ultimate strategy to purify and the purpose of the use of recombinant antigens should drive the selection of expression plasmids and hosts respectively.

11.5.4 Overexpression of recombinant proteins in *E. coli*

Once it is confirmed that the *E. coli* expression host has the expression plasmid of interest (a quick isolation of plasmid DNA and restriction enzyme digestion will suffice) a small-scale induction with 1 mM IPTG to evaluate levels of expression as well as the time of induction at which there is maximal expression.

An overnight culture of *E. coli*/pET23a-bosR is restarted in fresh medium (LB medium with 100μg/ml of ampicillin) and propagated at 37°C with shaking until the OD_{600} reaches 0.5. At this stage 1mM IPTG is added and samples collected at different intervals from 1 hr to 4 hr. The samples are prepared and analyzed by SDS-PAGE and stained by Coomassie blue to determine the optimum time at which there is maximal expression. In most cases it is around 3 to 4 hr while there are instances where there is increased expression even within 2 hr.

Several trouble shooting steps can be evaluated depending on the observed problems in terms of levels of overexpression. If the levels of expression is very low, the cultures following the addition of IPTG could be incubated at lower temperature such either 30°C or at room temperature. This is to prevent rapid accumulation of recombinant proteins that could result in increased toxicity to bacterial cells. Moreover, this will also be evident in the form of reduction in the OD_{600} measurement at different time points following addition of IPTG.

It is also possible that the recombinant proteins are deposited as inclusion bodies which would result in the preferential accumulation of the proteins in the bacterial pellet instead of in the soluble fraction. As part of the pilot experiments the proteins from the soluble fraction and the bacterial pellet should be analyzed separately. If the majority of proteins is in the soluble fraction the procedure described below using native buffers co be applied.

Once the pilot studies provides an indication as to the parameters best suited for maximal expression, a large scale culture of 1 to 10 liters should be made and processed for purification. The cultures at OD600 should be induced with appropriate concentrations of IPTG for the length of time determined from pilot studies at which time an aliquot needs to be saved for analysis at –20°C. The cultures should be centrifuged at >3000xg and the pellet subjected to high pressure disruption using a French Press at a pressure of 1000 psi. In the absence of the equipment needed for disruption using a French Press, the pellets can be subjected to one cycle of freeze –thaw at –80°C and sonicated using lysis buffer appropriate to either purification under native or denaturing conditions.

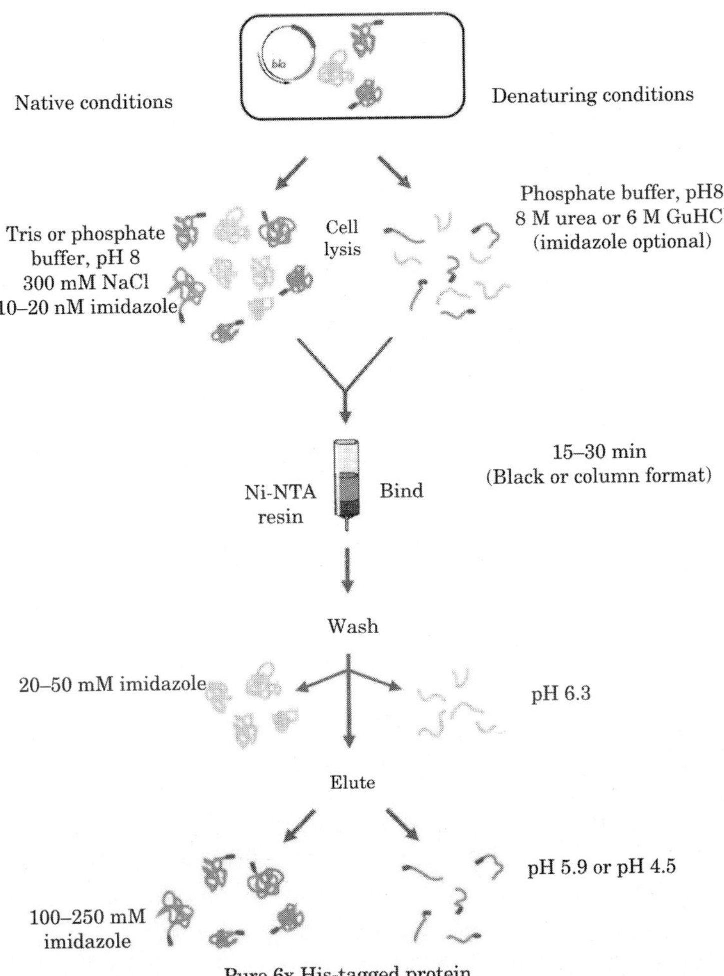

Fig. 11.7: Schematic representation of the purification of 6X-histidine tagged proteins using NiNTA beads as per manufacturers instructions adapted from 'The QIA expressionist ™' fifth edition, Qiagen, Valencia, CA, USA.

The lysates generated by either procedure should be centrifuged and an initial analysis for the levels of overexpression should be determined. If the recombinant proteins are present in sufficient amount in the supernatant, the sample could be processed for purification using the nickel affinity column chromatography. In the event the proteins are localized to the pellet, it is possible to disrupt the pellet using the denaturing buffers and subsequently renaturing the recombinant proteins using native elution buffers. The procedures used for affinity purification of 6X-Histidine tagged proteins are adapted from Qiagen as the procedure involves use of NiNTA beads. Other purification matrices are available and procedures have to be standardized as per the specifications of the beads.

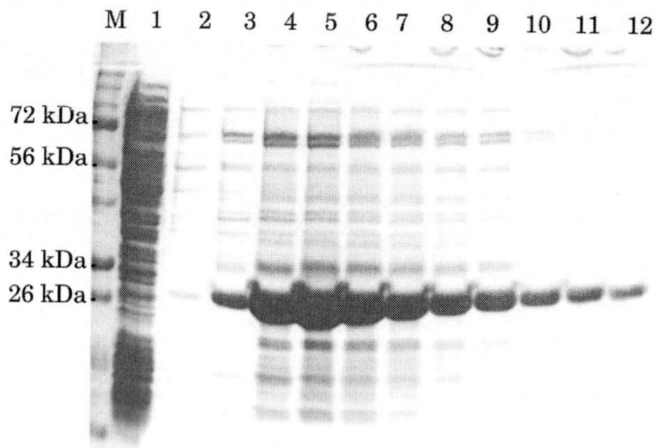

Fig. 11.8: Purification of recombinant BosR (rBosR). A bacterial protein from the spirochetal pathogen *Borrelia burgdorferi* was overexpressed as a recombinant protein with a C-terminal 6X-Histidine tag. The rBosR was purified using Nickel affinity column. Elution fractions were analyzed using SDS-12.5% PAGE and stained with Coomassie Brilliant Blue. Note the preferential enrichment of the recombinant proteins from a total lysate due to the presence of the 6X-Histidine tag. While there are other contaminating proteins in fractions depicted in lanes 4 to 8, there is a near homogenous purification of rBosR in fractions shown in lanes 10–12.

11.5.5 Purification of 6X-Histidine tagged proteins using NiNTA affinity columns

The NiNTA beads ~10ml (50% weight/volume in ethanol) is centrifuged at <500 g for 2 min in 50 ml centrifuge tube to remove the ethanol. The beads are washed 3 times in the lysis buffer (native or denaturing) depending on what was used during the disruption of the bacterial cells. The beads are then incubated with the supernatants containing the recombinant proteins are incubated at 4°C with shaking for 4hrs at which time the beads are washed by centrifugation with the wash buffer to remove non specific binding of proteins. Then the beads loaded on to a column and the bound 6X-Histidine tagged proteins are eluted using an elution that has 250 mM imidazole, which displaces the histidine bound to the beads. The volumes of the elution fractions are dependent on the concentration of the input proteins and usually ranges from 0.1 ml to 1 ml per tube. The purification of the 6X-Histidine tagged proteins is a well-established procedure providing good yields of recombinant proteins. As shown in Fig 11.8, there is a significant enrichment of the recombinant proteins (BosR, a 22kDa protein) containing the 6X-Histidine tag, which can be dialyzed against phosphate buffered saline, quantified, aliquoted and stored at –80°C until further use. The presence of the thrombin cleavage site between the C-terminal end of BosR and the 6X Histidine tag can also be used to cleave the mature BosR protein without the His tag if certain biochemical properties of recombinant protein require the removal of the tags useful for purification of recombinant proeins.

These procedures can be utilized for expression of either prokaryotic or eukaryotic proteins that do not have significant post-translational modifications. Even though there are several other strategies to generate recombinant proteins, use of *E. coli* as the expression host is still a very common practice. The same strategies could be employed using cDNA specific to VH fragments from B cells or hybridomas that make antibodies that have significant therapeutic or diagnostic values. This strategy is an important alternative to generation of mAbs without the limitations of species-specific segments that limit the use of mAbs for therapeutic purposes.

11.6 Production of Mono-specific Serum against Recombinant Proteins

Once the recombinant proteins are purified to homogeneity, the components of the elution buffer employed in the purification process should be removed by dialysis against phosphate buffered saline (PBS) at 4°C. The dialysis can be achieved by using dialysis membranes with molecular weight cut-off appropriate to the size of the recombinant protein. In most cases a 5000 Dalton cut off membrane is used to remove most of the constituent of the elution buffer by dialyzing against multiple changes of PBS. It is important to ensure that the purified proteins are not diluted during the dialysis procedure. This can be achieved by reducing the length of the dialysis tubing to limit the dilution process but at the same time there should be sufficient exchange for the replacement of the salts and other constituents of the elution buffer. An alternate procedure is to load the proteins on to Slide-A-Lyzer ™ dialysis cassettes with a molecular weight cutoff of 2 kDA and dialyze against PBS at 4°C overnight and with one or two changes of PBS. In addition it is also possible to use centrifugal filtration cartridges with 5 to 10K cutoff which will ensure removal of the constituents of the elution buffer and at the same time will also facilitate the concentration of the recombinant protein in the retentate. The retentate can then be dilute depending on the concentration of the protein required for functional analysis or generation of immune serum.

11.6.1 Immunization protocol for generation of mono-specific serum in BALB/c mice

1. The purified, concentrated recombinant proteins should be filter sterilized using a 0.22 micron syringe filter to remove any potential bacterial contaminants.
2. Determine the concentration of the recombinant protein using standard assays to determine the protein concentration. The commonly used

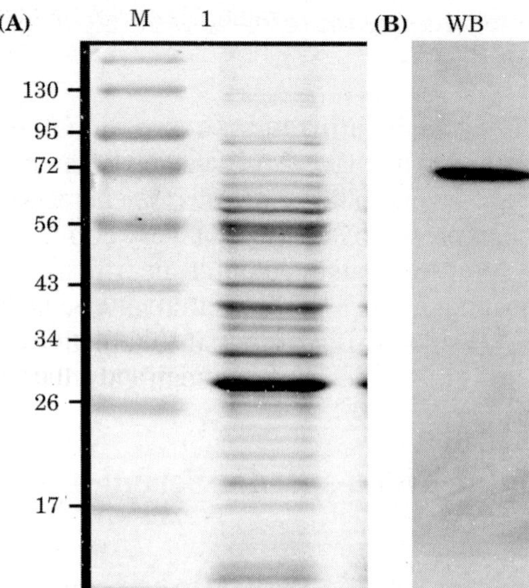

Fig. 11.9: (A) Coomassie blue stained gel depicting the proteins of *Borrelia burgdorferi* (Lane 1). The molecular weigh marker in kDa are indicated on the left. (B). Mono-specific serum generated against recombinant P66 recognizes a 66 kDa protein by western blot (WB) analysis consistent with the size of the protein used to generate the mono-specific serum in BALB/c mice. Note the robust detection of a single protein amongst several borrelial proteins and this methodology is a great alternative to Mabs as it provides a means to generate antibodies with specificity to multiple epitopes present within the same antigen. The blot was developed using HRPO-conjugated sheep anti-mouse antibodies and the reactivity detected by Enhanced Chemiluminescence.

procedure is the BCA assay (bicinchoninic acid; Pierce ™) which measures the protein concentration accurately and reliably within a short period of time.

3. Usually 6 to 8 week old (*n*=5) BALB/c female mice is immunized with at least 50 µg/mice of recombinant proteins emulsified in equal volume of Titermax Gold adjuvant and administered in small volumes subcutaneously (in 3 to 4 different areas). A second and third booster (25µg/mice) are giving via the same route after 2 and 3 weeks following the first injection. At week 4, a small amount of blood is collected from immunized mice and evaluated by ELISA based assay at to the levels of the titers induced compared to that of naïve mouse serum. If the antibody titers are sufficiently high, the animals are subjected to terminal bleeds following institutionally approved protocols. The mice are euthanized by CO_2 inhalation and the blood is collected following cardiac puncture using needles of appropriate gauge. The serum is separated by centrifugation of blood at 9000×g for 10 min. The serum each individual mice should be pooled and aliquots (in 50 to 100 µl volumes) should be stored at –20°C until use.
4. As shown in Fig. 11.9, the reactivity of the mono-specific serum could be as specific as monoclonal antibodies with the added advantage of having

immunoglobulins reacting to multiple epitopes as against just one that would be a monoclonal antibody. For example, recombinant P66, a 66 kDa borrelial protein classified as a porin was purified as described earlier. The purified protein was used to generate serum in BALC/c mice as described above. As shown in Fig. 11. 9B, there was reactivity to only one protein migrating at around 66 kDa in total lysates of *B. burgdorferi* indicating the specificity of the antibodies generated even though P66 does not appear to be a major protein in the total lysates (Fig. 11.10A). The generation of mono-specific serum with reactivity to a variety of recombinant proteins is helpful if the intended use of the serum is to immunoprecipitate the specific antigen and if the antigen exhibit extensive variation between different isolates and if the specificity of the epitope recognized is not an important criterion. While these antibodies are of multiple isotypes with broad range of reactivities to linear and conformational epitopes (depending on the purification of the recombinant antigens under native conditions retaining the overall structure of the protein), they tend to react with greater affinity. These antibodies are helpful as controls while standardizing protocols during development of diagnostic assays and for a variety of biochemical and research related purposes.

11.7 Anti-peptide Antibodies

One of the main advantages of generating mAbs is the ability to isolate hybridomas that would secrete antibodies that are specific to linear or conformational epitopes present on a particular protein used as the inducing antigen. Sometimes it is not possible to obtain mAbs specific to a linear or a conformation epitope that is of interest such as an one on the surface of a virus predicted to mediate viral interaction with a receptor on mammalian cells. Under these circumstances, an alternative approach would be to synthesize a short stretch of amino acids or peptides corresponding to an epitope on a given protein and use the peptide as an antigen to generate anti-peptide specific antibody.

Since the peptides are short and have a linear sequence, their capacity to induce a productive immune response is rather limited even though these epitopes could be immunodominant within the context of a large protein that is processed and presented to appropriate immune cells by the host major histocompatibility molecules.

The aforementioned problem could be circumvented by conjugating or coupling peptides with immunogenic carriers such as keyhole limpet hemocyanin (KLH). The conjugation of short peptides to KLH is a well-established procedure and enhances the immunogenecity of the short peptides significantly. Anti-peptide antibodies can then be derived from mice or rabbits using standard immunization procedures and evaluating the titers of the serum samples collected at different time-points post-immunization.

One of the caveats associated with the generating peptide-specific antibodies is that it is predominantly driven in the favor of linear epitopes rather than conformational epitopes. Since the immunogenetics of the host plays a critical role in the generation of immunodominant peptides, it rather difficult to assemble and synthesize peptides that would are similar to conformational epitopes that are derived from the processing and presentation of antigens within the context of the host immunogenetics.

Recently, a number of bioinformatics approaches have been developed to analyze individual proteins as well as the predicted protein sequences from entire genomes for immunodominant T cell epitopes. A similar approach has also been developed for predicting B cell epitopes where algorithms are generated on a variety of properties associated with particular class of proteins. These algorithms use predicted sequence in conjunction with three-dimensional structure of the proteins if available to derive at the best-bet B cell epitopes.

A number of parameters such as antigenicity, hydrophobicity, hydrophilicity, presence of exposed or flexible loops, secondary structure profiles, beta-turn structure analysis are combined to generate a subset of peptides that can be synthesized and evaluated for binding using serum form infected patients or animals to identify the immunodominant epitopes unique to a given pathogen. Moreover, other biochemical and biophysical characteristics of proteins such as post-translational modifications such as the presence of di-or tri palmytoic acid (lipoproteins) or sites for prenylation or addition of grenyl groups are also evaluated from the primary amino acid sequence to derive these B cell epitopes.

A number of advances have also been made specifically due to high-throughput three dimensional structure analyses of proteins to determine potential conformational epitopes. Analysis of peptides comprising of these conformational epitopes enhance the chance of generating antibodies with the potential to have the capacity to neutralize the interactions between a ligand and its cognate receptor and facilitate identification of neutralizing antibodies. In addition a battery of test such as in vitro neutralization analysis or evaluation of in vivo protective efficacy in naïve experimental models of infection with antibodies against conformational epitopes will add to the validation of use of these antibodies for therapeutic and diagnostic purposes.

The recent advances in the fields of proteomics especially with the expansion of the use of two-dimensional gel electrophoretic procedures and the rapid identification of proteins and peptides through mass spectrophotometric analysis have contributed to generation of antibodies against specific peptides increasing the efficacy and specificity of their use.

11.8 Plantibodies

Antibodies produced in plants are otherwise called as plantibodies and determinants derived from that can serve to induce an immune response are referred to as plantigens.

The use of antibodies as therapeutic agents was first established by Emil von Behring and Shibasaburo Kitasato in 1890. They used serum from animals injected or immunized with a non-lethal dose of a toxin and transferred the immune serum to naïve animals and established the principle of protective immunity conferred by the serum from immunized animals. They coined the term antibodies for the molecules in the serum that conferred the protective immunity. Since then a large body information has been accumulated that has provided the basis to develop strategies to generate antibodies as therapeutic agents against a variety of maladies such as infectious diseases, cancers and other inflammatory conditions that arise due to the increased concentrations of toxins or other proteins that induce these conditions. Obviously, methods to neutralize these components would mitigate their effects and in the process limit the deleterious effects of these antigens and the pathogens that cause the disease.

A commonly used approach to control one such problem, namely diseases caused by bacterial pathogens, is the use of antibiotics. While the use of antibiotics has provided a significant benefit in control of infectious diseases in humans and animals, there are several disadvantages in long term, extensive use of antibiotics especially in food animals. There is an alarming increase in the levels of resistance towards a broad array of antibiotics in a wide range of bacterial populations thereby limiting their utility as effective chemotherapeutic agents. Moreover, use of antibiotics as growth promoting agents in intensive animal husbandry, while beneficial in the short term for economic reasons, has serious implication for human health. Significant concentrations of antibiotics are present in milk, meat and other farm products resulting in the gradual development of resistance toward these agents and therefore making it necessary to develop additional chemotherapeutic agents. If alternate, economically viable strategies that reduce bacterial, viral and parasitic burdens in food animals is incorporated in the husbandry practices, there will be significant advantages in the form of safe food supply, reduced chances of acquiring resistance to antibiotics and reduced exposure to toxic intermediates from pesticides to name a few.

An important criterion for developing these strategies is the cost involved in developing, manufacturing and administration of antibodies or vaccines that reduce the economic losses incurred due to infectious diseases. One alternative that has not been completely exploited is the use of plants as a source of antibodies and as a delivery vehicle for administration of vaccines especially to food animals.

11.8.1 Advantages of using plants for generation of antibodies

1. Economically viable-easy to cultivate in large amounts and process the plants for large-scale purification of antibodies
2. Ability to engineer high concentration of antibodies in select compartment of plant cells
3. Appropriate post-translational modifications on antibodies facilitating use animals and humans
4. Ability to engineer antibodies as component of seeds
5. Easy storage and distribution for site of production to sites of consumption.

11.8.2 Disadvantages of using plants

1. Variability in the accumulation of enough concentrations of the products in various compartments
2. Plant products that have the potential to induce allergies in some individuals
3. A more reliable set of guideline for various down stream processing of products from plants are not readily available
4. Potential for pesticide and other plants related contaminants.

Most of the neutralizing antibodies that have been used for commercial applications have been in human diseases and there are only a limited set of technologies available to generate antibodies in plants even though there has been significant advances in the production of plant based vaccines. The lack of economic advantages for administering antibodies against infectious diseases in livestock even though there is a great potential for delivering recombinant antibodies produced in plants against pathogens of economic importance affecting the gastro-intestinal tracts of food animals that also cause human infections. The major goal is to administer antibodies orally with little or no purification thereby reducing the cost of production of these products. While a major hurdle has been the low concentration of the antibody molecules in the plant material, there have been several examples of use of plantibodies in variable levels of efficacy in providing protection. For example a dimeric protein specific to transmissible gastroenteritis virus (small immune protein–SIP) was generated using the ε-CH_4 domain of human IgE with the scFv antibodies specific to TGEV that has been stabilized using a linker sequence as described in *Chapter 10*. Crude plant extracts containing the fusion protein was administered to two-day piglets resulted in lower viral titers in the gut and lungs but the protection was not similar to that observed with monoclonal antibodies generated in mammalian hosts. A similar observation was also noted when CH_3 domain of IgA was fused to derive TGEV specific SIP that conferred reduced viral loads in the gut and lungs. Recombinant chicken IgA has been evaluated in passive immunization strategies against avian Coccidiosis caused by intracellular protozoan parasite belonging to the genus *Eimeria*. Moreover, recent studies have also revealed that the plant cells can be engineered to assemble secretory IgA complexes such as the dimeric IgA complex with the J-chain as well as its association with the chicken secretory component. These observations clearly demonstrate that plant cells could be engineered to successfully generate significant amount of antibodies, which could then be used without significant cost escalation towards their purification.

11.8.3 Strategies for expression antibodies in plants

1. There are several molecular biology methodologies directed at the transformation of plant cells and varies with the type of cells used
2. Appropriate plasmids with capacity to expression proteins in various compartments of the plant cells-use of specific target sequences to enhance localization of antibodies in select subcellular compartments
3. Selective expression of foreign proteins in tubers, seeds and chloroplasts
4. Expression of foreign proteins as fusion components of major plant proteins
5. Use of plant viral vectors to deliver that plasmids to appropriate locales in the plant cell.

It is beyond the scope of this chapter to go into the details of the molecular biology techniques involved in the expression of foreign protein in plant cells. While several of these techniques are similar to what has been described in *Chapter 10* and in the earlier components of this chapter, there are specific requirements for transformation and selection of transformants of plant cells.

REFERENCES

Barbas, C.F., Kang, A.S., Lerner, R.A, and Benkovic, S.J. (1991). Assembly of combinatorial antibody libraries on phage surfaces: the gene III site. Proc. *Natl. Acad. Sci. USA* **15**: 7978–7982.

Butler, M. and Dawson, M. (1992). Cell Culture Labfax. Oxford: BIOS Scientific Publisers. ISBN: 0121480607 (edn.).

Choi, K.S., Nah, J.J., Ko, Y.J., Kang, S.Y and Jo, N.I. (2005). Rapid competitive Enzyme-Linked Immunosorbent Assay for detection of antibodies to Peste des petits ruminants virus. *Clinical and Diagnostic Laboratory Immunology* **12**: 542–547.

Devlin, T.M. (1992). The textbook of biochemistry 3rd edition, Wiley-Liss Inc, NY.

Dong Li, Zai-Xin Liu, Pu Sun, Yong-Liang Li, Zeng-Jun Lu, Mei-Na Tian, Ying-Li Chen, Bao-Xia Xie, Hui-Fang Bao, Yuan-Fang Fu, Yi-Mei Cao, Ping-Hua Li, Xin-Wen Bai, Jia-Chuan Sun, Jian-Hong Guo, Xiang-Tao Liu and Qing-Ge Xie (2010). The efficacy of FMD vaccine reduced non-structural proteins with a mAb against 3B protein Veterinary Research Communication **34**: 445–457.

Kirschning, C.J, Dreher, S., Maass, B., Fichte, S., Schade, J., Köster, M., Noack, A., Lindenmaier, W., Wagner, H., Böldicke, T. (2010). Generation of anti-TLR2 intrabody mediating inhibition of macrophage surface TLR2 expression and TLR2-driven cell activation. BMC Biotechnology **10**: 31.

Kohler, G. and Milstein, C. (1975). Continuous culture of fused cells secreting antibodies of pre defined specificity. *Nature* **256**: 495– 497.

Koolman, J., and Rohm, K.H. (1996). Colour Atlas of biochemistry, Thieme, Stuttgart.

Kuroiwa, Y., Kasinathan, P., Choi, Y.J., Naeem, R., Tomizuka, K., Sullivan, E.J., Knott, J.G., Duteau, A., Goldsby, R.A., Osborne, B.A., Ishida, I., Robl, J.M. (2002). Cloned transchromosomic calves producing human immunoglobulins. *Nature Biotechnology* **20**: 889– 894.

Lawrence, P.K., Nelson, W. R., Liu, W., Knowles, D. P., Foreyt, W. J. and Srikumaran, S. (2008). $â_2$ integrin Mac-1 is a receptor for Mannheimia haemolytica leukotoxin on bovine and ovine leukocytes. *Veterinary Immunology and Immunopathology* **122**: 285–294.

Li, J. and Zhu, Z. (2010). Research and development of next generation of antibody-based therapeutics. Acta Pharmacologica Sinica **31**: 1198–1207.

Littlefield, J. W. (1964). Selection of Hybrids from matings of flibroblasts *in vitro* and their presumed recombinants. *Science*: **145**: 709–710.

Ming, Y., Clavijo, A., Li, M., Hole, K., Holland, H., Wang, H., Deng, Y.D. (2007). Identification of a major antibody binding epitope in the non-structural protein 3D of foot-and-mouth disease virus in cattle and the development of a monoclonal antibody with diagnostic applications. *J. of Immunological Methods.* **321**: 174–181.

Naessens.J., Scheerlinck.J.P., Buysscher, De E.V., Kennedy, D. and Sileghem, M. (1998). Effective *in vivo* depletion of T cell subpopulations and loss of memory cells in cattle using mouse monoclonal antibodies. Veterinary Immunology and Immunopathology **64**: 219–234.

Nancy, E.T., Katherine, M.F., Stalder, E.S. and Burgess, R.R. (2009). Identification, Production, and Use of Polyol-Responsive Monoclonal Antibodies for Immunoaffinity Chromatography. *Methods in Enzymology* **463**: 475–494.

Pontecorvo, G. (1976). Polyethylene glycol (PEG) in the production of mammalian somatic cells hybrids. *Cytogenet. Cell Genet.* **16** (1–5): 399–400.

Raj, G. D., Mathivanan, B., Matheswaran, K., Nachimuthu, K., and Davis, W.C. (2007). Lymphocyte subset distribution in apparently normal and single intradermal test-positive water buffaloes analyzed by flow cytometry. *Research in Veterinary Sci.* **82**: 34–38.

Raj, G. D., Ratnapraba, S., Matheswaran, K., Deshpande, M., Srikumaran, S., Nainar, A. M. and Nachimuthu, K. (2003) Development of an enzyme linked immunosorbent assay for estimation of buffalo immunoglobulins using anti-bovine light chain monoclonal antibodies. *Buffalo Journal* **1**: 83–90.

Raj, G. D., S. Sivakumar, K. Matheswaran, M. Chandrasekhar, V. Thiagarajan and K. Nachimuthu (2003). Detection of egg drop syndrome virus antigen or genome by enzyme-linked immunosorbent assay or polymerase chain reaction. Avian Pathology **32**: 545–550.

Saravanan, P., Sen, A., Balamurugan, V., Bandyopadhyay, S.K. and Singh, R.K. (2008). Rapid quality control of a live attenuated Peste des petits ruminants (PPR) vaccine by monoclonal antibody based sandwich ELISA. *Biologicals.* **36**: 1–6.

Schwaber, J. and Cohen, E.P. (1973). Human x mouse somatic cell hybrid clone secreting immunoglobulins of both parental types. *Nature* **244**: 444–447.

Seki, C., Robiolo, B., Periolo, O., Iglesias, M., D'Antuono, A., Maradei, E., Barros, V., Torre, La J., Mattion, N. (2009). Rapid methodology for antigenic profiling of FMDV field strains and for the control of identity, purity and viral integrity in commercial virus vaccines using monoclonal antibodies Veterinary Microbiology **133**: 239–251.

Singh, R.P., De, U.K., and Pandey, K.D. (2010). Virological and antigenic characterization of two Peste des Petits Ruminants (PPR) vaccine viruses of Indian origin. Comparative Immunology, Microbiology and Infectious Diseases **33**: 343–353.

Singh, R.P., Sreenivasa, B. P., Dhar, P. and Bandyopadhyay, S. K. (2004). A sandwich-ELISA for the diagnosis of Peste des petits ruminants (PPR) infection in small ruminants using anti-nucleocapsid protein monoclonal antibody. *Archives of Virology*. **149**: 2155–2170.

Srikumaran, S., Goldsby, R.A., Guidry, A. J., Haque, B., Onisk D. V. Srikumaran, P. (1987). Library of monoclonal bovine immunoglobulins and monoclonal antibodies to bovine immunoglobulins. Hybridoma **6**: 527–530.

Timberlake, K.C. (1992). Chemistry–5th Edition, Haper-Collins Publishers Inc, NY.

Towbin, H., Staehelin, T. and Gordon, J. (1979). Electrophoretic transfer of proteins from polyacrylamide gels to nitrocellulose sheets: procedure and some applications. PNAS 76 (9): 4350.doi:10.1073/pnas.76.9.4350. PMC 411572. PMID 38.

Vani, J., Nayak, R. and Shaila, M. S. (2007). Maintenance of antigen-specific immunological memory through variable regions of heavy and light chains of anti-idiotypic antibody. *Immunology.* **120**: 486–496.

Zhanga, D., Li, P., Qi Zhanga, Zhanga, W., Huanga, Y., Dinga, X. and Jianga, J. (2009). Production of ultrasensitive generic monoclonal antibodies against major aflatoxins using a modified two-step screening procedure. Analytica Chimica Acta **636**: 63–69.

SUGGESTED READING

Akerstrom, B., Brodin, T., Reis, K. and Bjorck, L. (1985). Protein G: A powerful tool for binding and detection of monoclonal and polyclonal antibodies. *J Immunol* **135**:2589–2592.

Alley, S.C., Okeley, N.M. and Senter, P.D. (2010). Antibody–drug conjugates: targeted drug delivery for cancer. *Current Opinion in Chemical Biology*: **14**: 529–537.

Anon, (1994). Legislative basis Directive 75/318/EEC–Production and Quality Control of Monoclonal Antibodies.

Anon, (1999). Monoclonal Antibody Production-*A Report of the* Committee on Methods of Producing Monoclonal Antibodies, Institute for Laboratory Animal Research, National Research Council, National Academy Press, Washington, DC.

Beck, C., Stiefel, H. and Stinnett, T. (1987). Cell-culture bioreactors. *Chem. Eng. Feb* **16**:121–129.

Beuvery, E.C., Griffiths, J.B. and Zeijlemaker, W. P. (1995). Animal Cell Technology: Developments Towards the 21st Century, Kluwer Academic Publishers, Dordrecht, Boston, London, 1207p., ISBN: 0–7923–3736–0.

Birch, J.R. and Lennox, E.S. (1995). *Monoclonal Antibodies: Principles and Applications* Wiley-Liss: New York, 344 p., ISBN: 0–471–05147–0.

Boi, C. (2007). Membrane adsorbers as purification tools for monoclonal antibody purification. *Journal of Chromatography* B, 848: 19–27.

Borrebaeck, C.A. (1995). *Antibody Engineering* Oxford University Press: New York, Oxford, 2nd ed., 390 p., ISBN: 0–19–509150–7. NAL call number: TP248.65 I49A57 1995.

Brodeur, B. and Tsang, P. (1986). High yields of monoclonal antibody production in ascites. *J Immunol Methods* **86**:239–241.

Capra, J.D. (1996) *Antibody Engineering* Chemical Immunology Series, Vol. 65, Karger: Basel, Switzerland; New York, NY, 200p., ISBN: 3–8055–6356–6.

Choi, K.S., Nah, J.J., Ko, Y.J., Kang, S.Y. and Jo, N.I. (2005). Rapid competitive Enzyme-Linked Immunosorbent Assay for detection of antibodies to Peste des petits ruminants virus. *Clinical and Diagnostic Laboratory Immunology* **12**: 542–547.

Chowdhury, P.S. and Wu, H. (2005). Tailor-made antibody therapeutics. *Methods* **36**: 11–24.

Cuesta, A.M., Sainz-Pastor, N., Bonet, J., Oliva, B. and lvarez-Vallina, L. A. (2010). Multivalent antibodies: when design surpasses evolution. *Trends in Biotechnology* **28**: 355–362.

Darby, C., Hamano, K. and Wood, K. (1993). Purification of monoclonal antibodies from tissue culture medium depleted of IgG. *J. of Immunol* **159**: 125–129.

Darwish, I.A. (2006). Immunoassay Methods and their Applications in Pharmaceutical Analysis: Basic Methodology and Recent Advances. *International J. of Biomedical Sci.* **2**: 356–372

de Geus, B. and Hendriksen, C. (1998). *In vivo* and *in vitro* production of monoclonal antibodies-Introduction. *Res Immunol* **149**:533–534.

De Leij, L., Poppema, S. and The, T. H. (1983) Cryopreservation of newly formed Hybridomas. *J. of Immunol Methods,* **62**: 69–72.

Dewar, V., Voet, P., Denamur, F. and Smal, J. (2005). Industrial implementation of *in vitro* production of monoclonal antibodies. *ILAR J.* **46**: 3–10.

Dhinakar Raj, G., Mathivanan, B., Matheswaran, K., Nachimuthu, K. and Davis, W.C. (2007). Lymphocyte subset distribution in apparently normal and single intradermal test-positive water buffaloes analyzed by flow cytometry. *Research in Veterinary Sci.* **82**: 34–38.

Dhinakar Raj, G., Sivakumar, S., Matheswaran, K., Chandrasekhar, M., Thiagarajan, V. and Nachimuthu, K. (2003). Detection of egg drop syndrome virus antigen or genome by enzyme-linked immunosorbent assay or polymerase chain reaction. *Avian Pathology* **32**: 545–550.

Ducry, L. and Stump, B. (2010). Antibody-Drug Conjugates: Linking Cytotoxic Payloads to Monoclonal Antibodies. *Bioconjugate Chem.* **21**: 5–13.

Dvorakova, H., Valicek, L. and Reichelova, M. (2005). Detection of mycoplasma contamination in cell cultures and bovine sera. *Vet. Med. – Czech,* **50**: 262–268.

Evans, T. and Miller, R. (1988). Large-scale production of murine monoclonal antibodies using hollow fiber bioreactors. *BioTechniques* **6**: 762–767.

Falkenberg, F., Weichert, H. and Krane, M. (1995). *In vitro* production of monoclonal antibodies in high concentration in a new and easy to handle modular mini fermentor. *J. of Immunol* **179**: 13–29.

Filpula, D. (2007). Antibody engineering and modification technologies. *Biomolecular Engineering* **24**: 201–215.

Gillette, R.W. (1987). Alternatives to pristane priming for ascitic fluid and monoclonal antibody production. *J. of Immunol Methods* **99**:21–23.

Harlow, E. and Lane, D. (1988). Antibodies: A laboratory manual. New York: Cold Spring Harbor Laboratory Press.

Hoekstra, D.S., Klappe, K., Hoff, H. and Nirg, S. (1989). Mechanism of fusion of Sendai virus: Role of hydrophobic interactions and mobility constraint of viral membrane proteins- effects of polyethylene glycol. *J. of Biol. Chem.* **264**: 786–792.

Hoffmann, P., Jiménez-Diaz, M., Weckesser, J. and Bessler, W. G. (1996). Murine bone marrow-derived macrophages constitute feeder cells for human B cell hybridomas. *J. of Immunol Methods* **196**: 85–91.

Jackson, L., Trudel, L., Fox, J. and Lipman, N. (1996). Evaluation of hollow fiber bioreactors; as an alternative to murine ascites production for small scale monoclonal antibody production. *J. of Immunol Methods* **189**: 217–231.

Jarvis, D.L. (2009). Baculovirus–Insect Cell Expression Systems. *Methods in Enzymology*, **463**: 192–218.

Klerx, J., Jansen Verplanke, C., Blonk, C. and Twaalfhoven, L. (1988). *In vitro* production of monoclonal antibodies under serum-free conditions using a compact and inexpensive hollow fibre cell culture unit. *J. of Immunol Methods* **11**: 179–188.

Knazek, R., Gullino, P., Kohler, P. and Dedrick, R. (1972). Cell culture on artificial capillaries. *Science* **178**: 65–67.

Köhler, G. and Milstein, C. (1975). Continuous cultures of fused cells secreting antibody of predefined specificity. *Nature* **256**: 495–497.

Koolman, J. and Rohm, K.H. (1996). *Colour Atlas of Biochemistry*, Thieme, Stuttgart.

Kozlowski, S. and Swann, P. (2006). Current and future issues in the manufacturing and development of monoclonal antibodies. *Advanced Drug Delivery Reviews* **58**: 707–722.

Kurkela, R., Fraune, E. and Vihko, P. (1993). Pilot-scale production of murine monoclonal antibodies in agitated, ceramic-matrix, or hollow-fiber cell culture systems. *BioTechniques* **15**: 674–693.

Li, D., Liu, Z.X., Sun, P., Li, Y.L., Lu, Z.J., Tian, M.N., Chen, Y.L., Xie, B.X., Bao, H.F., Fu, Y.F., Cao, Y.M., Li, P.H., Bai, X.W., Sun, J.C., Guo, J.H., Liu, X.T. and Xie, Q.G. (2010). The efficacy of FMD vaccine reduced non-structural proteins with a mAb against 3B protein. *Veterinary Research Communication* **34**: 445–457.

Li, J. and Zhu, Z. (2010). Research and development of next generation of antibody-based therapeutics. *Acta Pharmacologica Sinica* **31**: 1198–1207.

Linn, S. (2009). Strategies and Considerations for Protein Purifications. *Methods in Enzymology*, **463**: 10–19.

Löfblom, J., Feldwisch, J., Tolmachev, V., Carlsson, J., Ståhl, S. and Frejd, F.Y. (2010). Affibody molecules: Engineered proteins for therapeutic, diagnostic and biotechnological applications. *FEBS Letters* **584**: 2670–2680.

Lowa, D., O'Leary, R., Pujar, N.S. (2007). Future of antibody purification. *J. of Chromatography B*, **848**: 48–63.

Malviya, G., Conti, F., Chianelli, M. Scopinaro, F., Dierckx, R.A. and Signore, A. (2010). Molecular imaging of rheumatoid arthritis by radiolabelled monoclonal antibodies: new imaging strategies to guidemolecular therapies. *Eur J. of Nucl Med Mol Imaging* **37**: 386–398.

Marx, U. (1998). Membrane-based cell culture technologies: A scientifically and economically satisfactory alternative to malignant ascites production for monoclonal antibodies. *Res Immunol* **149**: 557–559.

Maurice, E., Salvana, T. and Salata, R.A. (2009). Infectious Complications Associated with Monoclonal Antibodies and Related Small Molecules. *Clinical Microbiology Reviews* **22**: 274–290.

Naessens, J., Scheerlinck, J.P., Buysscher, E.V., Kennnedy, D. and Sileghem, M. (1998). Effective *in vivo* depletion of T cell subpopulations and loss of memory cells in cattle using mouse monoclonal antibodies. *Veterinary Immunology and Immunopathology* **64**: 219–234.

Nam, K.S. (1991). Effective production of monoclonal antibodies against phospholipids by intrasplenic immunization method. *Korean Biochem. J.* **24**: 176–181.

Newsome, B.W. and Ernstoff, M.S. (2008). The clinical pharmacology of therapeutic monoclonal antibodies in the treatment of malignancy; have the magic bullets arrived? Br *J. of Clin Pharmacol* **66**: 6–19.

Nunez, R. (2001). Flow Cytometry Instrumentation. *Curr. Issues Mol. Biol.* **3** (2): 39–45.

Ohlin, M. and Borrebaeck, C.A. (1994). Flow cytometric analysis of the stability of antibody production by human × human × mouse heterohybridoma subclones. *J. of Immunol Methods* **29**: 75–82.

Okada, Y. and Murayama, F. (1965). Multinucleated giant cell formation by fusion between cells of two different strains. Exp. Cell Res. **40** (1): 154–158.

Olafsen, T. and Wu, A.M. (2010). Antibody Vectors for Imaging. *Semin Nucl Med* **40**: 167–181.

Pardue, R.L., Brady, R.C., Perry, G.W. and Dedman, J. R. (1983). Production of Monoclonal Antibodies In Vitro Immunization of Spleen Cells Against Calmodulin *J. of Cell Biology* **96**: 1149–1154.

Ritter, M.A. and Ladyman, H. M. (1995). *Monoclonal Antibodies:* Production, Engineering and Clinical Application, Postgraduate Medical Science Series Vol. No. 3, Cambridge University Press: New York, NY, 500 p., ISBN:0–521–47354–3. NAL call number: QR186.85 M6623 1995.

Rohrer, T. (2009). Antibody drug conjugates - Potent weapons for the oncology arsenal. *Chemistry Today* **27**: 5–10.

Rosaa, P. A. J., Azevedoa, A. M., Ferreiraa, I. F., Sommerfeldb, S., Bäcker, W. and Aires-Barros, M. R. (2009). Downstream processing of antibodies: Single-stage *versus* multi-stage aqueous two-phase extraction. *J. of Chromatography A*, **1216**: 8741–8749.

Saerens, D., Ghassabeh, G.H. and Myldermans, S. (2008). Single-domain antibodies as building blocks for novel therapeutics. *Current Opinion in Pharmacology* **8**: 600–608.

Saleem, M. and Kamal, M. (2008). Monoclonal antibodies in clinical diagnosis: A brief review application. *African J. of Biotechnology* **7**: 923–925.

Saravanan, P., Sen, A., Balamurugan, V., Bandyopadhyay, S.K. and Singh, R.K. (2008). Rapid quality control of a live attenuated Peste des petits ruminants (PPR) vaccine by monoclonal antibody based sandwich ELISA. *Biologicals* **36**: 1–6.

Seki, C., Robiolo, B., Periolo, O., Iglesias, M., D'Antuono, A., Maradei, E., Barros, V., La Torre, J. and Mattion, N. (2009). Rapid methodology for antigenic profiling of FMDV field strains and for the control of identity, purity and viral integrity in commercial virus vaccines using monoclonal antibodies. *Veterinary Microbiology* **133**: 239–251.

Sharkey, R.M., Rossi, E.A., McBride, W.J., Chang, C.H., Goldenberg, D.M. (2010). Recombinant bispecific monoclonal antibodies prepared by the dock-and-lock strategy for pretargeted radioimmunotherapy. *Semin Nucl Med* **40**: 190–203.

Singh, R.P., De, U.K., Pandey, K.D. (2010). Virological and antigenic characterization of two Peste des Petits Ruminants (PPR) vaccine viruses of Indian origin. *Comparative Immunology, Microbiology and Infectious Diseases* **33**: 343–353.

Singh, R.P., Sreenivasa, B.P., Dhar, P. and Bandyopadhyay, S.K. (2004). A sandwich-ELISA for the diagnosis of Peste des petits ruminants (PPR) infection in small ruminants using anti-nucleocapsid protein monoclonal antibody. *Archives of Virology* **149**: 2155–2170.

Stellwagen, E. (2009). Gel Filtration. *Methods in Enzymology*, **463**: 373– 385.

Thermo Scientific *Nalgene and Nunc Cryopreservation Guide.*

Thermo Scientific Pierce® Protein Purification Technical Handbook.

Thompson, N.E., Foley, K.M., Stalder, E.S. and Burgess, R.R. (2009). Identification, Production, and Use of Polyol-Responsive Monoclonal Antibodies for Immunoaffinity Chromatography. *Methods in Enzymology* **463**: 475–494.

Timberlake, K.C., (1992). Chemistry 5th Edn., Haper-Collins Publishers Inc, NY.

Trebak, M., Chong, J.M., Herlyn, D. and Speicher, D.W. (1999). Efficient laboratory-scale production of monoclonal antibodies using membrane-based high-density cell culture technology. *J. of Immunol Methods* **230**: 59–70.

UKCCR (1998). United Kingdom Co-ordinating Committee on Cancer Research. Guidelines for the Welfare of Animals in Experimental Neoplasia (Second Edition). 1998. *Br J. of Cancer* **77** (1): 1–10.

Underwood, P.A. and Bean, P.A. (1985). The influence of methods of production, purification and storage of monoclonal antibodies upon their observed specificities. *J .of Immunol Methods* **80**: 189–197.

Urh, M., Simpson, D. and Zhao, K. (2009). Affinity Chromatography: General Methods *Methods in Enzymology*, **463**: 418–435.

Yang, M., Clavijo, A., Li, M., Hole, K., Holland, H., Wang, H. and Deng, M.Y. (2007). Identification of a major antibody binding epitope in the non-structural protein 3D of foot-and-mouth disease virus in cattle and the development of a monoclonal antibody with diagnostic applications. *J. of Immunol Methods.* **321**: 174–181.

Zerbs, S., Frank, A.M. and Collart, F.R. (2009). Bacterial Systems for Production of Heterologous Proteins. *Methods in Enzymology.* **463**: 150–166.

Zhanga, D., Li, P., Zhanga, Q., Zhanga, W., Huanga, Y., Dinga, X. and Jianga, J. (2009). Production of ultrasensitive generic monoclonal antibodies against major aflatoxins using a modified two-step screening procedure. *Analytica Chimica Acta* **636**: 63–69.

GLOSSARY

Term	*Description*
Adjuvant	An immunological agent that increases the antigenic response
Affibody	Antibody mimetics that bind to target proteins or peptides with high affinity
Affinity	Strength of the reaction between a single antigenic determinant and a single combining site on the antibody
Affinity chromatography	A selective type of chromatography that uses the specific interaction between two molecules
Agglutination	Clumping of large particulate antigen following binding to a specific antibody
Allotype	Allelic variants within the constant regions
Amino acid	Building blocks of proteins
Analytical sensitivity	Is the smallest detectable amount of the analyte in question
Analytical specificity	Is the degree to which the assay does not cross-react with other analyte
Anti idiotype antibody	An antibody that is directed against the idiotype of another antibody, capable of mimicking the antigen
Antibody	A specific protein which is produced in response to an immunogen and which reacts with an antigen
Antigen	A substance that reacts with the products of a specific immune response
Antibody drug conjugate	mAbs attached to biologically active drugs by chemical linkers with labile bonds
Autoradiography	Is the direct exposure of film to beta particles or gamma rays
Avidity	Overall strength of binding of an antigen with many antigenic determinants and multivalent antibodies
Cell culture	Growth and maintenance of cells *in vitro*
Cell sorting	Separation of the cells of the desired type from a heterogenous population using specific markers
Chemiluminescence	Emission of light driven by a chemical reaction
Chimeric antibodies	Murine variable regions + human constant regions
Chromatography	Method used to separate or analyze complex mixtures by distribution between a stationary phase and a mobile phase which percolates through the stationary bed

Glossary (*Contd...*)

Term	*Description*
Calorimetry	Science of colour measurement
CDR	Complementarity determining regions, the variable domains of the heavy and light chains consist of three hypervariable regions each which actually bind to the epitope on the antigen
Cross reactivity	Ability of a paratope to react with more than one epitope
Cryopreservation	A process where cells are preserved by cooling to low temperatures
D value	Decimal reduction time is the time required at a certain temperature to kill 90% of the organisms being studied
Diafiltration	Similar to dialysis but involves forcing solutions through the membrane by pressure
Diagnostic sensitivity	Is the proportion of known infected reference animals that test positive in the assay
Diagnostic specificity	Is the proportion of uninfected reference animals that test negative in the assay
Dialysis	Separation technique that facilitates the removal of small, compounds from the protein of interest by selective diffusion through a semi-permeable membrane
DIVA	Differentiation of infected and vaccinated animals
Electrophoresis	Movement of charged molecules under the influence of an electric field
ELISA	Enzyme linked immunosorbent assay–most common form of immunoassay
ELISPOT	Used for detection and quantification of antibody producing cells
Epitope	That portion of an antigen that combines with the products of a specific immune response
FACS	Fluorescent activated cell sorting
Feeder cells	'Extra' cells to support the growth of newly formed hybridomas
Fermenter	Vessel in which the process of fermentation takes place
Flow through assay	Immunoassay using vertical flow of reagents, involves washing after every step (compare with lateral flow)
Fluorescence	Emission of light of longer wavelength, by a substance that has absorbed light of a different wavelength
Fluorography	Is the exposure of film by secondary light that is generated by the excitation of a fluor or a screen by a beta particle or a gamma ray
FP ratio	Fluorescent protein ratio used for conjugating fluorochromes to antibodies
Fragment crystallisable	The enzyme papain cuts the immunoglobulin in front of the hinge region into two parts: the Fab (fragment antigen binding) and the Fc (fragment crystallizable) part
Fragment variable	The minimum antigen-binding unit of an that consists of the associated variable domains of heavy and light chains
Frame work regions	Serves as a scaffold to hold the hyper variable regions of the antibody in position to contact antigen

Glossary (*Contd...*)

Term	*Description*
Fusion	Fusion of B lymphocyte and myeloma cells
Gating	Selecting populations of interests by defining their characteristics during flow cytometry
Gel filtration	Separation based on size as it passes through a gel filtration medium packed in a column, also called molecular exclusion or gel permeation chromatography
Genetic code	Rules for information encoded in genetic material to be translated into proteins
Hapten	A substance that is non-immunogenic but which can react with the products of a specific immune response
HAT medium	Hypoxanthine–Aminopterin–Thymidine selection method to differentiate parent myeloma cells from fused lymphocyte and myeloma cells
Humanized antibody	Murine CDR + human framework regions
Hybridoma	Fusion of B lymphocyte and myeloma cells that has the property of continuous growth
Idiotype	Consist of the unique combination of VH and VL which characterize a particular immunoglobulin's combining site
Immunoassays	Assays using the specific interaction between antigen and antibody
Immunogen	A substance that induces a specific immune response
Immunoglobulin	A protein produced by plasma cells playing a role in immunity, Antibody used in context of antigen, immuno globulins in general
Intrabodies	Intracellular antibodies targeted to specific subcellular compartments by fusion to specific signal peptides
Ion exchange chromatography	Use of a stationary solid phase to covalently attach anions or cations onto it
Isoelectrofocussing	Method that exploits the differences in isoelectric points of proteins for their separation
Isotype	Distinct forms of light or heavy chains which are present in all members of a species
Isotype switching	Change of the isotype of the antibody without changing the specificity of the antigen binding site
Knock out mouse	A genetically engineered mouse in which one or more genes have been switched off
Lateral flow assays	Immunoassay involving lateral flow of reagents, does not involve washing of unbound reagents, also called as immuno chromatography tests of simply strip tests
Limiting dilution	Separate cells from a heterogenous population from each other and grow as single, isolated cells in culture
Luminescence	Emission of light from a cool object
Lyophilization	A process in which water is removed from a product by freezing in vacuum, allowing ice to change directly from solid to vapor without passing through a liquid phase (sublimation), also called as freeze drying

Glossary *(Contd...)*

Term	*Description*
Micro filtration	Filtration process to remove contaminants from a fluid by passage through a microporous membrane
Monoclonal antibody	Antibody against a single epitope, isotype and affinity
Nude mouse	Mutated mouse that does not have a thymus
pH	Negative logarithm of hydrogen ion activity in a solution
pI	pH when there is no net charge on the protein making it immobile
Phage display technology	Displaying proteins or peptides on the surface of bacteriophage
Phagemids	A chimeric vector, a hybrid of filamentous phage M13 and plasmids
pKa	The negative logarithm of the acid dissociation constant, Ka
Plantibodies	Antibodies produced by genetically modified crops
Polyclonal antibody	Antibodies against multiple epitopes, isotypes and affinities
Polymerase chain reaction	An *in vitro* method of DNA amplification using specific primers
Precipitation	Clumping of soluble antigens following binding to a specific antibody
Protein tags	Peptide sequences genetically included in to a recombinant protein
Proteins	Polymer of amino acids joined by peptide bonds
Radio immunoprecipitation	Immunoprecipitation that uses an isotope-labeled antibody or an antigen
Ribosome display technology	A method for the selection and evolution of scFv
Single chain fragment variable	Is a fusion protein of the variable regions of the heavy and light chains of immunoglobulins connected with a short linker peptide
Single domain antibody	Single-domain antigen-binding derivatives of antibodies
Specificity	Ability of an individual paratope to react with only one epitope
Spectrophotometry	Measurement of how different wavelengths of light are absorbed
Stem cells	Cells with the potential to develop into many different types of cells in the body
Ultra filtration	A process wherein water and other small molecules, are driven through a semi permeable membrane by a trans membrane force such as centrifugation of high pressure
Veneering	Replacement of the surface of the nonhuman antibody with amino acids from a human antibody, also called resurfacing
Western blotting	The process of transferring protein from a gel to a micro porous membrane in an electrical field

APPENDIX - I

Table 1: Precipitation with $(NH_4^+)_2SO_4^{2-}$ based on % saturation

Values calculated according to Protein Purification, R. K. Scopes (Springer-Verlag, New York), Third Edition, p. 346, 1993.

	Final percent saturation to be obtained																
	20	**25**	**30**	**35**	**40**	**45**	**50**	**55**	**60**	**65**	**70**	**75**	**80**	**85**	**90**	**95**	**100**
Starting percent saturation	Amount of ammonium sulphate to add (grams) per liter of solution at 20 °C																
0	113	144	176	208	242	277	314	351	390	430	472	516	561	608	657	708	761
5	85	115	146	179	212	246	282	319	358	397	439	481	526	572	621	671	723
10	57	86	117	149	182	216	251	287	325	364	405	447	491	537	584	634	685
15	28	58	88	119	151	185	219	255	293	331	371	413	456	501	548	596	647
20	0	29	59	89	121	154	188	223	260	298	337	378	421	465	511	559	609
25		0	29	60	91	123	157	191	228	265	304	344	386	429	475	522	571
30			0	30	61	92	125	160	195	232	270	309	351	393	438	485	533
35				0	30	62	94	128	163	199	236	275	316	358	402	447	495
40					0	31	63	96	130	166	202	241	281	322	365	410	457
45						0	31	64	98	132	169	206	245	286	329	373	419
50							0	32	65	99	135	172	210	250	292	335	381
55								0	33	66	101	138	175	215	256	298	343
60									0	33	67	103	140	179	219	261	305
65										0	34	69	105	143	183	224	267
70											0	34	70	107	146	186	228
75												0	35	72	110	149	190
80													0	36	73	112	152
85														0	37	75	114
90															0	37	76
95																0	38

Table 2: Concentrations of commercially available acids

Acid	*Molecular (wt.)*	*Molarity (m)*	*Concentration (g/l)*	*% by (wt.)*	*Specific gravity*
Acetic acid	60.05	17.4	1045.0	99.5	1.05
Formic acid	46.02	23.4	1080.0	90.0	1.20
Hydrochloric acid	36.50	11.6	424.0	36.0	1.18
Nitric acid	63.02	15.99	1008.0	71.0	1.42
Perchloric acid	100.5	11.65	1172.0	70.0	1.67
Phosphoric acid	80.0	18.1	1145.0	85.0	1.70
Sulphuric acid	98.1	18.0	1766.0	96.0	1.84

Table 3: Greek Alphabets

Alpha	á	Beta	â
Gamma	ã	Delta	ä
Epsilon	å	Zeta	æ
Eta	ç	Theta	è
Iota	é	Kappa	ê
lambda	ë	Mu	ì
Nu	í	Rho	ñ
Sigma	ó	Tau	ô
Phi	ö	Chi	÷
Psi	ø	Omega	ù

Table 4: Abbreviations and molecular weight of amino acids

Amino acid	*Three letter abbreviation*	*One letter symbol*	*MW*
Alanine	Ala	A	89
Arginine	Arg	R	174
Asparagine	Asn	N	132
Aspartic acid	Asp	D	133
Cysteine	Cys	C	121
Glutamine	Gln	Q	146
Glutamic acid	Glu	E	147
Glycine	Gly	G	75
Histidine	His	H	155
Isoleucine	Ile	I	131
Leucine	Leu	L	131
Lysine	Lys	K	146
Methionine	Met	M	149
Phenyl alanine	Phe	F	165
Proline	Pro	P	115
Serine	Ser	S	105
Threonine	Thr	T	119
Trptophan	Trp	W	204
Tyrosine	Tyr	Y	181
Valine	Val	V	117

Table 5: The Genetic Code

FIRST POSITION	*2ND POSITION*								THIRD POSITION
U	UUU	Phe	UCU	Ser	UAU	Tyr	UGU	Cys	U
	UUC	Phe	UCC	Ser	UAC	Tyr	UGC	Cys	C
	UUA	Leu	UCA	Ser	UAA	End	UGA	End	A
	UUG	Leu	UCG	Ser	UAG	End	UGG	Trp	G
C	CUU	Leu	CCA	Pro	CAU	His	CGU	Arg	U
	CUC	Leu	CCC	Pro	CAC	His	CGC	Arg	C
	CUA	Leu	CCA	Pro	CAA	Gln	CGA	Arg	A
	CUG	Leu	CCG	Pro	CAG	Gln	CGG	Arg	G
A	AUU	Ile	ACU	Thr	AAU	Asn	AGU	Ser	U
	AUC	Ile	ACC	Thr	AAC	Asn	ACC	Ser	C
	AUA	Ile	ACA	Thr	AAA	Lys	AGA	Arg	A
	AUG	Met	ACG	Thr	AAG	Lys	AGG	Arg	G
G	GUU	Val	GCU	Ala	GAU	Asp	GGU	Gly	U
	GUC	Val	GCC	Ala	GAC	Asp	GGC	Gly	C
	GUA	Val	GCA	Ala	GAA	Glu	GGA	Gly	A
	GUG	Val	GCG	Ala	GAG	Glu	GGG	Gly	G

Table 6: Half life of radio nuclides

Radionuclide	*Symbol*	*Half life*
Tritium	^{3}H	12-43 years
Carbon	^{14}C	5730 years
Sulphur	^{35}S	87.4 days
Phosphorous	^{33}P	25.5 days
Chlorine	^{36}Cl	3.01×10^{5} years
Phosphorous	^{32}P	14.3 days
Iodine	^{131}I	8.06 days
Iodine	^{125}I	60 days
Cobalt	^{57}Co	270.5 days
Cobalt	^{58}Co	70.8 days
Selenium	^{75}Se	120 days
Mercury	^{197}Hg	64.4 hr
Mercury	^{203}Hg	47 days

Table 7: Conversion of RCF to RPM

$$RCF = \frac{r(2\eth N)^2}{g}$$

where

g - is earth's gravitational acceleration,

r - is the rotational radius,

N - is the rotational speed, measured in revolutions per unit of time.

This relationship may be written as

$$RCF = 1.118 \times 10^{-5}\ r_{cm}\ N^{2}{}_{RPM}$$

Table 7: *(Contd...)*

where

r_{cm} - is the rotational radius measured in centimetres (cm)
N^2_{RPM} - is rotational speed measured in revolutions per minute (RPM), and
G = (980.65 cm/sec^2) (3600 sec^2/minute^2) = 3530340 cm/minute^2

Table 8: Nomogram for converting maximum relative centrifugal force (RCF)to RPM

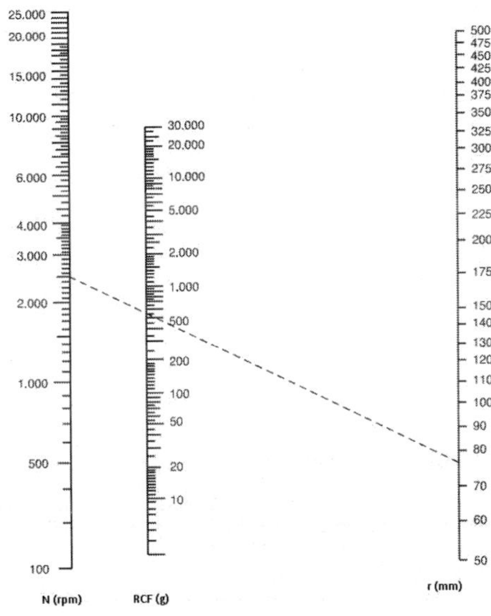

Table 9: Addresses of suppliers of BALB/c mice in India

http://www.ninindia.org/lab_animals.htm
Indents for animals may please be sent to:

Officer-in-charge
National Centre for Laboratory Animal Sciences
National Institute of Nutrition
Jamai Osmania
Hyderabad–500 007.
Telegram: NUTRITION
Fax: 040–2700 3317/2701 9074
Telephone: 040–2719 7201/202/205/207

For ordering the mice, the following information has to be specified:

(a) Your CPCSEA registration Number
(b) Your Institutional Animal Ethics Committee's approval for the animals required
(c) Species
(d) Strain
(e) Age and /or weight range
(f) No. of animals required
(g) Sex (orders for both male and females will be given preference)
(h) Date on which the animals are required
(i) Nearest airport
(j) Distance from the airport to the Institute
(k) Telegraphic code, Fax number and Telephone numbers
(l) Residence Telephone number of the officer ordering for the animals.

Table 10: Addresses of cell culture suppliers in India

Name and addresses of cell culture suppliers

ATCC–USA
American Type Culture Collection
P. O. Box No. 1549,
Manassas, VA 20108,
USA
tech@atcc.org

MTCC- India
Microbial Type Culture Collection
Institute of Microbial Technology,
Sector 39A,
Chandigarh – 160 036
Indiacurator@imtech.res.in

ATCC- India
American Type Culture Collection & Gene Bank
LGC Prochem India Pvt. Ltd.,
Unit No. 401-402,
Model Export Bhavan,
Plot No. 488B, VITC, 14th Cross,
2nd stage, Peenya,
Bangalore – 560 058
Indiain@lgcpromochem.com

NCCS- India
National Centre for Cell Science
NCCS complex,
University of Pune campus,
Ganesh Khind,
Pune – 411 007,
Maharashtra
India
www.nccs.res.in

Table 11: Companies in India offering mAb production as a contract research

Chromous Biotech Pvt. Ltd.
842, II Floor,
Sahakar Bhavan,
A block, Sahakarnagar,
Bangalore – 560 092

Mediclone Biotech Pvt. Ltd
Block-B, 36/37 OMR,
M.K. Srinivasan Nagar Main Road,
Perungudi,
Chennai – 600 096

Biotech Desk Pvt. Ltd.
4F 5, Ballad Estate,
Tarnaka,
Hyderabad – 500 017

Bangalore Genei
No. 6, VI Main,
BDA Industrial SuburbNear SRS Road,
Peenya, Bangalore – 560 058

Krishgen Biosystems
135/37 Zaveri Bazar,
Sonawala Bldg.,
2nd Floor,
Mumbai – 400 002

GenPro Biotech
3022, Sector-A,
Pocket B & C,
Vasant Kunj,
New Delhi – 110 070

Reliance Life Sciences,
Dhirubhai Ambani Life Sciences Center,
R-282, TTC Industrial Area of MIDC,
Thane-Belapur Road,
Rabale,
Navi Mumbai – 400 701

Imgenex India Pvt. Ltd.
E-5, Infocity, KIIT Post Office,
Bhubaneshwar – 751 024

Bioklone
Plot No. 14 and 15,
Golden Jubilee Biotech Park,
(Inside SIPCOT IT Park),
Siruseri, Navalur P.O.,
Kanchipuram District – 603 103

Agile Lifescience Technologies India Pvt. Ltd.
Shop No. 8/9/12,
Mona Lisa CHS,
Plot No. 50, Sector–19,
Airoli, Navi Mumbai – 400708

Genxbio Health Sciences (P) Ltd.
Flat. No.111, S-530,
Delhi – 110 092

Bhat Bio-tech India Private Ltd.
No. 11A, IV Cross Veerasandra Industrial Area
Electronics City, Bangalore–560 100
Life Technologies India Pvt. Ltd.
306, Agarwal City Mall,
Opposite M2K,
Pitampura, Delhi – 110034

Axiva Sichem Biotech
5531, Basti Harphool Singh,
Sadar Thana Road,
Delhi – 110 006

INDEX

D

E

F

G

H

I

K

L

M

N

O

P

Q

R

S

T

U

V

W

Z